The Early Modern Englishwoman:
A Facsimile Library of Essential Works

Series II

Printed Writings, 1641–1700: Part 1

Volume 4

Writings on Medicine

Advisory Board:

Margaret J.M. Ezell
Texas A & M University

Elaine Hobby
Loughborough University

Suzanne W. Hull
The Huntington Library

Barbara K. Lewalski
Harvard University

Stephen Orgel
Stanford University

Ellen Rosand
Yale University

Mary Beth Rose
University of Illinois, Chicago

Hilda L. Smith
University of Cincinnati

Retha M. Warnicke
Arizona State University

Georgianna Ziegler
The Folger Shakespeare Library

The Early Modern Englishwoman:
A Facsimile Library of Essential Works

Series II

Printed Writings, 1641–1700: Part 1

Volume 4

Writings on Medicine

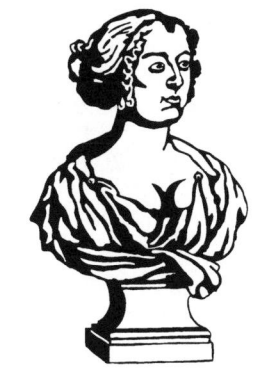

Selected and Introduced by
Lisa Forman Cody

General Editors
Betty S. Travitsky and Patrick Cullen

Ashgate

Aldershot • Burlington USA • Singapore • Sydney

The Introductory Note copyright © Lisa Forman Cody 2002

All rights reserved. No part of this publication may be reproduced, stored in a retrieval system, or transmitted in any form or by any means, electronic, mechanical, photocopying, recording, or otherwise without the prior permission of the publisher.

Published by
Ashgate Publishing Limited
Wey Court East
Union Road
Farnham
Surrey, GU9 7PT
England

RG
950
.W756
2002

Ashgate Publishing Company
Suite 420
101 Cherry Street
Burlington
VT 05401-4405
USA

Ashgate website: http://www.ashgate.com

British Library Cataloguing-in-Publication Data
The early modern Englishwoman : a facsimile library of
  essential works
  Part 1: Printed writings, 1641–1700: Vol. 4: Writings on
  medicine
  1. English literature – Early modern, 1500–1700   2. English
  literature – Women authors   3. Women – England – History –
  Renaissance, 1450–1600 – Sources   4. Women – England –
  History – Modern period, 1600 – – Sources   5. Women – Literary
  collections
  I. Cody, Lisa Forman   II. Travitsky, Betty S.   III. Cullen, Patrick
  Colborn
  820.8'09287

Library of Congress Cataloging-in-Publication Data
The early modern Englishwoman: a facsimile library of essential works. Part 1. Printed Writings, 1641–1700 / general editors, Betty S. Travitsky and Patrick Cullen.

See page vi for complete CIP Block 00–64297

The image reproduced on the title page and on the case is from the frontispiece portrait in *Poems. By the Most Deservedly Admired Mrs. Katherine Philips* (1667). Reproduced by permission of the Folger Shakespeare Library, Washington, DC.

ISBN 978-0-7546-0214-9

Transfered to Digital Printing in 2010

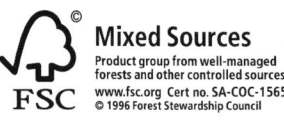

Mixed Sources
Product group from well-managed forests and other controlled sources
www.fsc.org Cert no. SA-COC-1565
© 1996 Forest Stewardship Council

Printed and bound in Great Britain by
MPG Books Group, UK

CONTENTS

Preface by the General Editors

Introductory Note

Jane Sharp
    The Midwives Book. Or the whole Art of Midwifry Discovered

Elizabeth Cellier
    To Dr.— An Answer to his Queries, concerning the Colledg of Midwives
    'A Scheme for the Foundation of a Royal Hospital'

Mary Trye
    Medicatrix, or The Woman-Physician

Appendix:
    The Mid-wives just Petition: Or, A complaint of the divers good Gentlewomen of that faculty

Library of Congress Cataloging-in-Publication Data
Writings on medicine / selected and introduced by Lisa Forman Cody.
    p. cm. – (The early modern Englishwoman. Printed writings, 1641–1700, Part 1 ; v. 4)
    Includes bibliographical references.
    Contents: The midwives book, or, The whole art of midwifry discovered / by Mrs. Jane Sharp – To Dr. — an answer to his queries concerning the Colledg of Midwives / Elizabeth Cellier – 'A scheme for the foundation of a royal hospital' ... / by Elizabeth Cellier – Medicatrix, or, The woman-physician / M. Trye – The mid-wives just petition, or, A complaint of the divers good gentlewomen of that faculty.
    ISBN 0-7546-0214-1
    1. Midwifery–Early works to 1800. 2. Women physicians–Early works to 1800. I. Sharp, Jane, Mrs. Midwives book. II. Cellier, Elizabeth, fl. 1680. To Dr. — an answer to his queries concerning the Colledg of Midwives. III. Cellier, Elizabeth, fl. 1680. 'Scheme for the foundation of a royal hospital' ... IV. Trye, Mary. Medicatrix. V. Cody, Lisa Forman VI. Mid-wives just petition. VII. Title: Midwives book. VIII. Title: To Dr. — an answer to his queries concerning the Colledg of Midwives. IX. Title: 'Scheme for the foundation of a royal hospital' ... X. Title: Medicatrix. XI. Series.

RG950 .W756 2000
618.2—dc21

00–64297

PREFACE
BY THE GENERAL EDITORS

Until very recently, scholars of the early modern period have assumed that there were no Judith Shakespeares in early modern England. Much of the energy of the current generation of scholars has been devoted to constructing a history of early modern England that takes into account what women actually wrote, what women actually read, and what women actually did. In so doing the masculinist representation of early modern women, both in their own time and ours, has been deconstructed. The study of early modern women has thus become one of the most important—indeed perhaps the most important—means for the rewriting of early modern history.

The Early Modern Englishwoman: A Facsimile Library of Essential Works is one of the developments of this energetic reappraisal of the period. As the names on our advisory board and our list of editors testify, it has been the beneficiary of scholarship in the field, and we hope it will also be an essential part of that scholarship's continuing momentum.

The Early Modern Englishwoman is designed to make available a comprehensive and focused collection of writings in English from 1500 to 1750, both by women and for and about them. The three series of *Printed Writings* (1500–1640, 1641–1700, and 1701–1750) provide a comprehensive if not entirely complete collection of the separately published writings by women. In reprinting these writings we intend to remedy one of the major obstacles to the advancement of feminist criticism of the early modern period, namely the limited availability of the very texts upon which the field is based. The volumes in the facsimile library reproduce carefully chosen copies of these texts, incorporating significant variants (usually in appendices). Each text is preceded by a short introduction providing an overview of the life and work of a writer along with a survey of important scholarship. These works, we strongly believe, deserve a large readership—of historians, literary critics, feminist critics, and non-specialist readers.

The Early Modern Englishwoman also includes separate facsimile series of *Essential Works for the Study of Early Modern Women* and of *Manuscript Writings*. These facsimile series are complemented by *The Early Modern Englishwoman 1500–1750: Contemporary Editions*. Also under our general editorship, this series will include both old-spelling and modernized editions of works by and about women and gender in early modern England.

New York City
2001

INTRODUCTORY NOTE

The four works presented here are the only known exclusively medical texts written by women during the Restoration, but they dramatically challenge generalizations once made about medical practice and female healers in this period. Early modern English medicine is sometimes generalized as having been strictly divided into a solely male and hierarchical system of three tiers. At the top, physicians took university degrees, advocated medical theories based on classical texts rather than observation and experimentation, and in practice avoided contact with their elite patients' bodies. At the bottom, apothecaries prepared drugs prescribed by physicians, but also dispensed advice to ordinary people unable to afford physicians' high fees. Surgeons were ranked in between the other two professions in terms of status, and performed the dramatic and dangerous, but sometimes heroically successful manoeuvres of sutures, amputations, lithotomies, and bonesetting. But viewing all medical practice as fitting into this formal tripartite scheme of male medicine ignores the reality of the seventeenth-century healing arts. In fact, women also practised medicine, but they did so almost entirely outside the three formal ranks. Until the 1970s, historians characterized these early modern female practitioners as ignorant and unskilled. Jane Sharp's *The Midwives Book*, Elizabeth Cellier's *To Dr. —*, and Mary Trye's *Medicatrix* helped overturn this assumption, instead revealing their female authors as learned not only in medical issues but also in the humanities and sciences more broadly. Historians now know that many seventeenth-century female practitioners, particularly urban midwives and a handful of recognized women surgeons, were highly literate and usually belonged to an upper-middle or upper socio-economic class.

Female healers were rarely permitted to join the ranks of surgeons and physicians, yet women may have been just as popular and successful in practice as male doctors. Even if they operated outside the formal medical institutions, women's medical practice within their families and neighbourhoods was taken for granted by contemporary diarists and observers. These contemporaries treated certain healing arts – from making poultices and teas to minding ill children – as natural extensions of housewives' proper domestic duties.

Perhaps the most obvious extension from the household to medical care was that of midwifery, and even male medical authors described attending routine deliveries, an activity particularly suited to women only. In the seventeenth century, even though several male doctors wrote works on pregnancy and childbirth, the vast majority of midwives were women, with male surgeons and physicians called only in obstetrical emergencies to try saving the life of the mother. The best and most recent historical scholarship shows that seventeenth-century midwives offered excellent care in the estimated 98 percent of deliveries which were normal, and that they even successfully negotiated many difficult cases (Wilson, 15–19, 33). Jane Sharp's *The Midwives Book* offers advice and observations on a par with many contemporary midwifery and gynaecological texts, all written by men.

Although (or perhaps because) contemporaries acknowledged women's 'natural' ability and success as midwives and healers, male physicians tried to check female practitioners (as well as those alternative male healers labelled 'quacks' and 'charlatans' who sold nostrums and claimed to perform medical miracles). In addition to trying to control all 'quacks', both male and female, some seventeenth-century physicians and surgeons also argued that ordinary midwives should be trained and regulated formally because attending all deliveries required proper medical knowledge. The most vocal of these medical regulators, in particular members of the Chamberlen family, had experience in obstetric emergencies themselves and asked that they be granted the right to examine and control female midwives, who, unlike their contemporary male practitioners, operated independently and beyond the reach of formal medical institutions. The midwife Elizabeth Cellier promoted an alternative model which would allow midwives largely to govern themselves as a 'Colledg of Midwives' paralleling the College of Physicians.

Mary Trye did not, as far as we know, practice midwifery. She did however treat smallpox, gout, syphilis, consumption, malarial 'agues', 'falling sickness', scurvy, stones and other common ailments by carrying on her father's work in 'physical chymistry'. Like her father, Trye proposed an alternative theoretical and practical framework to the dominant Galenic model promoted by the London College of Physicians. The chemical physicians followed Paracelsus and Helmont who argued that underlying chemical reactions directed the body's processes and its 'humours'; therefore healers should offer medicines rather than bleeding patients. Like her father, she also hoped that experimentally-based 'chymical physic' would triumph over the theories and phlebotomies endorsed by the College of Physicians.

History would realize Trye and Cellier's goals, but only centuries later. The basic logic of 'physical chymistry' would not displace the Galenic system entirely until the nineteenth century with modern organic chemistry and pharmaceutical science; British midwives would not be institutionalized as an independent, self-regulating profession until 1902.

Rather than presenting these authors' texts in chronological order, we begin with women's work as midwives and then move to the unique case of Mary Trye, 'physical chymist'.

Jane Sharp

Jane Sharp seems to have been a successful midwife, yet no biographical details of her life are yet known. If she was licensed by the Church of England as many other midwives were (a procedure partly used to help ensure that newborns were not baptised secretly as Catholics), her registration does not survive, but there are plausible reasons explaining her absence from these and other records. Since she published her work in 1671 as a 'Practitioner in the art of Midwifery above thirty years' Sharp was of a generation to seek licensing just when ecclesiastical licensing was suspended from 1642 to 1661 during the Civil War. Perhaps Sharp was a Catholic and thus would never have sought registration from the Anglican Church. Because Sharp fails to appear as a witness on the nearly five-hundred London midwifery certificates surviving from 1661 to 1699, it is likely she lived and practised outside the capital. Even though her publisher, Simon Miller, identified her as 'Mrs. Jane Sharp' on the title page of *The Midwives Book*, this may have been a courtesy title. The vast majority of seventeenth-century English midwives were married and had experienced pregnancy, but we cannot say for certain whether Sharp also was a wife and mother.

The Midwives Book

Jane Sharp's *The Midwives Book* is the first and only midwifery manual written by a woman in English before 1700. Her 1671 text of 418 pages was cited by other authors into the early eighteenth century. Sharp's text was edited, shortened to 244 pages, given new illustrations, and retitled *The Compleat Midwife's Companion* by John Marshall, a London printer in the early 1720s. Two printings of this text survive, a 'third edition' of 1724 and a 'fourth' of 1725. Although a second edition of Sharp's 1671 text has not yet been located, the third and fourth editions of that text are identical to each other except for their title pages. Elaine Hobby speculates that Marshall sold fewer copies of a 'second edition' of Sharp than he anticipated, so he reintroduced the same volume with newly-printed title pages for the third and fourth editions in 1724 and 1725. Marshall's editorial cuts are revealing and suggest that certain assumptions about the female reproductive body and humoural theory which Sharp and other Restoration authors reported were no longer as widely accepted. Marshall for instance cuts Sharp's description of the womb having seven cells (69–70), the theory of 'maternal imagination' causing monstrous births (117–118, 122–124), and several classical and humoural references throughout.

Jane Sharp's original 1671 text both resembles and differs from other contemporary works on obstetrics. Another fifteen texts on midwifery and gynaecology written by men, plus several more general works on sexuality and birth appeared between 1640 and 1700. Some, such as Mauriceau's *The Accomplisht Midwife* (1673), were written by male physicians presumably for midwives and male doctors interested in maternal anatomy, the stages of labour, and obstetric techniques. Other works, such as the pseudonymous *Aristotle's Master-Piece* (1690), presumably targeted a broader audience interested less in technical midwifery and more in descriptions of genitals, sexual pleasure, theories of conception, embryology, diet, and astrological impact on reproduction. Sharp's *The Midwives Book* resembles many of these works (particularly Culpeper's 1651 *Directory for Midwives*) in its physiological observations and explanations, its anecdotes and recommendations. Sharp's text combines Galenic, humoural theory, renaissance speculations about reproductive anatomy, widely circulated tales, and more straightforward midwifery techniques and recipes for remedies. Given its hundreds of pages on genital anatomy, conception, marriage, female diseases, folklore and various matters not immediately connected to the delivering of infants, the book seems designed as much for curious mothers and fathers as for midwives. *The Midwives Book* may surprise modern readers for its energetic depiction of sexual anatomy and female sexuality, but this reflects seventeenth-century beliefs. Because conception was the goal of marital sexual relations, Sharp makes recommendations to women and men that will make sex pleasurable and reproductively successful.

Unlike some male authors who cast aspersions on supposedly negligent midwives, Sharp generally vindicates her sex even though she explains that the 'many Miseries Women endure in the Hands of unskilful Midwives ... meerly for Lucres sake' have led her to publish the book in the first place. She argues that a good midwife must possess both speculative and practical knowledge; the 1671 text heavily emphasizes the former. Sharp says fairly little about routine deliveries, suggesting 'above all take heed you force not the birth till the time be come, and the Child come forward and appears ready to come forth' (199–200). Sharp describes the signs of dangerous pregnancies and parturition in more detail, but does not present specific case-studies as do contemporary male authors or the French midwife, Louise Bourgeois, author of the 1617 *Observations diverses* (translated in English as part of *The Compleat Midwife's Practice Enlarged* [1663]). Sharp suggests interventionist, surgical and pharmaceutical techniques for female midwives themselves to use instead of necessarily calling a male physician or surgeon in obstetrical emergencies.

From the seventeenth century onward, male doctors and many historians characterized early modern midwives as ignorant and meddlesome. Although the best, most recent historical scholarship has argued that *in practice* English midwives offered sensible and highly successful care, it must be admitted that the first edition of Jane Sharp's text may have partly contributed to the negative stereotype of female midwifery, both in its reliance on renaissance theories and its interventionist recommendations. To be fair, Sharp would not have been able to witness anatomical dissections, and like many male contemporary authors also lacking this knowledge, she reports centuries-old speculations about the seven chambers of the uterus, the power of pregnant women's imagination to shape the foetus in utero and other stories that anatomically-trained surgeons and obstetricians would attack by the early eighteenth century. Sharp's interventionist suggestions were primarily for the serious emergency, an understandable moment to command a midwife to cut. In short, Sharp's text is no less sophisticated than other contemporary texts, and if anything, shows that Sharp read widely, wrote well, and had certainly attended women in labour.

Like some other midwifery and gynaecological texts, *The Midwives Book* includes plates both of the mother's reproductive organs and the foetus in utero. The artist and engraver of the plates remain unidentified. The plates were possibly sold separately from the text, and are similar to images included in other midwifery texts of the seventeenth and early eighteenth century. Sharp's images are highly schematic, for instance showing the full-term foetus as floating in a balloon-like uterus.

The Folger Library's copy of Sharp has been chosen as the base copy because it is cleaner and more loosely bound than other existing copies. As with all other copies, the page numbers have been misprinted from page 305 to 321. The text itself on these pages is in proper order and sequence. The plate facing page 150 is from The Huntington Library, and is reduced in size to fit this facsimile volume.

Elizabeth Cellier

Aside from the dates of her birth and death, much more is known about Elizabeth Cellier, 'the Popish Midwife', than about Jane Sharp. English and Protestant-born,

Cellier converted to Catholicism and was married at least twice, the second time to Peter Cellier, a French Catholic merchant. The Celliers lived on Arundel Street in St Clement Danes, London and were connected socially to the city's elite and aristocratic Catholic community. Elizabeth Cellier gained notoriety for her involvement in a complicated, slightly farcical, political drama nick-named 'The Meal-Tub Plot' of 1679, an offshoot of the better-known and tragic 'Popish Plot' of 1678. Cellier was imprisoned for several months and tried for treason; she was acquitted, but then published a self defence entitled *Malice Defeated* (1680) which promptly led the authorities to try her for libel. This time she was unlucky, forced to pay a one thousand pound fine and stand in the pillory on three separate occasions. Cellier and her supporters published accounts of these events, while several others published satirical, misogynistic, and anti-Catholic attacks against her. In many of these pieces, Cellier's midwifery plays a key role. Sometimes her occupation is invoked metaphorically, but often too as evidence of either her feminine cunning or her matronly uprightness, depending on the pamphlet's stance.

Cellier gained public notice in 1687 and 1688 specifically as a midwife by proposing the creation of a 'Colledg of Midwives' which apparently won the approval of the Catholic James II, and predicting that the King's wife, Mary of Modena, would at last give birth to a son. The prediction came true, but in so doing apparently ended James's effective support of Cellier's proposed institution. James no doubt had more pressing concerns than supporting Cellier's plans since the birth of a Catholic heir jeopardized the Protestant succession to the throne. Public and parliamentary fears about this in part led to 'The Glorious Revolution' of 1688 which ultimately replaced James with his safely Protestant son-in-law and daughter, William and Mary. England was secured from a Catholic monarch, but the Catholic Cellier had apparently lost any chance of formally organizing her fellow midwives.

In the summer of 1687, Cellier sent James II a detailed administrative plan for training female midwives and supporting poor, pregnant women and abandoned children. She proposed a network of maternity hospitals and a foundling home in London which would be managed by a governess, twenty-four female midwives, and one man-midwife. Cellier's 'A Scheme for the Foundation of a Royal Hospital' remained unpublished in her day, and was first published in the 1744–1746 edition of *The Harleian Miscellany* and again in 1751 in *A Fourth Collection of Scarce and Valuable Tracts*. Cellier's original proposal was greeted favourably by the king, but it seems to have also generated some public discussion which led her to publish *To Dr.—*, a response to critics sceptical about an institution managed by female midwives.

Unlike male practitioners who belonged to the Royal College of Physicians and the Royal College of Surgeons, midwives lacked the formal structure of a chartered corporate body governing their training and practice. Nonetheless, seventeenth-century midwives still managed to create valuable networks among themselves. Urban midwives learned their trade through semi-formal apprenticeships, and they often sought ecclesiastical licensing after serving several years as a 'deputy' or assistant midwife. Yet this system of apprenticeship and church licensing was neither uniform nor universal. The Chamberlen family of surgeons made attempts to organize female midwives in 1617 and again in 1634 when a group of female midwives countered with their own petition to the Royal College of Physicians. All of these attempts to regulate midwifery failed.

To Dr.— and 'A Scheme for the Foundation of a Royal Hospital'

To Dr.—, printed in January of 1688, is actually Cellier's second essay proposing a midwifery college, but it is the only one of the two published in her day. Six months before she published this pamphlet, she had sent her proposal, 'A Scheme', to James II. Cellier's plan to organize the midwives into a pedagogical and regulated corporation was not the first made during the century, but it was the first made by an individual woman. The plan was designed to remedy irregularities in the training and licensing of midwives and to generate substantial revenues for a building, facilities, and its organizer by charging one thousand midwives five pounds membership each and another thousand midwives fifty shillings each. Most of all, Cellier's plan would have offered midwives regular access to anatomical knowledge and to monthly pedagogical demonstrations.

Historians have offered different explanations for Cellier's publishing *To Dr.—* on 16 January 1688. The unnamed doctor-recipient of the tract has been assumed to be Hugh Chamberlen, one of Cellier's neighbours in St Clement Danes and a member of the powerful Chamberlen family which had tried to regulate and control female midwives earlier in the century. Some historians have suggested that Hugh Chamberlen engineered the 1687 plan and used Elizabeth Cellier as a female front to gain support among London's midwives. Others have suggested that the college and cradle-hospital were her own design, and that publishing the tract as a learned reply to either real or imagined queries from Chamberlen was for publicity.

In either case, *To Dr.—* mostly attempts to legitimate the notion of a female corporation of midwives through historical precedent. Using Biblical passages, examples from Greek antiquity, Roman London and European lore, Cellier argues that corporations of midwives existed 'some Hundreds, if not Thousands of Years before you can prove one of Physicians'. As Helen King has insightfully shown, Cellier creatively rewrote history to align stories of the Greek midwife Agnodike with Cellier's own political adventures.

Several copies of *To Dr.—* survive, some of which have a title-page that appears to have been printed during the eighteenth century. The copy from the Folger Library has been chosen for reproduction here because it is loosely bound, generously trimmed, and very clean compared to other copies. Cellier's name is spelled 'Celleor' in this tract, but 'Celier' and 'Cellier' in other pamphlets.

Cellier's 'A Scheme for the Foundation of a Royal Hospital' describes the structure of her midwives' college. Here she explains that the thousands of maternal and infant deaths over the previous decades were caused 'for want of due skill and care, in those women who practice the art of midwifery'. Her plan thus included a two-pronged attack on maternal and infant mortality. First, a college for teaching, examining, and regulating midwives would train midwives to manage parturition more successfully, and second, 'a Cradle-Hospital' would house orphaned, abandoned and illegitimate babies who might otherwise die. According to Cellier in *To Dr.—*, 'in September last [1687], our Gracious Soveraign was pleased to promise to unite the Midwives into a Corporation, by His Royal Charter, and also to found a *Cradle-Hospital* to breed up exposed Children, to prevent the *many Murders, and the Executions which attend them*'.

Elizabeth Cellier's 1687 manuscript proposal sent to James II remained unpublished in her day, but was first printed in *The Harleian Miscellany* (1744–1746) and again in

A Fourth Collection of Scarce and Valuable Tracts (1751). The version of 'A Scheme' reproduced here is from the William Andrews Clark Library's copy of *A Fourth Collection of Scarce and Valuable Tracts* (volume 2, 243–249).

Mary Trye

Mary Trye was the only child of Thomas O'Dowde, a fairly well-known healer and scientific speculator of the 1660s. Dates of her birth and death are unknown, but she reveals in *Medicatrix* that she began practicing medicine at her father's side in London in 1663; she describes having successfully treated the full-range of common, but deadly early modern diseases by using his medicines for over a decade. She moved to Warwick to practice medicine sometime after the 1665 plague, then returned to London to set up shop in Pall-Mall in 1674 and published her only known work the following year. Trye was her married name, and she mentions having several children.

Medicatrix

Accounting for Trye's life-work as a healer and for the characteristics of *Medicatrix* requires describing her father's work and contemporary squabbles among scientists and doctors in some detail. Thomas O'Dowde, an Irishman of elite birth and a loyal supporter to the crown throughout the Civil War, was impoverished and frequently imprisoned during the Interregnum. His fortunes greatly improved with the Restoration when he began treating syphilis and other virulent diseases with special chemical medicines prepared in his 'laboratory'. Along with some thirty other experimenters, O'Dowde gained the favour of Restoration courtiers in 1664 for an alternative medical college, based on 'chymical physic' and modelled on the principles of the Royal Society. O'Dowde and his colleagues based their experimental and practical work on Paracelsian and Helmontian medicine in opposition to the Galenic model promoted by the College of Physicians. In concrete terms, this meant that the chemical physicians emphasized pharmaceutical solutions while the Galenicists tended to bleed their patients. According to other contemporaries and their own publications, by 1665 the chemical physicians had gained widespread popularity in London with both elites and the populace before the arrival of that year's epidemic plague. When the plague did strike, the chemical physicians stayed in the city working in pesthouses, while the Galenic physicians fled, refusing to administer to the sick. O'Dowde, his wife, and several of his colleagues perished for their commitment, and so did public faith in 'chymical physic'.

Although physical chemistry was somewhat discredited for its inability to save more lives, this alternative practice continued to be attacked by some members of the College of Physicians who were threatened by other medical sects and also the widespread popularity of the Royal Society. The Warwick physician and author of several medical and political treatises, Henry Stubbe, continued the controversy, accusing the chemical physicians and Royal Society of promoting popery in his 1670 *Campanella Revived*. As Stubbe's work had specifically attacked her father, Trye published *Medicatrix* as a sharp rebuttal partly vindicating his memory and lancing

Stubbe, but also more subtly justifying her own newly-established medical practice in London.

Mary Trye may have known Stubbe personally as they both practised in Warwickshire contemporaneously; the dozens of pages she spends refuting him and comparing him pejoratively to Cicero imply that she had more disagreements with Stubbe than the few sentences referring to her father in *Campanella* would imply. Trye's clever comparisons between Stubbe and Plutarch's Cicero rhetorically deflate Stubbe (and by extension other physicians opposed to the Royal Society) as '*Verbalists*' forever puffing words rather than observing nature or truly healing the sick as she and her fellow '*Medicinalists*' do.

Trye exploits the traditional dualism between cerebral males, the masters of words, and females, the authorities over concrete, practical matters. From the beginning of her text Trye acknowledges female medical-authorship as unique, sarcastically quipping to Stubbe that she will 'give him ... a reasonable measure of sense, which I believe is as much, and more, then he expects from a Woman; he will be so kind as to excuse me for the vacancy of those Masculine Capacities he himself glories in: And the rather, because he well understands, that such fine things, as are prettily term'd Philosophical in him, will scarce be thought rational in me' (5). Such asides are clearly not self-deprecating, but rather foils to help build Trye's authority (and her father's memory) as *real* healers, practitioners truly observing nature, experimenting with medicinal solutions, administering and healing the sick instead of fomenting religious divisions and pompously invoking Galen.

Historians have so far only briefly mentioned Trye's work as merely a defence of her father's life and work, but this misses the subtlety of *Medicatrix* and its likely ulterior motives. Although more than half the text attacks Stubbe and hagiographically recounts her father's life, other portions build an argument for her observationally-based chemical preparations and medical practice in opposition to the College of Physicians' emphasis on Galenic theories, supposed verbal nonsense, and practice of bleeding.

Curiously, neither Trye in *Medicatrix* nor her father, Thomas O'Dowde, in his *The Poor Man's Physician* of 1665 (Wing 0139A), actually describes what chemical preparations are so medicinally successful. According to a broadside advertising O'Dowde's treatise (Wing 0139cA), the chemical physicians seem to have prescribed vomits, enemas and other therapies designed to jar the body's humours, not unlike the methods of regular physicians. The motive behind Trye's text may have been mostly to attract customers to her mysterious medicines and healing services. Unlike Jane Sharp who offered pharmaceutical recipes which midwives and mothers could actually follow, Trye keeps her ingredients to herself. By recalling her father's valiant attempts to save plague victims and counterpoising him with the troublesome Henry Stubbe, and by attaching her own methods to those of the very popular Royal Society, Trye may not explicitly say much about herself, but she implicitly advertizes herself as a learned, accomplished medical hero newly arrived in London and ready for business.

The copy of Mary Trye's *Medicatrix* from the Cambridge University Library in Cambridge, England has been chosen as the base copy because it is consistently the clearest surviving copy. Because it is tightly bound with narrow gutters, twenty-seven pages have been substituted from the copy at the National Library of Medicine in

Bethesda, Maryland. There are small discrepancies between the two copies, most notably in their slightly different title pages.

Appendix

The Mid-wives just Petition

Although seventeenth-century metropolitan midwives came from a disproportionately elite socio-economic class, they were also depicted in contemporary satirical sources as bawdy and outspoken. And though midwives were often shown to be sympathetic to fellow women, they were sometimes characterized as financially motivated. *The Mid-wives just Petition* of 1643 nicely captures the stereotype of the midwife's varied traits: strong, articulate, humane, and also earthy and a little covetous. Although such historians as Doreen Evenden consider *The Mid-wives just Petition* a serious proposal to Parliament made by London's midwives, the pamphlet's gently satirical tone suggests that it may have been a spoof, one of many mock-petitions published during the Civil War. *The Mid-wives just Petition* of 1643 was reprinted in 1646 as *The Mid-wives just Complaint* with slight modifications in the final paragraph reflecting that year's diplomatic and military situation.

The copy chosen here is the 1643 version from the William Andrews Clark Library at the University of California, Los Angeles.

References

Wing C1663 [Cellier], *M2005* [anon.], *T3174* [Trye]
Cellier, Elizabeth (1745), 'A Scheme for the Foundation of a Royal Hospital', in *Harleian Miscellany*, vol. 4, London: T. Osborne
Cody, Lisa Forman (1999), 'The politics of reproduction: from midwives' alternative public sphere to the public spectacle of man-midwifery', *Eighteenth-Century Studies* 32
Cook, Harold J. (1986), *The Decline of the Old Medical Regime in Stuart London*, Ithaca: Cornell University Press
Cook, Harold J. (1987), 'The society of chemical physicians, the new philosophy, and the restoration court', *Bulletin for the History of Medicine* 61
Cook, Harold J. (1989), 'Physicians and the new philosophy: Henry Stubbe and the virtuosi-physicians', in Roger French and Andrew Wear (eds), *The Medical Revolution of the Seventeenth Century*, Cambridge: Cambridge University Press
Cressy, David (1997), *Birth, Marriage, and Death: Ritual, Religion, and the Life-Cycle in Tudor and Stuart England*, Oxford: Oxford University Press
Eccles, Audrey (1982), *Obstetrics and Gynaecology in Tudor and Stuart England*, London: Croom Helm
Evenden, Doreen (2000), *The Midwives of Seventeenth-Century London* (Cambridge Studies in the History of Medicine), Cambridge: Cambridge University Press
Evenden, Doreen (1993), 'Mothers and their midwives in seventeenth-century London', in Hilary Marland (ed.), *The Art of Midwifery: Early Modern Midwives in Europe*, London: Routledge
Evenden, Doreen (1998), 'Gender differences in the licensing and practice of female and male surgeons in early modern England', *Medical History* 42

George, Margaret (1988), *Women in the First Capitalist Society: Experiences in seventeenth-century England*, Urbana: University of Illinois Press

Hobby, Elaine (ed.) (1999), 'Introduction', in Jane Sharp, *The Midwives Book, Or the Whole Art of Midwifry Discovered*, Oxford: Oxford University Press

Hunter, Lynette and Sarah Hutton (eds) (1997), *Women, Science and Medicine 1500–1700: Mothers and Sisters of the Royal Society*, Phoenix Mill, UK: Sutton Publishing

King, Helen (1993), 'The politick midwife: models of midwifery in the work of Elizabeth Cellier', in Hilary Marland (ed.), *The Art of Midwifery: Early Modern Midwives in Europe*, London: Routledge

Laqueur, Thomas (1990), *Making Sex: body and gender from the Greeks to Freud*, Cambridge: Harvard University Press

Marland, Hilary (ed.) (1993), *The Art of Midwifery: Early Modern Midwives in Europe*, London: Routledge

Porter, Roy and Leslie Hall (1995), *The Facts of Life: the creation of sexual knowledge in Britain, 1650–1950*, New Haven: Yale University Press

Sharp, Jane (1671), *The Midwives Book*, London: Simon Miller

Thomas, Henry (1953), 'The Society of Chymical Physitians: an echo of the great plague of London, 1665', in E. Ashworth Underwood (ed.), *Science, Medicine and History*, London: Oxford University Press

Wilson, Adrian (1995), *The Making of Man-midwifery: Childbirth in England, 1660–1770*, Cambridge: Harvard University Press

LISA FORMAN CODY

Jane Sharp's *The Midwives Book* (*STC* S2969A) is reproduced by permission of the Folger Library (219594). The first figure, set between pages 150 and 151 has been substituted, by permission, from the copy at The Huntington Library. The text block of the original measures 70 × 120 mm.

Readings where the Folger copy is unclear:

145.1	piss
145.2	but the
145.3	vessel to
145.4	blood, to
145.5	to hold
145.6	in the
145.7	from
145.8	and
145.9	child
145.10	requires,
145.11	muscles
145.12	open
145.13	but
145.14	business,
145.15	when we
145.16	the
145.17	childs
145.18	of the
145.19	Yard, but
145.20	because it
145.21	After for-
145.22	moves not,
145.23	time he
145.24	time af-
145.25	fully
152.1	cause there

The Midwives Book.

THE MIDWIVES BOOK.

Or the whole ART of
MIDWIFRY
DISCOVERED.

Directing Childbearing Women
how to behave themselves

In their { Conception, Breeding, Bearing, and Nursing } of CHILDREN.

In Six Books, *Viz.*

I. An Anatomical Description of the Parts of Men and Women.

II. What is requisite for Procreation: Signes of a Woman being with Child, and whether it be Male or Female, and how the Child is formed in the womb.

III. The causes and hinderance of conception and Barrenness, and of the paines and difficulties of Childbearing with their causes, signes and cures.

IV. Rules to know when a woman is near her labour, and when she is near conception, and how to order the Child when born.

V. How to order women in Childbirth, and of several diseases and cures for women in that condition.

VI. Of Diseases incident to women after conception: Rules for the choice of a nurse; her office; with proper cures for all diseases Incident to young Children.

By Mrs. *Jane Sharp* Practitioner in the Art of MIDWIFRY above thirty years.

London, Printed for *Simon Miller*, at the Star at the West End of St. Pauls, 1671.

THE
MIDWIVES BOOK.
Or the whole Art of
MIDWIFRY
Discovered.

Directing Childbearing Women
how to behave themselves

TO HER
MUCH ESTEEMED,
AND
EVER HONOURED FRIEND,
THE LADY
ELLENOUR TALBUTT,
BE THESE
My Poor and Weak Endeavours
Humbly Presented
BY
Madam
An Admirer of Your
Vertue and *Piety*,
Jane Sharp.

To her
UNASSUMED
AND
MUCH ESTEEM'D FRIEND,
THE LADY
EN UE TAHITI,
THESE
Poetical Wish Endeavors
Are humbly Inscribed
by

Maria

A Votary of Pure
Friendship.

TO THE
MIDWIVES
OF
ENGLAND.

Sisters.

I Have often sate down sad in the Consideration of the many Miseries Women endure in the Hands of unskilful Midwives; many professing the Art (without any skill in Anatomy, which is the Principal part effectually necessary for a Midwife) meerly for Lucres sake. I have been at Great Cost in Translations for all

Books

Books, either French, Dutch, or Italian of this kind. All which I offer with my own Experience. Humbly begging the assistance of Almighty God to aid you in this Great Work, and am

Your Affectionate Friend

Jane Sharp.

THE

THE CONTENTS

Of the several

CHAPTERS.

BOOK. I.

OF the necessity and usefulness of the Art of Midwifry. Page 1.
CHAP. I. *A brief description of the Generative parts in both Sexes, and first of the Vessels in Men appropriated to Generation* p. 5.
CHAP. II. *Of the Seed-preparing Vessels* p. 6.
CHAP. III. *Of the Vessels that make the Change of the Red Blood into a white substance like Seed.* p. 8.
CHAP. IV. *Of the Cods, or rather the Stones contained therein.* p. 10.
CHAP. V.

The Contents.

CHAP. V. *Of the Carrying Vessels* p. 14.
CHAP. VI. *Of the Vessels for Seed* p. 16.
CHAP. VII. *Of a Mans Yard* p. 18.
CHAP. VIII. *Of the Nut of the Yard* p. 27.
CHAP. IX. *Of the Muscles of the Yard* p. 28.
CHAP. X. *Of the Generative parts in Women* p. 33.
CHAP. XI. *Of the Womb* p. 38.
CHAP. XII. *Of the likeness of the Privities in both Sexes* p. 40.
CHAP. XIII. *Of the Privy passage in the Secrets of the Female Sex* p. 41.
CHAP. XIV. *Of the Seed-preparing Vessels in Women* p. 54.
CHAP. XV. *Of the Seed-carrying Vessels in Women* p. 58.
CHAP. XVI. *Of Womens Stones* p. 60.
CHAP. XVII. *Of the Womb or Matrix* p. 63.
CHAP. XVIII. *Of the fashion of the Womb, and the parts of which it is made* p. 73.

BOOK. II.

CHAP. I. **W**hat things are required for the *Procreation of Children* p. 87.
CHAP. II. *Of true Conception* p. 92.

CHAP. III.

The Contents.

CHAP. III. *Signes that a Women hath conceived, and whether it be a boy or Girle* p. 102.

CHAP. IV. *Of false Conception, and of the Mole, or Moon calf* p. 106.

CHAP. V. *Of the Causes of Monstrous Conceptions* p. 116.

CHAP. VI. *Of the resemblance, or likeness of Children to Parents* p. 120.

CHAP. VII. *Of the sympathy between the Womb and other parts* p. 125

CHAP. VIII. *How the Child grows in the Womb, and how the parts of it are successively made* p. 132.

CHAP. IX. *Of the Posture the Child lieth in the Womb.* p. 153.

BOOK. III.

CHAP: I. *What hinders Conception, and the causes of Womens Barrenness* p. 163.

CHAP. II. *Of the great pain and difficulty of Child-bearing, with the signes, cause, and Cure* p. 166.

BOOK.

The Contents.

BOOK IV.

CHAP. I. Rules for Women when near their labour   p.187.
CHAP. II. To know the fit time when the child is ready to be born   p.205.
CHAP. III. What must be done after the woman is delivered   p.210.
CHAP. IV. When and how to cut off the Child's Navel-string, and what is the consequent thereof   p.212.
CHAP. V. What is best to bring away the Secundine or After-birth   p.217.
CHAP. VI. Of the great pains and throws some Women suffer after they are delivered   p.219.
CHAP. VII. Of the Cholick some women are afflicted with in the time of their travel   p.220
CHAP. VIII. Of Womens miscarrying or Abortment, with the Signs thereof   p.221.

BOOK. V.

CHAP. I. How Women in Childbirth must be governed   p.228.
CHAP. II. Of the loosness of the Womb   p.236.
CHAP. III. Of Feavers after Child-bearing   p.243.
CHAP. IV. Of Womens Vomiting   p.248.
CHAP. V.

The Contents.

CHAP. V. Of Womens diseases in general p. 250.
CHAP. VI. Of the Green Sickness or white Feaver p. 266.
CHAP. VII. Of the straitness of the Womb p. 299.
CHAP. VIII. Of the largeness of the Womb p. 285.
CHAP. IX. Of the Terms in Women. p. 288.
CHAP. X. Of the overflowing of the Courses, and immoderate Flux thereof p. 296.
CHAP. XI. Of the Whites or Womans disease, from corruption of Humours p. 302.
CHAP. XII. Of the swelling and puffing up of the Body, especially the Belly and Feet of Women after delivery p. 308.
CHAP. XIII. Of Cold, Moist, Hot, Dry, and all the several distempers of the Womb p. 313.

BOOK. VI.

CHAP. I. Of the Strangling of the Womb, and the effects of it, with the Causes and Cure p. 317.
CHAP. II. Of the Falling Sickness p. 328.
CHAP. III. Of Womens Breasts and Nipples, the Diseases incident to the same, with their Cures. p. 336.
CHAP. IV.

The Contents.

CHAP. IV. *Neceſſary Directions for Nurſes* p. 351.
CHAP. V. *Inſtructions in the choiſe of Nurſes* p. 360.
CHAP. VI. *Of the Child.* p. 372.
CHAP. VII. *Diſcoveries of the ſeveral Diſeaſes incident to Children, with the Cure* p. 377.

THE MID-WIVES BOOK.

BOOK. I.

The Introduction.

Of the necessity, and Usefulness of the Art of Midwifry.

THe Art of *Midwifry* is doubtless one of the most useful and necessary of all Arts, for the being and well-being of *Mankind*, and therefore it is extremely requisite that a *Midwife* be both fearing God, faithful, and exceeding well experienced in that profession. Her fidelity shall find not only a reward here from man, but God hath given a special example of it, *Exod.* 1. in the Midwives of *Israel*, who were so faithful to their trust, that the Command of a King could not make them depart from it, viz. *But the Mid-*

wives

wives feared God, and did not as the King of Egypt commanded them, but saved the men children alive. Therefore God dealt well with the Midwives; and because they feared God, he made them Houses.

As for their knowledge it must be twofold, *Speculative*, and *Practical*, she that wants the knowledge of Speculation, is like to one that is blind or wants her sight: she that wants the Practice, is like one that is lame and wants her legs, the lame may see but they cannot walk, the blind may walk but they cannot see. Such is the condition of those Midwives that are not well versed in both these. Some perhaps may think, that then it is not proper for women to be of this profession, because they cannot attain so rarely to the knowledge of things as men may, who are bred up in Universities, Schools of learning, or serve their Apprentiships for that end and purpose, where Anatomy Lectures being frequently read, the situation of the parts both of men and women, and other things of great consequence are often made plain to them. But that *Objection* is easily answered, by the former example of the Midwives amongst the *Israelites*, for though we women cannot deny, that men in some things may come to a greater perfection

fection of knowledge than women ordinarily can, by reason of the former helps that women want; yet the holy Scriptures hath recorded Midwives to the perpetual honour of the female Sex. There being not so much as one word concerning *Men-midwives* mentioned there that we can find, it being the natural propriety of women to be much seeing into that Art: and though nature be not alone sufficient to the perfection of it, yet farther knowledge may be gain'd by a long and diligent practice, and be communicated to others of our own sex. I cannot deny the honour due to able *Physicians*, and *Chyrurgions*, when occasion is: Yet we find even that amongst the *Indians*, and all barbarous people, where there is no Men of Learning, the women are sufficient to perform this duty: and even in our own Nation, that we need go no farther, the poor Country people where there are none but women to assist (unless it be those that are exceeding poor and in a starving condition, and then they have more need of meat than Midwives) the women are as fruitful, and as safe and well delivered, if not much more fruitful, and better commonly in Childbed than the greatest Ladies of the Land. It is not hard words that perform the work, as if none underſtood the Art that cannot underſtand Greek. Words are but the ſhell, that we ofttimes break our Teeth with them to come at the kernel, I mean our brains to know what is the meaning of them; but to have the ſame in our mother tongue would ſave us a great deal of needleſs labour. It is commendable for men to imploy their ſpare time in ſome things of deeper Speculation than is required of the female ſex; but the Art of *Midwifry* chiefly concern us, which, even the beſt Learned men will grant, yielding ſomething of their own to us, when they are forced to borrow from us the very name they practiſe by, and to call themſelves *Men-midwives*. But to avoid long preambles in a matter ſo clear and evident, I ſhall proceed to ſet down ſuch rules, and method concerning this Art as I think needful, and that as plainly and briefly as poſſib'y I can, and with as much modeſty in words as the matter will bear: and becauſe it is commonly maintain'd, that the Maſculine gender is more worthy than the Feminine, though perhaps when men have need of us they will yield the priority to us; that I may not forſake the ordinary method, I ſhall begin with men, and treat laſt of my own ſex,

ſo

so as to be understood by the meanest capacity; desiring the Courteous Reader to use as much modesty in the perusal of it, as I have endeavoured to do in the writing of it, considering that such an Art as this cannot be set forth, but that young men and maids will have much just cause to blush sometimes, and be ashamed of their own follies, as I wish they may if they shall chance to read it, that they may not convert that into evil that is really intended for a general good.

CHAP. I.

A brief description of the Generative parts in both sexes; and first of the Vessels in Men appropriated to procreation.

THere are six *parts* in Men that are fitted for *generation*.

1. The Vessels that prepare the matter to make the seed, called *the preparing Vessels*.

2. There is that part or Vessel which works this matter, or transmutes the blood into the real desire for *seed*.

3. The *Stones* that make the *Seed* fructifie.

4. There are Vessels that conveigh the *Seed* back again from the *Stones* when they have concocted it.

5. There are the seminal or *Seed-Vessels* that keep or retain the *Seed* concocted.

6. The *Yard*, that from these *containing Vessels*, casts the seed prepared into the Matrix.

CHAP. II.

Of the Seed-preparing Vessels.

1. The *Vessels* that prepare the matter to make the *Seed* are four, two *Veins* and two *Arteries*, which go down from the small guts to the Stones; they have their names from their office, which is to fit that matter for the work, which the Stones turn into Seed that is made fruitful by them, though it be a kind of Seed or blood changed into a white substance before it comes to the Stones.

It will be needful that you should know that the fountain of *blood* is the *Liver*, and not the *Heart*, as was anciently supposed, and the Liver by the Veins disperse the blood

blood through the Body. The two *Arteries* that prepare the matter, arise both from the great *Artery* or Trunk that is in the *Heart*, and is the beginning of all the *Arteries*, for the *Arteries* rise from the *Heart*, as the *Vein*, do from the *Liver*; but the two *Veins* for preparation of Seed, are one on the right the other on the left side; the right Vein proceeds from the great hollow Vein of the *Liver*, a little below the beginning of the *Emulgent Vein*; but the left Vein springs commonly from the root of the *Emulgent Vein*, yet it hath been seen to have a branch that comes to it from the Trunk of the hollow Vein. Of these two *Veins* and *Arteries* there is one *Vein*, and one *Arterie* of each side; these two Veins in the middle part, pass streight through the Loins, and they repose upon the Lumbal Muscle, having only a thin skin, that comes betwixt them, and there they divide and scatter themselves into the skinny parts that are near adjoining. All these Veins and Arteries so descending, are called *Seed-preparing Vessels*, and they are covered with a skin that comes from the *Peritonæum*, the *Vein* lies uppermost, and the *Artery* under it. The lower part of these two *Veins* goes beyond the *Midriff* to the *Stones*, and descends

with

with a little *Nerve*, and that *Muscle* which holds up the *Stones*, through the doubling of the *Midriff*, but they pass not through the *Peritonæum*, and when it comes near the *Stones* an *Artery* joins with it, and then are these Vessels with that skin that comes from the *Peritonæum* twisted together as the young twigs of Vines are, and so pass they to the end of the *Stones*. These two *Arteries* have their beginning from the great *Artery* a little below the *Emulgent*, and so they go downwards till they join with the two *Veins* formerly mentioned; the two Veins they prepare and carry the natural Blood to make *Seed* of; the two *Arteries*, they carry the *vital Spirits* or vital blood.

CHAP. III.

Of the Vessels that make the change of red Blood into a white substance like Seed.

These Vessels, as you heard before, are also four, two *Veins* and two *Arteries*, that at their first descending keep near one to the other, carrying their different blood,

one

one from the Liver the other from the Heart, as fit matter for the *Stones* to make *Seed* of; but before they come at the Stones, they twist one with the other, sometimes the *Veins* going into the *Arteries*, and sometimes again the *Arteries* going into the *Veins*, thus they joyn their forces, the better to prepare the matter for the use of the *Stones*, and after that they part again, which things are full of delight for a Man to behold, that he may the more admire the excellency of the works of the great God that hath so wonderfully made Man. The two *Veins* and two *Arteries*, after they have joyned with many ingraftings and twistings together, appear but two *Bodies* crumpled like the *tendrels of a Vine*, white and pyramidal, and rest one upon the right, the other on the left Stone, piercing the very tunicles of the Stones with very small veins, and so disperse themselves all through the bodies of the Stones. The substance of these vessels is betwixt that of the stones and that of the Veins and Arteries, being neither wholly kernels, nor wholly skinny; their office is, by their several twistings, to mingle the vital and natural blood together which they contain, and by vertue they borrow from the Stones, to change the colour of red blood into a matter that is white, prepared immediately

ately for the Stones to make Seed of.

CHAP. IV.

Of the Cods, or rather the Stones contained therein.

THE Cods is as it were a purse for the Stones to be kept in with the seminary Vessels, and this purse is divided in the middle with a thin membrane, which some call the seam, and may be seen on the outside of the Cods, making a kind of wrinkle that runs all along the length of it, and just in the middle: This member suffers many kinds of diseases and distempers, the property of it is to be dilated and extended, by which means there arise sundry Ruptures, the Watry Uly, the windy, the Humoral, the Fleshy, and the watry ruptures, and all this happens by reason of too much repletion of the vessels of seed caused by much grosse or watry bloud. Within this pursy and sobbing and chaking of the stones which are two whole kernels like to the kernels of womens paps, their figure is Oval, and therefore some call them Eggs.

The substance of the Stones hath neither blood

blood in it nor feeling, yet they feel exqusitely by reason of the pannicles, and each stone hath two Muscles sticking to their pannicles, to lift them up that they hang not too loose. They are temperately hot and moist, but the bloud that flowes to them is very hot, by which means they draw as a Limbeck the matter of seed from the whole Body. Physicians place them amongst the Principal parts for the Generation and the preservation of mankind. They are fastned to all the Principal parts by Veins, Arteries, and Pannicles, they are subject to mulplicity of diseases and distempers. They are wrapt up in three several Coats, the outermost is the purse or Cod common to them both; it differs from other skin that covers the Body, because other skin is smooth, this is wrinkled, that it may observe the motions of the stones, to extend or shrink with them, when they ascend, or descend: they ascend in time of copulation, but in all violent heats, or Feavers, or weakness, or in old age, the stones hang down, which is alwayes a very strong sign of much damage in sickness. The second Coat wraps up the stones as the first purse doth, but the second wraps them nearer, and is not so wide as the first; and though the fleshy pannicle from which it springs be thinner here than any where else,

yet

yet it is full of small arteries and veins, that carry in vital & natural bloud to keep the stones warm, which are of themselves a very cold part. The third Coat immediately wraps in the Stones, and is white, thick, and strong to preserve the soft and loose substance of the Stones. Some persons there are, yet not many, and those Monsters in nature, that have but one stone, and some three stones, but one stone is oftener than three; and unlesse it be some great failing in Nature, I rather think that the other stone lyeth up close within the Body, as sometimes both stones do, and do not come down into the Cod till such an age, or at certain times as is proved by experience, where the stones lie within, and come not down; such persons are more prone to venery, because the stones are kept warmer than when they appear; yet the stones are tyed with strings that are long and slender, which are Muscles that hang by on both sides, to keep the stones from being overstretched or oppressing the passage of the the seminal Vessels; if any ill chance befall the stones then these Muscles are exceeding sensible of pain and subject to swell by reason of it. The left stone is the biggest, and therefore some think more femals are begotten than males, and the right is the hotter and breeds the stronger Seed, and therefore it is generally

main-

maintained, that Boyes are begotten from the right ftone, but Girles with the left. Thofe that have hotteft ftones are moft prone to Venery: and their ftones are longer and harder, and they are more hairy about thofe parts efpecially. The right ftone is the hotteft in all, becaufe it receives more pure and Vital blood from the hollow Vein and the great Artery than the left doth, which receives onely a watry bloud from the Emulgent Vein. But both of them have an innate quality to make Seed, and without the Stones no procreation can be; as we fee that fuch as are gelded lofe the faculty of Generation, though they want nothing elfe but their ftones. The fubftance of the ftones is very like to the Seed it felf, moift, white and clammy. There is yet another Veffel, or conduit belonging to the ftones, which is called the Veffel of ejecting, or cafting forth of the Seed, it comes from the head of the ftones to the root of the yard overthwart the ftones in a fmall body like a Silkworm, by one end the carrying veffel elutes the ftones, and carries forth the feed, from the other end the cafters forth of the Seed paffeth and defcends to the bottom of the ftones, and bends back again and is knit to the preparing Veffels, and returns to the head of the ftones, and fo goes upward till it touch the bone of the fmall guts, keeping

clofe

close to the preparing vessels, till it pierce the production of the Hypogastrium or lower belly, which is the upper part of the place where the hair grows above the Privities; it reacheth from the Navil to that hair, and so it runnes from thence through the hollowness of the hip and sides between the bladder and the straight gut, till it come as far as the forestanders, and so fixeth it self, where it ends at the root of the Yard where it begins; so long as it remains amongst the Coats of the stones, it is full of many windings forward and backward, but near the end it hath many little Bladders like Warts.

CHAP. V.

Of the carrying Vessels.

THe carrying Vessels on both sides, are certain small bladders, united between the Bladder and the right Gut, the last of them, with the seminary Vessels, by a little pipe ends in the forestanders: These carry and conveigh the seed that is first fully concocted in the stones, by the great heat of them by reason of the vital blood that is brought to them, to the seminary Vessels which are to hold the Seed,

till

till there is cause to cast it forth. They are but two white nervous sinews, obscure, hollow Pipes, they rise from the Stones to the Belly not far from the preparing Vessels, from the hollow of the belly they return and go to the backside of the bladder; betwixt that and the right gut, and near the neck of the bladder they are joyned to the Vessels for Seed, which are like a Honey-comb; these Honey-combs or hollow Cells have an oyly matter in them, for they attract the fatty substance from the Seed, and that they send forth into the urinary passage chiefly in the act of carnal copulation, lest the thin skin of the Yard, which is very quick of feeling should be hurt by the sharpness of the Seed. The carrying Vessels fall at last into the vessels ordain'd to the Seed till there is use for it. The carriers strengthen the vessels for the seed, and are storehouses for it, that the whole store be not wasted in one act; you shall find in some persons enough to serve for severall acts of copulation. They are hollow and round to contain the more Seed, and they are full of membranes that they may be shortned or lengthened as the Seed is more or less in quantity, and are full of meanders and turnings, that the seed pass not away without a mans will.

CHAP

CHAP. VI.

The Vessels for seed.

THe Vessels for Seed are such as you call kernels in your meat, we call them here forestanders; they are two little stones seated at the root of the Yard, a little above the sphy-aster of the the bladder, they are wrapt up with a skin that covers them, they seem to be round, but they are flat behind, and before, they are loose and spongy as kernels usually are, and white, and hard, in some persons more or less, they having a quick feeling to stir up delight in Copulation; they have some small pipes which open into the common pipes through which the Seed passeth into the Yard: these kernels or forestanders being pressed by the lower muscles of the Yard, besides the oyly fat substance they defend the urinary passage by, they also defend the Vessels that carry the seed to them, lest by much standing and stretching of the Yard the carriers of seed should be hurt; they have another use also, for lying between the bladder and the right gut, they serve for cushions for the vessels to rest upon, to keep them from violent pressing, and this is the cause why those that are costive and cannot easily go to stool, when they strain to do their business, they press those kernels and sometimes void some Seed, and also must needs make some water, more or less when they go to stool. These kernels compass the vessels that carry the seed, and through the midst of these passeth the water or Urine pipe, or common passage both for seed and Urine, or conduit of the Yard. At the mouth of this conduit where the carrying vessels meet with it, there is a thin skin that keeps the vessels for seed that are like a spunge in nature, that they shed not forth the seed against mens will. But this skin is full of holes, which open by the violent heat and motion in Copulation, and so the seed finds its way out, for it is a thin spirit, and the rather by reason of motion, and passes like Quicksilver through a piece of leather; there are no more holes to be seen in this skin than in a piece of leather, unless it be seen in some persons after death, who were in their lifetime troubled with a great running of the Reins as it is called, but properly an involuntary shedding of the Seed, because these holes are become so great, that the subtile seed cannot be kept back by it; the reins are to part the Urine from the blood, and to send that to the bladder by the conduits of Urine, but not to send forth seed or to provide it,

the

that is the work of the stones as I said. Yet by communication of parts, if the reins be much offended, the seminary parts cannot perform their office as they should, but an involuntary shedding of Seed will follow, untill such time as the reins be strengthened and cured. I shall give onely one observation and so conclude this Chapter: And that is a warning to all that cut for the stone in the bladder, of what age soever they be who are cut; oftentimes in drawing forth the stone they so rend and tear the seed vessels, that such persons are never able to beget Children, they may hatch the Cuckows Eggs, and keep other mens if they please, but they shall never get any themselves; these kernels are a hard and spungy substance near as great as a Walnut.

CHAP. VII.
Of a mans yard.

The Yard is as it were the Plow wherewith the ground is tilled, and made fit for production of Fruit; we see that some fruitful persons have a Crop by it' almost every year, onely plowing up their own ground, and live more plentifully by it than the Countryman can with all his toil and cost: & some there are that plow up other mens ground, when they can find such lascivious women that will pay them

them well for their pains, to their shame be it spoken, but commonly they pay dear for it in the end, if timely they repent not. The Yard is of a ligamental substance, sinewy and hollow as a spunge, having some muscles to help it in its several postures. The Yard and the Tongue have more great Veins and Arteries in them than any part of the Body for their bigness; by these porosities, by help of Imagination the Yard is sometimes raised, and swels with a windy spirit only, for there is a natural inclination and force by which it is raised when men are moved to Copulation, as the motion is natural in the Heart and Arteries; true it is that in these motion is alwayes necessary, but the Yard moves only at some times, and riseth sometimes to small purpose. It stands in the sharebone in the middle as all know, being of a round and long fashion, with a hollow passage within it, through which passe both the Urine and Seed; the top of it is called the Head or Nut of the Yard, and there it is compact and hard, & not very quick of feeling, lest it should suffer pain in Copulation; there is a soft loose skin called the foreskin which covers the head of it, and will move forward and backward as it is moved; this foreskin in the lower part only in the middle, is fastned or tyed long ways

C 2   to

to the greater part of the Head of the Yard by a certain skinny part called the string or bridle. It is of temperament hot and moist, & it is joined to the middle of the share bone, and with the Bladder by the Conduit pipe that carrieth the Urine, & with the brain by Nerves and Muscles that come to the skin of it, to the Heart and Liver by Veins and Arteries that come from them. The Yard hath three holes or Pipes in it, one broad one and that is common to the Urine and Seed, and two small ones by which the Seed comes into the common long Conduit pipe; these two Arteries or Vessels enter into this pipe in the place called the *Perinæum*, which in men is the place between the root of the Yard and the Arsehole or Fundament, but in a woman it is the place between that and the cut of the neck of the womb; from those holes to the Bladder, that passage is called the neck of the Bladder, and from thence to the head of the Yard is the common pipe or channel of the Yard. The Yard hath four Muscles, two towards the lower part on both sides, one of them near the channel or pipe of the Yard, and these are extended in length, and they dilate the Yard and raise it up, that the Seed may with ease pass through it: two other muscles there are that come from the root of it

near

near the share bone that comes slanting toward the top of the Yard in the upper part of it, when these are stretched the Yard riseth, and when they slacken then it falls again, and if one of these be bent and the other be not, the Yard bends to that muscle that is stretched or bent.

If the Yard be of a moderate size, not too long, nor too short, it is good as the Tongue is, but if the Yard be too long, the spirits in the seed flee away; if it be too short, it cannot carry the Seed home to the place it should do.

The Yard also serveth to empty the Bladder of the water in it, and that is easily proved by a Louse put into the pipe of the Yard, which by biting will cause one to make water when the Urine is suppress. The foreskin was made to defend the Yard that is tender, and to cause delight in Copulation; the *Jews* were commanded to cut it off. Many diseases are incident to the Yard, but a priapisme or standing of the Yard continually by reason of a windy matter, is a disease that properly belongs to this part, and is very dangerous sometimes.

The Yard of a man is not bony, as in Dogs, and Wolves, and Foxes; nor gristly, for then it could not stand and fall as need is; it is made make of Skins, Brawns, Tendons, Veins, Arteries, Sinews, and great Ligaments; yet not so full of Veins but it may be emptyed and filled again, nor so full of Arteries as to beat alwayes, yet you shall find it beat sometimes; it consists not of Nerves for they are not hollow enough for the passages, but it is compounded of a peculiar substance that is not found in any other part of the body; the place of it, as I said, begins at the share-bone, and it is fast knit to the Yard between the Cods and the Fundament, so that there is a seam that comes up along the Cods and parts them in the midst between the Stones. The Yard is not perfectly round, but is somewhat broad on the back or upperside, it differs a little in some from others; the situation of it is so peculiar to Men, that they have herein a preeminence above all other creatures. Some men, but chiefly fools, have Yards so long that they are useless for generation. It is generally held, that the length or proportion of the Yard depends upon cutting the Navel string, if you cut it too short and knit it too close in Infants it will be too short, because of the string that comes from the Navel to the bottom of the bladder, which draws up the Bladder and shortnes the Yard: and this beside the general opinion,

stands

stands with so much reason, that all *Midwives* have cause to be careful to cut the Navel string long enough, that when they tye it, the Yard may have free liberty to move and extend it self, alwayes remembring that moderation is best, that it be not left too long, which may be as bad as too short. There are six parts to be observed of which the Yard consists: 1. Two sinewy bodies. 2. A sinewy substance to hold up the two side Ligaments and the urinary passage. 3. The Urinary passage it self. 4. The Nut of the Yard. 5. The four Muscles; and 6. The Vessels.

The two sinewy bodies are really two though they are joined together, they are long and hard, within they are spongy and full of black blood, the spongy substance within seems to be woven network, and is made of numberless Veins and Arteries, and the black blood that is contained in them is full of spirits. Motion and leisure in Copulation heats them, and makes the Yard to stand, and so will imagination; the hollow weaving of them together was to hold the spirits as long as may be that the Yard fall not down before it hath performed the work of nature. These side ligaments of the Yard where they are thick and round,

spring

spring from the lower part of the share-bone, and not the upper part as *Galen* supposed. At the beginning they are parted and resemble a pair of Horns or the Letter Y, where the common pipe for Urine and Seed goes between them. It is thus manifest that the greatest part of the Yard is made of two sinewy parts, one of them of each side, and they both end at the top of the head of the Yard, they come from two beginnings and lean upon the hip under the share-bone, and so run on to the Nut of the Yard. Also their substance is double, the outside is sinewy, hard and thick, the inside black, soft, loose, spongy and thin, they are joined by a thin and sinewy skin, which is strengthened by some slanting small Veins placed there like to a Weavers Shuttle; they are parted at their first rising to make way for the water pipe, but they are joined about the middle of the share-bone, and there they lose near a third part of their sinewy substance.

The use of these two sinewy bodies that make the yard, is for the vital spirits to run through the thin parts of them and fill the Yard with spirits, and they are so thick and compact, and strong on the outside, that they hinder these spirits from breaking
suddenly

suddenly away, for should they flee out, the Yard will stand no longer but presently fall down.

In the inside of the substance of the Yard which is wrapt about by the outward sinewy substance there is seen a thin and tender artery coming from the root of the Yard, and runs quite through the whole loose substance of it: Besides these there is a Conduit pipe placed at the lower part of the Yard that serves both for Seed and Urine to be put forth by, as common to them both, and it runs through the middle of the foresaid two sinewy bodies, and is of the same substance with them, and is loose and thick, soft and tender, and runs equally in all respects from the neck of the bladder to the top of the Yard, only it is something larger where it begins than where it ends at the top of the Nut. This pipe at first, as I said, hath three holes where it riseth from the neck of the bladder, that in the middle is wider than the other two pipes or holes are which stand on both sides of it, and which are derived from the passage that comes from the Seed Vessels, and they carry the Seed into this great pipe. In this great pipe where it is fastened to the Nut of the Yard, and with the two sinewy

newy bodies, there is a little hollow place wherein when a man is troubled with the running of the Reins by reason of the Pox, some corrupt Seed or sharp matter lyeth, which occasions great pains and Ulcers, and sometimes the Chirurgeon is forced to cut off the top of the Yard; and sometimes from these Ulcers there will grow a piece of flesh in the Yards passage for Urine, which hinders the Urine that it cannot come forth till that piece of flesh be taken away by conveighing something into that Urinary passage that may eat it off. There is one thing more worth taking notice of by Chirurgions; concerning this pipe or Urinary passage, that from the place where it begins and goes forward from the neck of the bladder to the spermatick Vessels and forestanders, that there is a thin and very tender skin which is of a most acute feeling, and to stir up delight in the act of Venery, and it will make the Yard stand upon any delightsome thoughts or desires. If the Chirurgions be not careful when they thrust the springs in near that place, they will soon break this skin and undoe their Patient. This common pipe comes from the neck of the bladder, that is, it begins there, but it doth not take its being from it; for boyl the bladder

der of any creature, and it will part from it whereby it is plain, that it is only join'd to it, and so runs on to the Nut of the Yard.

CHAP. VIII.

The Nut of the Yard.

THe Nut is a piece of soft thin brawny flesh, that it may do no hurt to the Womb when it enters; it is full of spirits and blood, very quick and tender of feeling, yet will endure to be touched; the skin of it is very pure thin skin; and if it be broken or rub'd off, it will soon grow again; but if the body of it be hurt in the fleshy part, or once lost, it will never grow again; it is a little sharp at the end, and made like to a top, that it may enter the better; it is fastened as I told you, to the foreskin or the lower part with a ligament or bridle, which is sometimes so streight tied, and is so strong, that it will pull the head of the Yard backwards when it stands; but it is usually broken, or gives way the first time that a man lyeth with a woman, for the combate is then doubtless so furious, that a man feels no pain of it by reason of the

abundance

abundance of pleasure that takes it off, otherwise doubtless the part is so quick of feeling, that no man were able to endure it.

CHAP. IX.

The Muscles of the Yard.

A Muscle is an Instrument for voluntary motion, for without that no part were in a capacity to move it self. There is a little Book lately set forth and is well worth the reading, concerning the reason of the motion of the Muscles. Of these Muscles the Yard hath four, two on each side to give motion to it. These Muscles are a fibrous flesh to make up their body; they have sinews for feeling, veins for nourishment, Arteries for vital blood, a skin to cover them, and to part one Muscle from another, and all of them from the flesh, you may if you please easily discern them in a leg of a Rabbit. Of each side of the Yard, one of these Muscles is shorter and thicker than the others are, and they serve to raise the Yard and to make it stand, and are therefore called raisers or erecters; the other two are longer and smaller, and they open the lower part of the

Urinary

Urinary pipe both when men make water, and when they cast forth the Seed, and are therefore called hasteners, because they dispatch and hasten the work; one pair of these Muscles comes from a part of the hip near the beginning of the Yard; besides that they raise the Yard to make it stand, they also bend the fore part of the Yard to be thrust into the womb, so that all things are so exactly fitted by nature, that a blind man cannot miss it. The two longer Muscles come from the sphincter of the Fundament, and are of a more fleshy substance; and are full as long as the Yard, under which they go downward ending at the side of the water pipe about the middle of the Yard; were it not for these large Muscles to open the conduit pipe, the passage would be stopt by repletion of nervy bodies, both when men should make water, or cast out the Seed: They also hold the Yard firm, that it lean not to either side, and serve farther to press forth the Seed out of the forestanders, all helping to the sudden and forceable casting it out in time of Copulation, lest the spirits fly away and the Seed prove unfruitful.

There are all manner of Vessels in the Yard, as Veins, Nerves, Arteries, yet *Columbus* tells us, that *Vesalius* a great *Anatomist*, maintains

tains that there is neither Vein, nor Nerve in it, which is very false, for there are some Veins and Arteries to be seen in the outward skin of the Yard, others are within, and there the Arteries are far more than the Veins, and are dispersed through the whole body of the Yard. The right Artery runs to the left side of it, and the left to the right side, the veins that appear on the outside of it, and on the foreskin, come from the under belly; and these Veins do swell with a frothy blood when the Yard begins to stand.

It hath also two sinews, the lesser of the two goes upon the skin, the greater upon the muscles and body of the Yard. These sinews scatter themselves from the marrow of that bone which is called the holy bone, and they pass quite through the Yard, and cause exceeding great delight when the Yard stands, and they prick forward in the action of Venery.

The Yard is stretched and made to swell by reason of fulness of Seed and plenty of wind, and therefore all windy meats, as Pulse, Beans, and Pease and the like, will make the Yard stand, and sometimes they cause a priapisme or continual standing of the Yard, which will be more troublesome
t ha$

than if it should never stand at all. It is not to be imagined what pains some have undergone, who by indiscreet taking of *Cantharides* have fallen into this grievous distemper, wherefore I would wish men to take heed lest they pay for it at last, for the Proverb is commonly true, sweet meat must have sour sawce. Sometimes the bladder is full of urine, and the veins are very hot which make the Yard to rise.

The Yard is placed betwixt the thighs, that it may stand the stronger to perform its work with all the force a man is able, and at the lower end of it to add more strength it is more fleshy, and that flesh is musculous, and besides that it hath two muscles as I said on both sides to poise it equally when it stands, they are indeed but small muscles yet they are exceeding strong.

The skin of the Yard is long and loose that it may swell or slack as the Yard doth, and the foreskin of that skin sometimes covers the head of the Yard, and sometimes goes so far back that it will not come forward again. This skin in time of the Venerious action, keeps the mouth of the womb close that no cold air get in, yet some think the action migh be better performed without it; the *Jews* indeed were commanded to be Circumcised, but now Circumcision avails not & is forbidden by the Apostle. I hope no man will be so void of reason and Religion, as to be Circumcised to make trial which of these two opinions is the best; but the world was never without some mad men, who will do any thing to be singular: were the foreskin any hindrance to procreation or pleasure, nature had never made it, who made all things for these very ends and purposes.

The top of the Nut hath a hole for the Urine and Seed to come forth by, and nature hath made a little round circle at the bottom of the Nut, with a fit jetting out from the body of the Yard, and when the Yard casts the Seed into the Womb, the neck of the womb with her own slanting fibres lays hold of it and embraceth it, and by this circle the Seed is kept in the womb that it cannot fly out again. The Nut of the Yard, when it is half covered with the foreskin, looks like an Acorn in the Cup, and therefore some call it *Glans*, which in Latin signifies an Acorn, in this Acorn or Nut of the Yard lyeth all the pleasure of Copulation, so that if the Nut were gone, many think there could be no more tickling or moving in the Seed, but all fruitful Copulation would be lost, or at least there would be no pleasure in the act of Generation, though the Stones might

might move a desire to it by transmitting of the Seed which is made by them. Let men be careful then how they enter too far, for it will be hard to say which were the greater loss, of the Stones or the Nut.

CHAP. X.

Of the Generation or Privy parts in Women.

MAn in the act of procreation is the agent and tiller and sower of the Ground, Woman is the Patient or Ground to be tilled; who brings Seed also as well as the Man to sow the ground with. I am now to proceed to speak of this ground or Field which is the Womans womb, and the parts that serve to this work: we women have no more cause to be angry, or be ashamed of what Nature hath given us than men have, we cannot be without ours no more than they can want theirs. The things most considerable to be spoken to are, 1. The neck of the womb or privy entrance. 2. The womb it self. 3. The Stones. 4. The Vessels of Seed. At the bottom of the womans belly is a little bank called a mountain of pleasure near the well-spring, and the place where the hair coming forth shews Virgins to be ready for procreation, in some far younger than others; some are more forward at twelve years than some at sixteen years of age, as they are hotter and riper in constitution. Under this hill is the springhead; which is a passage having two lips set about with hair as the upper part is: I shall give you a brief account of the parts of it, both within and without, and of the likeness and proportion between the Generative parts in both sexes.

CHAP. XI.

Of the Womb.

THe Matrix or Womb hath two parts, the great hollow part within, and the neck that leads to it, and it is a member made by Nature for propagation of children. The substance of the concavity of it is sinewy, mingled with flesh, so that it is not very quick of feeling, it is covered with a sinewy Coat that it may stretch in time of Copulation, and may give way when the Child is to be born; when it takes in the Seed from Man the whole concavity moves towards

wards the Center, and embraceth it, and toucheth it with both its sides. The substance of the neck of it is musculous and gristly with some fat, and it hath one wrinkle upon another, and these cause pleasure in the time of Copulation; this part is very quick of feeling. The concavity or hollow of it is called the Womb, or house for the infant to lie in. Between the neck and the Womb there is a skinny fleshy substance within, quick of feeling, hollow in the middle, that will open and shut, called the Mouth of the Womb and it is like the head of a Tench, or of a young Kitten; it opens naturally in Copulation, in voiding menstrous blood, and in child-birth; but at other times, especially when a woman is with Child, it shuts so close, that the smallest needle cannot get in but by force.

The neck is long, round, hollow, at first it is no wider than a mans Yard makes it, but in maids, much less. About the middle of it is a Pannicle, called the Virgin Pannicle, made like a net with many fine ligaments and Veins, but a woman loseth it in the first act, for it is then broken. At the end of the neck there are small skins which are called fore-skins; within the neck, a little toward the share bone, there is a short entrance, whose

orifice

orifice is shut with certain fleshy and skinny additions, whereby, and by the aforesaid foreskin, the air coming between, they make a hissing noise when they make water.

The figure of the concavity of the Womb is four quare, with some roundness, and hollow below like a bladder.

There is towards the neck of the Womb on both sides a strong ligament near the hanches, binding the womb to the back, they are like a Snails horns, and therefore are called the horns of the womb.

About these horns there is one Stone on each side, harder and smaller than Mens stones, and not perfectly round, but flat like an Almond; Seed is bred in them, not thick and hot as in Men, but cold Watry seed.

These Stones have not one purse to hold them both as Mens stones have, but each of them hath a covering of its own that springs from the *Peritoneum*, binding them about, the horns and each of them hath a small muscle to move them by.

The foresaid Seed-Vessels are plainted in these Stones, and are called preparing Vessels, descending from the Liver Vein, the great Artery and the Emulgent Veins; then there are other Vessels called carriers, that continually
dilate

dilate themselves and proceed as far as the concavity of the womb, where it is joyned to the neck, and they carry the Seed to the hollow of the Womb.

The many Orifices of these Vessels are called Cups, the menstruous blood runs forth by them, and the Infant suck's its nutriment from them by the Veins and Arteries of the Navel, that are joyned to these Cups.

A Woman hath no forestanders, for a womans Vessels are soft, and do not hurt the stones as they would do in Men because they are so hard.

The whole Matrix considered with the stones and Seed Vessels, is like to a mans Yard and privities, but Mens parts for Generation are compleat and appear outwardly by reason of heat, but womens are not so compleat, and are made within by reason of their small heat.

The Matrix is like the Yard turned inside outward, for the neck of the womb is as the Yard, and the hollow of it with its receivers, and Vessels, and *Stones*, are like the Cods, for the Cods turned in have a hollowness, and within the womb lye the Stones and seed Vessels, but Mens stones and Vessels are larger.

The place of the cut of the Matrix is between

tween the Fundament and the share-bone, and the place between both Arteries, is called the *Peritoneum.*

The neck from the cut by the belly goeth upward as far as the womb, and the place of it is between the right Gut and the bladder; all these are placed at length in the cavity of the belly.

The womb is small in Maids, and less than their bladder, neither is the hollow compleat, but groweth bigger as the body doth. In Maids of ripe years it is not much bigger than you can comprehend in your hand; unless when they come to be with Child, yet it grows by reason of their courses. The sides of it are fleshy, hard, and thick, but when a Woman is with Child it is stretched out and made thin and seems more sinewy, and then it riseth toward the Navel more or less according as the Child is in bigness.

It hath but one hollow Cell, yet this at the bottom is in some manner divided into two, as if there were two wombs fastened to one neck.

For the most part Boys are bred in the right side of it, and Girles in the left.

It joyns to the Brain by Nerves, to the Heart by Arteries, to the Liver and Lightes by Veins, to the right Gut by Pannicles, to the

bladder

bladder by the neck of it; which neck is short, and comes not forth as Mens do; it is joyned to the hanches by the hornes, the concavity of it is loose every way, and therefore it will fall to the sides, and sometimes it will come all forth of the body by the neck of it. Perhaps it is no error to say the Wombs are two, because there are two cavities like two hollow hands touching one the other, both covered with one Pannicle, and both end in one channel; No Man that sees a womb can well discern it unless he be well skiled in the Aspects, concerning limbs, and shadows, whereby Physicians are much helped in many practices as well as other Artificers.

The womb by reason of that which flows to it, is hot and moist. It is of great use to cleanse the body from superfluous blood, but chiefly to preserve the Child.

It is subject to all diseases, and the whole womb may be taken forth when it is corrupted, as I have seen, and yet the woman may live in good health when it is all cut away. In the year of our *Lord* 1520, upon the 5th. of *October*, *Domianus* a *Chirurgion*, cut out a whole womb from one called *Gentil*, the wife of *Christopher Briant* of *Millan*, in the presence of many Learned Doctors, and other Students: and that woman did afterwards follow her ordinary

dinary business, and as she and her Husband confest and reported, she kept company with her husband, and cast forth Seed in Copulation, and had her monthly courses as she was wont to have before.

CHAP. XII.

Of the likeness of the Privities of both sexes.

But to handle these things more particularly, Galen saith that women have all the parts of Generation that Men have, but Mens are outwardly, womens inwardly.

The womb is like to a mans Cod, turned the inside outward, and thrust inward between the bladder and the right Gut, for then the stones which were in the Cod, will stick on the outsides of it, so that what was a Cod before will be a Matrix, so the neck of the womb which is the passage for the Yard to enter, resembleth a Yard turned inwards, for they are both one length, onely they differ like a pipe, and the case for it; so then it is plain, that when the woman conceives, the same members are made in both sexes, but the Child proves to
be

be a Boy or a Girle as the Seed is in temper; and the parts are either thrust forth by heat, or kept in for want of heat; so a woman is not so perfect as a Man, because her heat is weaker, but the Man can do nothing without the woman to beget Children, though some idle Coxcombs will needs undertake to shew how Children may be had without use of the woman.

CHAP. XIII.

Of the secrets of the Female sex, and first of the privy passage.

SEven things are here to be observed: 1. The Lips. 2. The Wings. 3. The Clitoris. 4. The passage for Urine. 5. The four fleshy Knobs. 6. The membrane, or sinewy skin that joynes these four fleshy knobs together. 7. The neck of the womb.

The Lips, or Laps of the Privities are outwardly seen, and they are made of the common coverings of the body, having some spongy fat, both are to keep the inward parts from cold, and that nothing get in to offend the womb; some call this the womans modesty, for they are a double door like Flood-
gates

gates to shut and open: the neck of the womb ends in this, and it is as it were a skinny addition, for covering of the neck, answering to the foreskin of a Mans yard. These Lips which make the fissure of the outward orifice, are long, soft, of a skinny and fleshy substance; in some kind spongy and like kernels, with a hard brawny fat under them, and they are covered with a thin skin; but in those women that are married, they lye lower and smoother than in maids; when maids are ripe they are full of hair that grows upon them, but they are more curled in women than the hair of Maids. They that have much hair and very young are much given to venery.

The wings appear when the Lips are parted, and they are made of soft spongy flesh, and the doubling of the skin, placed at the sides of the neck, these compass the Clitoris, and are like a Cocks Comb. These wings besides the great pleasure they give women in Copulation, are to defend the Matrix from outward violence, and serve to the orifice of the neck of the womb as the foreskin doth to a mans Yard, for they shut the cleft with lips as it were, and preserve the womb from cold air and all injuries: and they direct the Urine through the large passage, as between two walls, receiving it from the bottom of

the

the cleft like a Tunnel, and so it runs forth in a broad stream and a hissing noise, not so much as wetting the wings of the Lap as it goes along; and therefore these wings are called *Nymphs*, because they joyn to the passage of the Urine, and the neck of the womb, out of which as out of Fountains, whereof the *Nymphs* were called Goddesses, water and humours do flow, & besides in them is all the joy and delight of *Venus*. Those parts that are seen without are the Lips, the slit, and the groin, but so soon as the Lips are divided there are three slits to be seen, the greatest is the outmost and is first seen, and there are two less slits between the wings, which serve to close up the parts the more firmly. But that which is the great and long slit, is made by the Lips, and bends backward toward the Fundament from the share-bone downward toward the slit of of the buttocks, and the more backward it goes the deeper and broader it is, and so it makes a trench like a Boat, and ends in the welt of the orifice of the neck of the womb.

The *Clitoris* is a sinewy hard body, full of spongy and black matter within it, as it is in the side ligaments of a mans Yard, and this *Clitoris* will stand and fall as the Yard doth, & makes women lustfull and take delight in Copulation, and were it not for this they would
have

have no defire nor delight, nor would they ever conceive. Some think that *Hermaphrodites* are only women that have their Clitoris greater, and hanging out more than others have, and fo fhew like a Mans Yard, and it is fo called, for it is a fmall exuberation in the upper, forward, and middle part of the fhare, in the top of the greater flit where the wings end. It differs from the Yard in length, the common pipe, and the want of one pair of the mufcles which the Yard hath, but is the fame in place and fubftance; for it hath two finewy bodies round, without thick and hard, but inwardly fpongy and full of holes, or pores, that when the fpirits come into it, it may ftretch, and when the fpirits are diffipated it grows loofe again; thefe finews as in a Mans Yard, are full of grofs black vital blood, they come from both the fhare-bones and join with the bones of the Hip, they part at firft, but join about the joining of the fhare-bones, and fo they make a folid hard body of the Yard; and the end is like the Nut, to which is joined a fmall mufcle on each fide. The head of this counterfeit Yard is called *Tentigo*, and the Wings joining cover it with a fine skin like the foreskin; it hath a hole, but it goes not through, and Veffels run along the

back

back of it as upon a Mans Yard; commonly it is but a small sprout, lying close hid under the Wings, and not easily felt, yet sometimes it grows so long that it hangs forth at the slit like a Yard, and will swell and stand stiff if it be provoked, and some lewd women have endeavoured to use it as men do theirs. In the *Indies*, and *Egypt* they are frequent, but I never heard but of one in this Country, if there be any they will do what they can for shame to keep it close.

The *Clitoris* in Women as it is very small in most, serves for the same purpose as the bridle of the Yard doth, for the womans stones lying far distant from the Mans Yard, the imagination passeth to the spermatical Vessels by the Clitoris moving and the lower ligatures of the Womb, which are joyned to the carrying Vessels of the Seed, so by the stirring of the Clitoris the imagination causeth the Vessels to cast out that Seed that lyeth deep in the body, for in this and the ligaments that are fastened in it, lies the chief pleasure of loves delight in Copulation; and indeed were not the pleasure transcendently ravishing us, a man or woman would hardly ever die for love.

I told you the Clitoris is so long in some women that it is seen to hang forth at their

Privities

Privities and not only the Clitoris that lyeth behind the wings but the Wings also, for the Wings being two skinny Caruncles, on each side one, joyn almost at first, arising from a welt or gard of the skin, of a ligamental substance in the back part the slit of the neck; and they ly hid betwixt the two Lips of the Lap: they alwayes almost touch one the other, and they go up to the end where the share-bone meets, and when they joyn they make a fleshy rising and cover the Clitoris with a foreskin and so they rise to the top of the great cleft. They are longer from the middle upward, and sometimes they will hang forth a little at the great slit without the lips with a blunt corner; yet they are threesquare, like that part of a Cocks Comb that hangs down under his throat both for form and colour; they are soft and spongy, partly fleshy, and partly skinny. In some Countries they grow so long that the Chirurgion cuts them off to avoid trouble and shame, chiefly in *Egypt*; they will bleed much when they are cut, and the blood is hardly stopt; wherefore maids have them cut off betimes, and before they marry, for it is a flux of humours to them, and much motion that makes them grow so long. Some Sea-men say that they have seen *Negro* Women go stark naked

naked, and these wings hanging out.

 Besides these, under the *Clitoris* and above the neck is the passage of the womans water, for the Woman makes not water through the neck of the womb, nor is it a common passage for Urine and Seed as in men, but it is only for Urine, therefore they that will cast an injection into the womans cleft to stop their water from coming forth too much upon any occasion concerns their bladder, must take heed they thrust not the spring into the mouth of the Matrix instead of the passage of the bladder.

 Near this are four Caruncles or fleshy knobs, in form like to Mirtle berries, they are round in maids, but they flag and hang down as soon as their maidenhead is lost, the uppermost of them is forked and largest, that it may admit the neck of the urinary passage; the other three are below this on the sides; they all serve to keep off air or any thing may offend the neck of the womb.

 Maids have these fleshy knobs joyned together by a sinewy skin interwoven with many small veins, and with a hole in the middle, and through that their Courses pass, it is about the bigness of a mans little finger in such as are grown up; this is that skin so much talked of, and is the token of Virginity ty wheresoever it is, for the first act of Copulation breaks it; some think that it is not found in all maids, but doubtless that is false, else it could have been no proof of Virginity to the *Israelites*. Yet certain it is that it may be broken before Copulation, either by defluxion of sharp humours, especially in young maids, or by thrusting in of Pessaries unskilfully to provoke the Terms, and many other ways.

The four fleshy knobs with this are like a Rose half blown when the bearded leaves are taken away, or this production with the Lap or privity is like a great Clove-gille-flower new blown, thence came the word deflowred.

The *Arabians* thought this skin called *Hymen* was the joining of five Veins together as they are placed on both sides; but that is rejected.

Termelius thought the sides of the womb stuck together and were parted by Copulation; there are many other opinions needless to trouble the Reader with. Whatsoever it is, there are certain Veins in it which bleed in the breaking of it; and the *Hebrew* maids were more careful to keep it unbroken, than the *French* and *Italian* are; or else *Columbus* would not say it is seldom found;

and

and *Laurentius* professeth he never could find it.

It lieth alwayes hid in the middle of the great cleft, and is peculiar no doubt to all maids, it is as long as the little finger and is broad in the middle, and is compassed about with a round hollowness, the fashion of it is round, but it ends in a point that hath a hole in it so long as the top of the little finger may be put into it; it is partly fleshy and partly skinny; there are also four skins, like Mirtle berries, as I said, at every corner of the bosome one, and there are also four membranes or skins that tie these together, and they go not slanting, but they run all right downward, from the inside of the said bosome, and are each of them placed in the distance between the foresaid fleshy skins, and with them they are almost equally stretched out; but both these and they are in several bodies shorter or larger, and the orifice at the end of them wider or smaller, the hole is then straitest when the fleshy skins are nearest joined together; for this cause some maids suffer not so much pain to lose their Maidenhead as others do; for when the Yard first enters the neck of the womb, the fleshy membranes and caruncles are torn up, and the caruncles are so stret-

E   ched

ched that a man would think they were never join'd together; some Vessels are opened by this means, & by reason of the pain puts maids to a squeek or two, but it is soon over; the younger the maids are the greater the pain, because of the dryness of the part, but they lose less blood in the act because of the smalness of the Vessels: the elder they are, by reason of their courses that have often flowed, the moisture is more and the pain less, by reason of the wetness and looseness of the *Hymen*, but the Flux of blood is greater, because the Vessels are greater, and the blood hath gotten a fuller passage thither; some pain there will be for all this but not much; yet if they have their Courses then running, or have had them some three or four daies before, the membranes are so dilated by the moisture of those parts that the pain is far less; which hath been a reason why some persons have been jealous of their new married Wives without a cause, thinking they had lost their Maidenheads before. It is best therefore for maids new married to keep their honour, and not to suffer any man to touch them during the time they have their monthly Terms. Besides that it is forbidden severely by the Law of God; and Physicians know, that those Children that are begotten

begotten during the time of separation will be Leprous, and troubled with an incurable Itch and Scabs as long as they live.

Also next to their caruncles lieth the outward cleft of the neck, and is placed as it were in the Trench of the great cleft, and is full of wrinkles and like a narrow valley leads the way by a round cavity into the inmost parts, and causeth the outward orifice of the neck of the womb, by which the Yard enters, to provoke the womans parts to give forth their Seed, and to cast in his own. There is a skinny ligament also in the back parts of the outward orifice of the neck which is strait in Maids, and is covered by the Trench, but in women that have born Children it is large and loose, and a certain sign, as well as the former, that Virginity is lost.

The neck of the womb is the distance between the Privy passage, and the mouth of the womb, into this the mans Yard enters in time of Copulation. It is eight inches long if the Woman be of a reasonable stature.

The substance of the Matrix is fleshy without, but skinny and all wrinkled within, that it may be able to retain the Seed, & that it may stretch exceedingly in Childbirth.

The neck of it stands directly betwixt the Urinary passage and the right Gut; which are the two great sinks of the body, that vain Man should not be over proud of his beginning.

It hath two membranes, and if you cut them you shall see a spongy flesh between them, such as is found in the five ligaments of the Yard, and it contains vital spirits, and causeth it to swell in the time of Copulation, and is full of numberless twigs of small Veins and Arteries.

The neck of the womb is the third part of it, and into it, as I said, the mans yard passeth, it is a passage within the passage of the *Peritoneum* called the Bason or Laver, placed between the right Gut and the bladder, and it is whiter than the superficies of the bottom; the cavity is deep, but the mouth or entrance is much narrower, it reacheth from the inward mouth of the womb to the outward mouth or lips of the Privities. It is a fit sheath to receive the Yard, and is long, that by it the mans Seed may be carried to the orifice of the Womb; it grows longer or shorter in time of Copulation, and wider and narrower, as the mans Yard is, so it swells more or less, is more open and more shut

shut; the length and wideness cannot be limited, because it is fit for any Yard: yet I have heard a *French* man complain sadly, that when he first married his Wife, it was no bigger nor wider than would fit his turn, but now it was grown as a Sack; Perhaps the fault was not the womans but his own, his weapon shrunk and was grown too little for the scabbard.

The neck of the womb is continued with the bottom of it, yet it hath a diverse substance from it, for it is sinewy and skinny that it may with more care be enlarged or contracted, not become too hard nor too soft.

The substance of it is spongy and fungous, like that of a mans Yard, that when there is Copulation, it may close about the Yard, which it doth by reason of many small Arteries which fill up the passage with spirits and make it become narrower. Wherefore in women that are lustfull, it swels in that time of desire, and the caruncles strut out, and the hole grows very strait.

In young maids it is more soft and delicate, but it grows every day harder as they grow elder; after many Children, and in old women it becomes hard like a gristle, by reason it is so often worn and by the Courses flowing forth.

It is smooth when you stretch it, and slippery, but otherwise full of wrinkles, unless it be where it ends in the Lap. In the entrance of the passage and in the fore part, there are many round folds and plaights, which cause the more pleasure in *Venus* action, by the attraction of the Nut of the Yard. In young women these folds are smoother and narrower, and the passage straiter, that it will scarce admit a finger to go in, yet through this do pass not onely the Menstruous blood, but also corrupt humours in those that have that disease is called the *Whites*.

CHAP. XIV.

Of the Vessels preparing Seed in Women.

AS in Men so in Women, the Seed vessels are either preparing or carrying Vessels. The Preparing vessels are neither more nor less than they are in Men; for they are just four, two Veins and two Arteries; and they arise as they do in men, for the right Vein is derived from the pipe of the great Liver vein under the Emulgent, but the left comes from the Emulgent on the left side: both the Arteries

teries come from the trunk of the great Artery, yet I do not say that there is no difference between these in men and women, for then it had been needless to go over this subject any more.

The differences are chiefly two; 1. Because womens passages are shorter, these vessels are shorter in women than they are in men, for womens stones lye in their bellies, but mens hang without in their Cods, but womens Vessels have by far more windings and turnings, hither and thither, out and in, than mens have, that the matter they bring may be better prepared; their windings up and down prove that they are not shorter, if they had room to go any farther as they have in Men.

It is worth observing, that you may know that the Vessels of the womb have union and communion one with the other, both the Veins & the Arteries; for the vital and natural blood are mingled to perform this great work, and it is thus brought to pass. The spermatick Veins passing by the side of the womb joyn with the foresaid Arteries, and then they make this mixture, and this is easily proved; for if you blow up the Seed Vein with a hollow pipe or quill, you shall see all the Vessels of the womb to swell at the same time, and to

E 4 be

be blown up with it; which is enough to confirm that they are all mingled and united.

These four Vessels bring the Seed from all parts of the body, that they may fit it & make it ready for Natures use. The right vein comes from the trunk of the hollow Liver vein, below the Emulgent vein, nigh unto the great hollow bone: but the left vein comes from the left Emulgent vein, for the great Artery is seated on this side by the hollow vein, and that Artery beats & throbs continually; and if the left Seed vein had come from the Trunk of the hollow vein as the right doth, it must have past over the great Artery, and then the never ceasing beating of the Artery would have broken this thin Vein, if nature had not provided the foresaid remedy against it. The Arteries both of them have the same beginning as they have in men, for they come from the Trunk of the great Artery, near the great bone under the Emulgent vein, and they are filled with vital blood, as the two Veins are with natural blood. Yet they do not fall out of the *Peritonaeum* as the Arteries of men do, nor do they reach the share-bone, because women have no reason to cast their Seed out of themselvs, but onely into their own womb, which is but a short way; nor do these Arteries interweave or

grow

grow together till they come into their stones; but with some variation again they are divided; for in women they are supported with fat membranes, & so brought to the Stones; yet by the way as they come they inoculate the Veins with the Arteries, and after that they branch into two parts, and the one part makes the Seed vessels; and that which is called *Corpus varicosum*, affording to the Cods and stones some small twigs for to feed them; but the other part is carried to the skin that cleaves to the bottom of the Matrix, and supplieth the higher part of its bottom with nourishment, and feeds the Infant in the womb also with blood: and moreover by these Vessels the monthly Terms are voided forth, especially of such women that are not with Child; but in Men they are all wrought up into one body which is called *Corpus varicosum*.

The difference that they make in shortness from the same Vessels in men, may be for this reason also, because the womans Seed doth not need so strong and great preparing as mens Seed doth; nor could their Vessels have been kept within the womans belly, had they not been made shorter than mens. But it is admirable to consider how strangely these Vessels are infolded and wrapt up one within the other to prepare the Seed: Yet because

womens

womens ſtones are but ſmall their Seed veſſels needed not to be great; ſo that ifthey have any Proſtates, ſaith *Galen*, to keep the Seed in, they are ſo ſmall they can hardly be diſcerned.

CHAP. XV.

Of the Seed-carrying Veſſels in Women.

THeſe veſſels that carry the Seed come from the lower part of the ſtones, they are on each ſide one, and are propt up by the ligaments of the womb, they are white and ſinewy, they do not go directly to the womb, but with many windings, and turnings, becauſe the way is ſhort, they are broad near the ſtones, then they grow leſs, and again when they come to the womb they are enlarged, they go to the horns of the womb and there they end, and by thoſe horns they paſs into the womb, this may be plainly ſeen in other Female creatures as well as in women though with much difference.

Theſe veſſels in their twiſtings are like to the Seed bladders as are in men, full of wrinkles, & in the midſt they have a hole or mouth like to
a Trum-

a Trumpets mouth, and it is curled up like Vine tendrils, they are more folded together than in Men, becaufe they are not to pafs through the *Peritoneum*, for womens ftones do not hang forth as mens do. Alfo they do not come from the ftones prefently to the neck of the bladder as with men, but they go from the ftones to the womb, and when they come to the fides of it, called the horns, there they part, and one part which is larger and fhorter enters into the middle of the horns of his own fide, or very near it, and there it delivers in, and fo into the cavity of the womb, Seed perfectly concocted; but the other part which is longer though it be narrower, paffeth along by the fides of the womb to the neck of it on both fides, and below the innermoft mouth of the womb they are implanted under the neck of it into the forestanders, which are not fo plain to be feen as they are with men, yet thefe hold the Seed there, till it is the time of Copulation, and then they caft it forth, for thus women great with Child do fpend their Seed, and not by opening the innermoft mouth of the womb as fome falfely think; for fo foon as a woman conceives, the mouth of the womb is moft exactly fhut clofe, yet they can lye with men all that while; and fome women before
others,

others, will take more pleasure, and are more desirous of their Husbands company than before, which is scarce seen in any other female creatures besides, most of them being fully satisfied after they have conceived; but it was needful for man that it should be so, because polygamy is forbidden by the Laws of God.

CHAP. XVI.

Of Women stones.

Women have need of stones to concoct and digest their Seed as well as men; the use of stones in both sexes is to make Seed fruitful, for if either the stones of the man or woman be out of temper they must needs be barren and unfruitful, nor is there any greater sign of health than when the stones are well; and of this Jugement was that great Physician *Hippocrates*.

There are many differences betwixt the stones of both sexes. 1. In place, because women are colder than men, their stones are kept within their lower belly to keep them warm and to make them fruitful, and they lye on either side of the womb, above the bottom, when women are not with Child; but when they are with Child, these stones lye near the
place

place where the hanch-bone, and the holy-bone join, and they are contained in loose skins coming from the *Peritoneum*, which skins cover also half the Stones, and they lie upon the Muscles of the Loins within the *Abdomen*.

2. Womans Stones have no Cod to hold them as Mens have; they have but one skin to cover them, for lying within the body they need no more; but mens Stones have four several skins to keep them warm because they hang without their bellies. Also the Cod or rather coat for the Stones, is softer, and thinner than the mans, and cleaves fast to them, that it seems to be the same body with them; this coat also receives the Vessels of blood, and wrapping them fast keeps the blood from shedding forth.

3. Womens Stones are not so thick, nor great, nor round, nor smooth, nor hard as mens are; but they are small and uneven, and broad and flat both before and behind; whereas mens are oval, smooth, large, round and equall; the upper side of womens Stones are so unequal that they resemble small kernels of the Kall joined together and they are long and hollow with small textures in them, and they are full of a watry humour like very thick Whey when Women are in good

good health, but when they are sickly they seem like bladders full of a clear watry humour, and sometimes of a yellow colour like Saffron, and will stink, so that it oftentimes causeth the strangling of the Mother, which Midwives call fits of the Mother.

4. Their Stones are also colder and moister, and so is their Seed, and therefore women have no Beards on their faces because of the coldness of their Stones.

5. They have no forestanders.

Mans Seed is the agent and womans Seed the patient, or at least not so active as the mans. *Aristotle* denyed that women had any seed at all; and *Jovianus Pontanus* would prove this by the Moon, which *Aristotle* likeneth to women in act of Procreation, who held that the Moon doth nothing but bring moist matter for the Sun to work upon in things below, but Hermetick Philosophy will prove, that the moisture the Moon brings, hath an active principle as well as the Sun: and so doubtless women are not only passive in Procreation, but active also as well as the man though not in so high a degree of action: her seed is more watry, and mans seed full of vital spirits, more condensed, thick and glutinous; for had the womans seed been as thick as the mans, they could never have

been

been so perfectly mingled together.

CHAP. XVII.

Of the Womb it self or Matrix.

THe Womb is that Field of Nature into which the Seed of man and woman is cast, and it hath also an attractive faculty to draw in a magnetique quality, as the Load-stone draweth Iron, or Fire the light of the Candle; and to this seed runs the Womans blood also, to beget, nourish, encrease and preserve the Infant till it is time for it to be born; for the natural and vegetable Soul is virtually in the Seed, and runs through the whole mass, and is brought into act by the Virtue and heat of the Woman that receives the Seed, and by the forming faculty which lies hid in the Seed of both Sexes, and in the disposition of the womb both Seeds are well mingled together at the same time in all parts of the body, I mean as to the parts made of Seed, but as for the parts made with blood, they are made at several times, as they can sooner or later procure nourishment and spirits. The parts therefore next the Liver are sooner made than those that are far from it,

and

and those are first made that the mothers blood first runs to, that is first the Navel Vein, and that being first made, by that the blood is carried to other parts.

The Womb is like a Bottle or Bladder blown when the Infant is in it, and it lieth in the lower belly, and in the last place amongst the entrails by the water course, because this is easily enlarged as the child grows in the Womb; and the child is by this means more easily begot, and the Woman delivered of it; nor is it any hindrance to the parts of nutrition while the woman continues with Child; but had the Womb where the Infant lieth, been seated in the middle or upper belly, the child would have been soon stifled, for the womb could not have stretched wider according to the growth of the Child, because the bones that compass the upper belly would have hindered it.

The hollow part of the belly where the Womb lieth is called the Bason, and it is placed between the Bladder and the right Gut; the bladder stands before it, and is a strong membrane to defend it, and the right Gut lieth behind it, as a pillow to keep off the hardness of the backbone, so that the womb lieth in the middle of the lowest belly to ballance the body equally, and to contain the womb:

Womb: the Bason is larger in women than in men, as you may see by their larger buttocks. As the child grows, the bottom of the womb which lieth uppermost, lying at liberty and not tyed, grows upward towards the Navel, and so leans upon the small Guts, and so fills all the hollow of the Flancks when women are near the time to bring forth.

The Womb is fastened and tied partly by the substance of it, and also by four ligaments, two above, and two beneath, but the bottom is not tied neither before, nor behind, nor above, but is free and at liberty, that it can stretch as need requires in Copulation, or Child-bearing, and it hath a kind of animal motion to satisfie its desire. *Galen* saith, that the sides are fastened to the hanch-bone, by membranes, & ligaments, coming from the muscles of the Loyns, and interwoven oft-times with fleshy fibres, and carried to other parts of the womb to hold it fast.

The neck of the womb is tied, but not every side, to the parts that lie near it; at the sides it is loosely tied to the *Peritoneum* by certain membranes that grow to it, and on the back part it is fastened with thin fibres, and a little fat to the right Gut and the holy-bone, it lieth upon that fat all along that passage, and it grows into one with the Fundament, above the Lap, to which it is joined before; if the Fundament chance to be ulcerated within, the dung hath been seen to fall out at the Lap.

The fore part is knit to the neck of the bladder, and because the wombs neck is broader than the neck of the bladder, some part of it is fastened by membranes coming from the *Peritoneum* to the share-bone; from hence it happens that when the womb is inflamed, the Woman hath a great desire to go to stool and to make water, but cannot.

The lower strings that fasten the Womb are two also, called the horns of the womb; they are sinewy, round, reddish, and hollow, chiefly at their ends, like to the husky membrane; and sometimes this hollowness is full of fat; these horns come from the sides of the Womb, and at their first coming forth they touch the Seed-carrying Vessels. When these productions are stretched too much, as they are ofttimes in hard labour in Childbirth, there happens to women a rupture as well as to men, but they may be cured by cutting and strong ligatures.

Fleshy fibres are joined to these productions after they come forth of the *Abdomen*, and they are small Muscles called holders up, in Women they belong not to the Stones as they do in men, because they join in men to the Seed Vessels. When these ligaments come at the share-bone, they change into a broad sinewy slenderness, mingled with a membrane which toucheth and covers the fore-part of the share-bone, and upon this the *Clitoris* cleaveth and is tied, which being nervous, and of pure feeling, when it is rubbed and stirred it causeth lustful thoughts, which being communicated to these ligaments, is passeth to the Vessels that carry the seed. Yet these holders up serve for other uses, for as they are Muscles that hold up the Stones in men, so they hold up the womb in women that it may be kept form falling out at the Lap.

The parts then of the womb are two; The neck or mouth, and the bottom: The neck is the entrance into it, which will open and shut like a purse; for in the act of Copulation it receives the Yard into it, but after conception the point of a Bodkin cannot pass; yet when the time comes for the Child to come forth, it will open and make room enough for the greatest child that is conceived: This made *Galen* wonder, and so should we all, to consider how fearfully and wonderfully *God* hath made us as the *Psalmist* saith;

The Works of the Lord are wonderful, to be sought out of all those that take Pleasure therein.

The form of the womb is exactly round, and in maids it is no bigger than a walnut, yet it will stretch so after conception, that it will easily contain the child and all that belongs to it; it is small at first to embrace the Seed that is but little cast into it. It is made of two skins, an outward, and an inward skin, the outward is thick, smooth, and slippery, excepting those parts where the Seed Vessels come into the womb; the inward skin is full of small holes.

It is far different from the Matrix of beasts, which *Galen* knew not, for the *Grecians* in those daies held it an abomination to dissect any man or woman though they were dead; all the knowledge of *Anatomy* they learned, was by dissecting Apes and such Creatures that were the most like to mankind, but the inside of men or women they saw not, and so were ignorant of the difference between them. Whence it is confirmed, that they knew not the seat of some diseases so well as we do, and therefore must need fall short of the cure; nor would they use the means to find out what disease they died of, which true *Anatomy* would have made known to them, and would have been a great furtherance

ance to preserve others that were sick of the same diseases that others died of before.

It hath been much and long disputed how many Cells are in the womb: *Mundinus* and *Galen* say there are seven several Cells, and that a woman may, by reason of so many places distinct one from the other, have seven Children at a birth, and many midwives are of this opinion, but none that ever saw the womb can think so; for there is but one hollow place, unless Men will say that those holes where the seed vessels come into the womb are places for Children to be conceived in. They that maintain seven Cells in the womb, say a woman may have seven Children at a birth, three Boys, three Girls, and one *Hermaphrodite*; others say a woman can have but two Children at once because nature hath given her but two breasts, she may as well go but two Miles because she hath but two legs, but it is usual for women to have three at one birth: In *Egypt* the place is so fruitful they have sometimes five or six at a birth. *Aristotle* tells us of one woman, that at four births brought forth twenty perfect living Children: but *Albertus Mignus* tells us of one woman who miscarryed of two and twenty perfect Children at once, and of another that had one hundred and fifty at once, and every one of them as big as a Mans little finger, but believe him that will: yet the story of *Margeret* Countefs of *Holfteed*, whofe Tomb is faid to be in a Monaftery in *Holland*, is much towder, to have had three hundred and fixty four living Infants born at a birth all living, & Chriftned. But to let this pafs, and come to what we know.

How comes it to pafs that Twins are conceived at the fame time, if the womb have no more but one Cell?

Empedocles faith, the caufe is plenty of feed that is fufficient to make more than one Child. *Afclepiades* afcribes it to the ftrength of the feed ejected: And *Ptolomy* to the pofition of the Starrs when Children are begot.

That twins are begot at the fame act of Copulation is held by all Antient and modern Writers, for the feed fay they being not caft into the womb all at once, divides in the womb, and makes more Children; another reafon they give is, that the womb, when it hath received the Seed, fhuts fo clofe that no more Seed can enter.

I anfwer to the firft queftion, That the beginning of conception is not fo foon as the feed is caft into the womb, for then a woman would conceive every time fhe receives it. But the perfect mixing of the feed of both sexes is the beginning of conception, and it is hard to believe, that the womb that is so small at first, that it will hardly hold a Bean, and having but one Cell, can mingle the man and womans seed together exactly in two places at the same time, and it is certain it shuts so close that no place is left for the air to enter in.

Second Answer, The womb doth not shut so close presently but that superfluous seed may come forth, and after conception the pleasures of *Venus* will open the womb at any time, for it opens the Muscles willingly in such cases; nor do all Authors agree that Twins are begotten at the same time, for all the *Stoick* Philosophers hold that they are begotten at several times, and if you read the Treatise of *Hermes*, he will tell you, that Twins are not conceived at the same minute of time; for if they were conceived at once, they must be born at once, which is impossible. Some may object, that the Treatise of *Hermes* speaks not to a minute, but if it be true to a Sign ascending, it must be true to a Degree, and to a minute, and Second.

All Authors allow of a *superfetation*, that is, the woman may conceive again when she hath conceiv'd of one Child before she be delivered of that. So *A'cumena* in *Plautus Amphitrio*, is said

said to have brought forth *Hercules* at seven Moneths, and *Iphyclus* three moneths after. *Hippocrates* tells us of a woman of *Larissa* who was delivered of two perfect living Children at forty days distance one from the other. *Avicenna* holds, that all women that have their Terms after conception, may conceive again before the first be born; and if they can conceive so long after again before the first be delivered, much rather sooner when the womb is not filled with the growth of the first. But to end this dispute we read *Gen.* 4. 2. That *Eve conceived again and bare his brother Abel*; the Original signifies, she conceived upon conception, *and bare his brother Abel*. And in the Treatise of *Hermes* you shall find a reason why two Children may be conceived a moneth asunder and yet born about the same time, and a woman may miscarry of one of them, and yet go her full time with the other, as *Hippocrates* shews in his Book *De natura Pueri*: Nay he relates of women that brought forth two Children at one birth, and a third fifteen weeks after. Let then Midwives take heed that they do not force the second Child before its time, especially if there be no great flux of bloud, nor signs of labour appearing.

Question. Why do women desire Copulation when they have already conceived, and beasts do not?

Pappea the Daughter of *Agrippa* a *Roman*, a lustful lass answered, because they are beasts. Some say it is a vertue and prerogative given to women, but they are those that call Vice Vertue. The truth is that *Adam's* first sin lyeth heavy upon his posterity, more than upon beasts, & for this the curse of *God* follows them, and inordinate lust is a great part of this curse, & the propagation of many Children at once is an effect of this intemperance. *Hippocrates* forbids women to use Copulation after conception; but I may not wrong the Man so much. But these are the fruits of Original sin, for which we ought to humble our selves in the presence of *God*, and pray earnestly for his assistance against the effects of it.

CHAP. XVIII.

Of the fashion and greatness of the Womb, and of the parts it is made of.

The womb is of the form of a Pear, round toward the bottom and large, but narrow by degrees to the neck, the roundness of it makes it fit to contain much, and it is therefore

fore less subject to be hurt. When women are wth Child the bottom is broad like a bladder, & the neck narrow; but where they are not wth Child the bottom is no broader than the neck. Some womens wombs are larger than others, according to the age, stature, and burden that they bear; Maids wombs are small and less than their bladders; but womens are greater, especially after they have once had a Child, and so it will continue. It stretcheth after they have conceived, and the larger it extends the thicker it grows.

It hath parts of two kinds; The simple parts it is made of, are Membranes, Veins, Nerves, and Arteries.

The compound parts are four; the mouth, the bottom, the neck, and the Lap or lips. The membranes are two as I said, one outward and the other inward, that it may open and shut at pleasure; the outward membrane is sinewy, and the thickest of all the membranes that come from the *Peritoneum*; it is strong and doubled, and cloaths the womb to make it more strong, and grows to it on both sides: The inward membrane is double also, but can scarce be seen but in exulcerations of the womb. When the woman conceives it is thick and soft, but it grows thicker daily, and is thickest when the time of birth is. Fibres
of

of all kinds run between these membranes, to draw and keep the Seed, and to thrust forth the burthen; and the flesh of the womb is chiefly made up of fleshy Fibres.

The three sorts of Fibres for Seed do plainly appear after women have gone long with Child, those that draw the seed are inward, and are not many, because the Seed is most cast into the womb by the Yard, the thwart Fibres are strongest, and most, and they are in the middle, but the Fibres that lye transverse are strong also, and lye outward, because it is great force that is required in time of delivery.

The Veins & Arteries that pass through the membranes of the womb come from divers places, for two Veins and two Arteries come from the Seed Vessels, and two veins and two Arteries from the vessels in the lower belly, and run upward, that from all the body, both from above and under, blood of all sorts might be conveighed, to bring nourishment for the womb, and for the infant in it; also they serve as Scavengers to purge out the Terms every moneth. The twigs of the Vein that is in the lower belly, mingle in the womb with the branches of the Seed veins, and the mouths of them reach into the hollow of the womb, and they are called cups; through these comes

more

more blood alwaies than the infants needs, that the Child may never want nutriment in the womb, and there may be some to spare when the time comds for the Child to be born; but after the birth, this blood comes not hither but goes to the Breasts to make Milk; but at all other times it is cast out monethly what is superfluous, and if it be not it corrupts and causeth fits of the Mother; yet they come oftner from the Seed corrupted, and staying there than they do from blood.

It is not onely blood is voided by the Terms, but multitude of humours and excrements, and these purgations last sometimes three or four days, sometimes a week, and young folk have them when the Moon changeth, but women in years at the full of the Moon; which is to be observed, that we may know when to give remedies to Maids whose Terms come not down, for we must do it in the time when the Moon is new or ready to change, and to elder women about the time that Nature useth to send them forth, because a Physician is but a helper to nature, and if he observe not natures rules he will sooner kill than cure.

The sinews of the womb are small but many, and interwoven like Net-work, which makes it quick of feeling; they come to the

upper

upper part of the bottom from the branches of the Nerves of the sixth Conjugation, which go to the root of the ribs, and to the lower part of the bottom, and to the neck of the Womb from the marrow of the Loins, and the great bone. Thus they by their quick feeling cause pleasure in Copulation, and Expulsion of what offends the part; they are most plentiful at the bottom of the Womb, to quicken and strengthen it in attracting and embracing the seed of man.

There is but one continued passage from the top or Lap to the bottom of the Womb; yet some divide it into four parts; namely into the upper part, or bottom, for that lieth uppermost in the body. 2. The mouth or inward orifice of the neck. 3. The neck. 4. The outward Lap, Lips, or Privity.

The chief part of these, which is properly the Womb or Matrix, is the bottom; here is the Infant conceived, kept, formed, and fed until the rational Soul be infused from above, and the Child born; The broader part or bottom is set above the share-bone that it may be dilated as the Child grows, the outside is smooth and

overlaid

overlaid with a watry moisture: there is a corner on each side above, and when Women are not with Child the seed is poured out into these, for the carrying Vessels for seed are planted into them: They are to make more room for the Child, and at first it is so small that the Parents seed fills it full, for it embraceth it, be it never so little, as close as 'tis possible; the bottom is full of pores, but they are but the mouths of the Cups by which the blood in Child-bearing comes out of the Veins of the womb, into the cavity. The corners of the wombs bottom are wrinkled, the bottom is softer than the neck of it; yet harder than the Lap and more thick. From the lower part of the bottom comes a piece an inch long like the Nut of the mans Yard, but small as ones little finger, and a Pins point will but enter into it, but it is rough to keep the Seed from recoiling after it is once attracted, for when the parts are over slippery, the humours are peccant, and those women are barren. *Hippocrates* faith, that sometimes part of the kall falls between the bladder and the womb and makes women fruitless.

This part may well be reckoned for another part of the womb, for it lieth between
the

the beginning of the bottom and the mouth, & there is a clear passage in it. The womb hath two mouths, the inward mouth and the outward, by the inward mouth the bottom opens directly into the neck, this mouth lyeth overthwart like the mouth of a Place, or the passage of the Nut of the Yard; the whole Orifice with the slit transverse is like the *Greek* Letter *Theta* Θ: it is so little and narrow that the Seed once in can scarce come back, nor any offensive thing enter into the hollow of the womb. The mouth lies directly against the bottom, for the Seed goeth in a streight line from the neck to the bottom.

The womb is alwayes shut but in time of generation, and then the bottom draws in the Seed, and it presently shuts so close that no needle, as I said, can find an entrance, and thus it continues till the time of delivery, unless some ill accident, or disease force it to open; for when women with child are in Copulation with men, they do give seed forth, but that seed comes not from the bottom, as some think, but by the neck of the womb. It must open when a child is born so wide as to give passage for it by degrees, because the neck of the womb is of a compact thick substance, and thicker when the birth

is

is nigh; wherefore there cleaves to it a body like glew, and by that means the mouth opens safely without danger of being torn or broken, and as often as the passage is open it comes away like a round crown, and Midwives call it the Rose, the Garland, or the Crown. If this mouth be too often and unreasonably opened by too frequent coition, or in over moist bodies, or by the whites, it makes women barren, and therefore Whores have seldom any Children; it is the same reason if it grow too hard, or thick, or fat, also the Cancer and the Schirrhus; two diseases incurable, which happen but seldom till the courses fail, are bred here.

Thus I have as briefly and as plainly as I could, laid down a description of the parts of generation of both sexes, purposely omitting hard names, that I might have no cause to enlarge my work, by giving you the meaning of them where there is no need, unless it be for such persons who desire rather to know Words than Things.

BOOK.

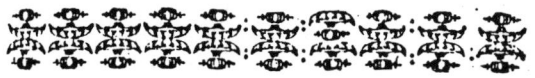

BOOK II.

CHAP. I.

What things are required for the procreation of Children.

I Have in the former part made a short explanation of the parts of both sexes, that are needful for this use, but yet some think that there is no need of describing the parts of them both, because some have written that the Generative parts in men, differ not from those in women, but in respect of place and situation in the body; and that a woman may become a man, and that one *Tyesias* was a man for many years, and after that was strangely metamorphos'd into a woman, and again from a woman to a man, and that in regard he had been of both sexes, he was chosen as the most fit

G   Judge

Judge to determine that great question, which of the two Male or Female find most pleasure in time of Copulation. Some again hold that man may be changed into a woman, but a woman can never become a man; but let every man abound in his own opinion, certain it is, that neither of these opinions is true: for the parts in men and women are different in number, and likeness, substance, and proportion; the Cod of a man turned inside outward is like the womb, yet the difference is so great that they can never be the same; for the Cod is a thin wrinkled skin, but the womb at the bottom is a thick membrane all fleshy within, and woven with many small fibres, and the Seed-Vessels are implanted so that they can never change their place; and moreover their Stones are for shape, magnitude, and composition too different to suffer a change of the sex; so that of necessity there must be a conjunction of Male and Female for the begetting of children. Insects and imperfect creatures are bred sundry wayes, without conjunction; but it is not so with mankind, but both sexes must concur, by mutual embracements, and there must be a perfect mixture of Seed issueing from them both, which vertually contain the Infant that must be formed from them. *God* made all things

things of nothing but man must have some matter to work upon or he can produce nothing.

The two principles then that are necessary in this case are the seed of both sexes, and the mothers blood; the seed of the Male is more active than that of the Female in forming the creature, though both be fruitful, but the female adds blood as well as seed out of which the fleshy parts are made, & both the fleshy and spermatick parts are maintain'd and preserv'd. What *Hippocrates* speaks of two sorts of Seed in both kinds, strong and weak seed, hot and cold, is to be understood only of strong and weak people, and as the seed is mingled, so are Boys and Girls begotten.

The Mothers blood is another principle of Children to be made; but the blood hath no active quality in this great work, but the seed works upon it, and of this blood are the chief parts of the bowels and the flesh of the muscles formed, and with this both the spermatical and fleshy parts are fed; this blood and the menstrual blood, or monthly Terms are the same, which is a blood ordained by Nature for the procreation and feeding of the Infant in the Womb, and is at set times purged forth what is superfluous; and it is an excrement

crement of the last nutriment of the fleshy parts, for what is too much for natures use she casts it forth; for women have soft loose flesh and small heat, and cannot concoct all the blood she provides, nor discuss it but by this way of purgation. The efficient cause of this purging, are the Veins that are burdened with this superfluity of the remaining blood, and desire to be discharged of it. Yet nature keeps an exact method and order in all her works; and therefore she doth not send this blood out but at certain periods of time, *viz.* once every month, and that only in some persons: generally maids have their terms at fourteen years old, and they cease at about fifty years; for they want heat and cannot breed much good blood nor expel what is too much; yet those that are weak sometimes have no courses till eighteen or twenty; some that are strong have them till almost sixty years old, fulness of blood and plenty of nutriment in diet brings them down sometimes at twelve years old: but commonly in *Climacterical* or twice seven years they break forth, heat and strength making way for them, and then maids will not be easily ruled, for their passages grow larger, the humours flow, and they find a way by their own thinness of parts, being helped by

the

the expulsive faculty. Men about the same age begin to change their faces and to grow downy with hair, and to change their notes and voices; Maids breasts swell; luftful thoughts draw away their minds, and some fall into Confumptions, others rage and grow almost mad with love.

The time of the courses is not so exact that it can be certainly determined by us who are not of Natures Cabinet counsel. Sometimes sharp corroding humours force the passage before it is time, and sometimes the blood is so thick that it cannot break forth. Lusty and Menlike women send them forth in three days, but idle persons and such as are always feeding will be seven or eight days about it; but there is a mean between them both that proportions the time accordingly, four dayes will be sufficient; but the quantity of blood that is cast out is more or less, considering the circumstance of age, temperament, diet, and nature of the blood, and that different according to the seasons of the year: the places by which it comes forth are the Veins, and the bottom of the womb, for the veins come from under the belly, and send branches to the bottom and to the neck of the womb, and when women are with Child, the superfluous blood runs out by the veins of the neck;

but maids and such as are not with Child, send this blood forth by the womb it self; by this blood the seed conceived increaseth, and when the Child is delivered, then it returns to the breasts for to make Milk as we hinted at before. Though the blood be a necessary cause, and nothing will be done without it that comes to perfection, yet the seed is the Principal cause in this building; for the seed is the workmaster that makes the Infant, and therefore the stones that make this seed must needs be Principal parts, though some exclude them, making only the Heart, the Brain, and the Liver, to be of the first rank; but the stones may in some sort be put in the first rank, not onely to make the body fruitful, but to work a change in the whole; Take away a Mans stones and he is no more the same man, but growes cold of constitution though he were never so hot before, and is subject to Convulsion fits, also their voice grows shrill and Feminine, and their manners and dispositions are commonly naught. *Eunuchs* may live without them, and it hath been an approved cure for the Leprosy in former times; but *Hppocrites* tells us, that the stones are the strength and vigour of Manhood, and that a convulsion of the stones threatneth Death, and the firmness or looseness of them is a great

sign

sign of good or evil, and that applications to the stones are very effectual to the strengthning of the body. It is then very needful for all to keep the Organs of procreation pure, and clean, that they may send forth good seed to make the work perfect, and that Children may be long lived, which they cannot well be, nor of sound constitutions, if they are begotten from corrupt Seed or unnatural blood. *Alchymists* lay the cause of all Childrens diseases on the Seed of the Parents; as plants have not the causes of their destruction from the Elements, but from their own Seed; as also we see, that when the Plague or any Epidemical disease rageth, all are not infected, because they have not that matter in them that will so soon take as it doth with others. That therefore the matter may be fit for the work of nature, there are two things very useful, good diet moderately taken, and conveniet labour and exercise of body. Ill diet causeth ill blood, and excess in meat or drink choakes the natural heat, causeth raw, crude humours, which will never make good blood, and ill blood will never make good seed, for every part hath its natural propriety to change the nutriment into its own likeness, as the Breasts change blood into Milk, the stones change it into seed alwayes suppoling such-previous preparations that are needful, or it cannot be done as it should be.

Temperance in eating and drinking will make both Parents and Children to be long lived, and there is as much difference between good and bad nourishment, as there is between pure Fountain water, and ditch water; but temperance is not to be understood as if there were a set proportion for all alike, for it is according to every ones constitution, what is too much for one Man or woman may be, too little for another; it is then such a quantity of meat or drink that the stomach can well master and digest for the feeding of the body. Those that work hard must eat more than Schollars that follow their studies, for the work of the stomach is called off by the intention of the mind, their meat must be less, and of easier digestion.

They that live in hot climates, or near the Sun have not so strong stomachs, as in colder regions, nor is it with us all one in Summer and winter, but every man or woman of years, by good observation may know his own temper, and what quantity will best agree with him; and so if he be not a fool he may be his own Physician.

Youth and age cannot feed alike, Children are often feeding because they want both for
growth

growth and nourishment, but old age not near so much; sick and healthful differ in the same kind.

I never could endure that preposterous way that most persons observe to the destruction of their Friends, that when they are sick they will never let them alone but provoke them to eat, whereas fasting is the better Doctor, so it be not out of measure.

The causes of great eating and drinking beyond the bounds of nature, are a liquorish appetite, and a fancy beyond reason: But having found out the causes, I shall prescribe some remedies withal. It is easy to know when you have eat or drank too much, or what agrees not with you; when you find nature charged with it, and is not able to digest it, vapours rising from the stomach that is glutted will choak the brain, and cause defluxions and multitudes of diseases: if you be sleepy after meat and drink, you have taken too much, for moderation makes a Man cheerful and not sleepy. Also refrain from all meats and drinks that agree not with your constitution, for they will never breed good blood, but if you have done amiss in surfeiting your self, or over eating, or using any thing that agrees not with you; remember that nature abhors all sudden changes; and therefore

fore you must not withdraw all at once but by degrees till you can bring your selves safely to a moderation. This intemperance of Parents is the cause that many Children die before their time; for what is too much can never be well concocted, but turns to ill and raw humours, and if the stomach turn the food into crude juyce, or chyle, the Liver that makes the second concoction can never mend it, to make good blood; nor can the third concoction of the stones to turn that blood into seed, make good seed of ill blood; for what is bad in the first concoction, the second concoction, nor third can ever rectify, but if the chyle be good, blood and seed will be good.

But you must know that nothing furthers good concoction more than moderate labour, for it stirs up natural heat; whereas idle persons breed crude humours. And therefore *Lycurgus* the *Lacedemonian* Law-giver commanded Maids to work, for saith he, this keeps their bodies in good temper, and free from crudities, and when they come to marry, their Children will be strong. There's as much difference between labour and sloth, as between the earth in Summer and Winter; in Summer the Sun by its heat makes it fruitful, in Winter it is chill for want of the Suns heat;

heat; Convenient labour sends the spirits to all parts of the body; when the Elements are unequally divided, death follows, so the better the spirits are distrubuted to the seed, the better will the seed be, and your Children the stronger, which is no small effect of moderate exercise, when sloth is the cause of their hasty dissolution: moderate labour open the pores of the body, and by sweat or insensible transpiration sends forth all fuliginous, and smoky vapours that choke the spirits and cause divers maladies; we find all this to be true in reason, and experience confirms it; for Countrey people that work hard digest what they eat, and their Children are usually strong and long liv'd. But Citizens and such as refuse to labour and live idle lives, I do not say all, I hope there will be the fewer, for what I have taken the pains to write now for their better instruction and reformation: then will Men wonder no longer what becomes of so many Children as are born in the City? one can hardly find as many living as are born in half a years time; I am perswaded not so many can be found to have lived to seven years of age. They that love their Children will take my advice, and they and their Children will have good cause to thank me for it; and besides the avoiding the mischiefs of intemperance to them-

themselves and posterity, they shall find the blessing of *God* upon them, as a great reward of this vertue of moderation, and the poor will have just cause to pray for me and them; for what is wastfully spent by the riotous, may be charitably bestowed upon their poor neighbours that stand in need of it.

CHAP. II.

Of true conception.

TRue Conception is then, when the seed of both sexes is good, and duly prepared and cast into the womb as into fruitful ground, and is there so fitly and equally mingled, the Man's seed with the womans, that a perfect Child is by degrees framed; for first small threads as it were of the solid and substantial parts are formed out, and the womans blood flowes to them, to make the bowels and to supply all parts of the infant with food and nourishment.

Conception is the proper action of the womb after fruitful seed cast in by both sexes, and this Conception is performed in less than seven hours after the seed is mingled, for nature

ture is not a minute idle in her work, but acts to the utmost of her power; it is not copulation, but the mixture of both seeds is called conception, when the heat of the womb fastens them; if the woman conceives not, the seed will fall out of the womb in seven daies, and abortion and conception are reckoned upon the same time.

The Seeds of both must be first perfectly mixed, and when that is done, the Matrix contracts it self and so closely embraceth it, being greedy to perfect this work, that by succession of time she stirs up the formative faculty which lieth hid in the seed and brings it into act, which was before but in possibilty, this is the natural property of the womb to make prolifick Seed fruitful, it is not all the art of man that setting the womb aside can form a living child.

To conceive with child is the earnest desire if not of all yet of most women, Nature having put into all a will to effect and produce their like. Some there are who hold conception to be a curse, because *God* laid it upon *Eve* for tasting of the forbidden fruit, *I will greatly multiply thy conception* : but, forasmuch as encrease and multiply, was the blessing of *God*, it is not the conception, but the sorrow to bring forth that was laid as a curse.

We

We see that there is in women so great a longing to conceive with child, that ofttimes for want of it the womb falls into convulsions and distracts the whole body.

The womb as I said is fast tied at the neck and about the middle, but the bottom hangs lose, so that it doth ofttimes fall into strange motions. The natural motion of it comes from the moving faculty, but the unnatural motions from some unhealthful and convulsive cause; which is most commonly bred in it for want of conception, and not bearing of children; we see no women ordinarily that are better in health, than those that often conceive with child, and some are so fruitful that they conceive with many children about the same time; so that considering his magnitude, surely no creature multiplies more than man, for he hath a priority in this blessing above the beasts. Twins are frequent, and sometimes two or three children at one birth, are not the same thing with superfetation, when children are got again before the first be delivered; you must not think divers Cells in the womb to be the cause of this multiplicity of children; for there is no such thing in the womb to be the cause of this multiplicity of children; for there is no such thing in the womb, but only one line that parts one side

from

from the other; but such women have larger wombs than others, and so the seed divided finds place to form more children than one, if their be sufficient strength in the several parts of the seed to do it. Yet when Twins are begotten, they have no more than one cake, called *Placenta*, that both their Navel vessels are received by; though they have different *Secundines* or Coats that cover them. It may be discerned, but with some difficulty, that a woman will have more than one child, by their heavy burden and slow motion, also by the unevenness of their bellies; and that there is a kind of separation made by certain wrinkles and seams to shew the children are parted in the womb; and if she be not very strong to go through with it in her Travel, she is in danger both she and her children. If the twins be both boys or both girls they will fare the better. Yet one is found by frequent examples to be more lusty & longer liv'd than the other, be they both of one sex, or one a boy the other a girl, that which is strongest entreaseth, but the weaker decayes or fails by reason of the prevailing force of the other.

Sometimes the woman conceives again a long time after her conception, the womb opening it self by reason of great delight in the action; though it were shut so close as

no

no air could enter: for the Matrix attracts and makes room for it. And this may fall out not only for once but at a third Copulation, that a woman may have one mischance and two children yet no twins. It may be discerned by the several motions of the Infants, but the mother is in great danger of her life by losing of so great a quantity of blood as she must needs lose at two births in so short a compass of time. It is most dangerous to spurr nature to delivery before her period, wherefore in such cases leave it to the work of nature, using only *Corroboratives*, and some such remedies as may facilitate her progress therein. But women may avoid this mischief that often happens, if they will rest themselves content when they have once conceived.

But that Story which I touched before, seems to me to be but a meer Romance; of *Margaret* Countess of *Henneberge*, and sister to *William* King of the *Romans*, as some writers record; that when she was forty years old, she was delivered at one birth successively of as many children as there are daies in the year, namely three hundred sixty five; the one half boys and the other half girls, and the odd child was divided to both sexes, an *Hermaphrodite*, partly male, partly female:

and

and that the cause of this miracle was from a curse of her sister, some say a poor beggar woman at her door, laid upon her for her causeless jealousie; and farther it is constantly reported, that these children were all baptized living at the Church of *Lardune* in *Holland* near the *Hague*, and the boys were all called *Johns*, the girls *Elizabeths*; there were two Silver Basons that they were Christned in, and *Guido* the *Suffragan* of *Utrecht* keeps them for to shew to strangers, and one of these Basons, as it is reported, was brought for a present to King *Charles* the second, before he came from thence; and they say farther, that presently after they were baptized, the mother and all her children died. Some write of another Countess in *Frederick* the eleventh's daies, who had five hundred boys at one birth.

But to leave this and to proceed to the causes of Conception: Notwithstanding that *God* gave the blessing generally to our first Parent, and so by consequent to all her succeeding generations, yet we find that some women are exceeding fruitful to conceive; and others barren that they conceive not at all; *God* reserving to himself a prerogative of furthering and hindering Conception where he pleaseth, that men and women may more earnestly

earnestly pray unto *God* for his blessing of Procreation, and be thankful unto him for it: so *Psal.* 127. 3. the *Psalmist* tells us, *Loe Children, and the fruit of the Womb are an heritage and gift that cometh from the Lord.* So *Hannah* pray'd in the first of *Samuel*, and gave thanks when *God* had heard her prayer. Some women are by nature barren, though both they themselves and their husbands are no way deficient to perform the acts of Generation, and are in all parts, as perfect as the most fruitful persons can be: Some think the cause is too much likeness and similitude in their complexions, for *God* having framed an Harmonious world, by a due disposing of contraries, they that are too like of constitution can never beget any thing; this I confess is hard to find, that they should agree in all respects, no difference of complexion at all; yet sometimes Physicians judge barrenness proceeds from too great similitude of persons; but I should rather think from some disproportion of the Organs, or some impediment not easily perceived; else how comes it to pass that some that have continued barren many years, at last have proved fruitful. I remember a story that I heard of a Watch-maker, who had an excellent Watch that was out of tune and he could never make it go true, what the

faul

fault was he could not find, at length he grew so angry that he threw the watch against the wall, and took it up again, and then he found it goe exceeding true; and by that means he came also to know the cause of the former defect, for indeed it proved to be nothing else but some inequality in the Case of the watch, which by throwing it against the wall, accidentally was amended; wherefore a small matter sometimes will remove the impediment if we can but find what it is.

Some say again the cause of barrenness is want of love in man and wife, whose Seed never mixeth as it should to Procreation of children, their hatred is so great; as it is recorded of *Eteocles* and *Polynices* two *Theban* Princes who killed each other, and when their bodies were afterwards burn'd, (as the manner of burial was in their daies, to preserve only their ashes in a pot,) as if the hatred still continued in their dead bodies, the flames parted in the midst and ascended with two points; and this extream hatred is the reason why women seldom or never conceive when they are ravished, and it proves as ineffectual as *Onan's* Seed when he spilt it upon the ground. The cause of this hatred in married people, is commonly when they are contracted and married by unkind Parents for some sinister ends against their wills; which makes some children complain of their Parents cruelty herein all the daies of their lives; but as Parents do ill to compel their children in such cases, so children should not be drawn away by their own foolish fanties, but take their Parents counsel along with them when they go about such a great work as marriage is, wherein consists their greatest woe or welfare so long as they live upon the earth.

Another cause that women prove barren is, when they are let blood in the arm before their courses come down, whereas to provoke the Terms when they flow not as they should, Women or Maids ought rather to be let blood in the foot, for that draws them down to the place nature hath provided, but to let blood in the arm keeps them from falling down, and is as great a mischief as can be to hinder them; wherefore let the Terms first come naturally before you venture to draw blood in the arm, unless the cause be so great that there is no help for it otherwise. The time of the courses to appear for maids is fourteen or thirteen, or the soonest at twelve years old; yet I remember that in *France* I saw a child but of nine years old that was very sickly until such time as she was let

blood

blood in the arm, and then she recovered immediately; but this is no president for others, especially in our climate, blood-letting being the ordinary remedy in those parts when the Patient is charged with fulness of blood, of what age almost soever they be.

There is besides this natural barrenness of women, another barrenness by accident, by the ill disposition of the body and generative parts, when the courses are either more or fewer than stands with the state of the womans body, when humours fall down to the womb, and have found a passage that way and will hardly be brought to keep their natural rode; or when the womb is disaffected, either by any preternatural quality that exceeds the bounds of nature, as heat or cold, or dryness, or moisture; or windy vapours.

Lastly, There is barrenness by inchantment, when a man cannot lye with his wife by reason of some charm that hath disabled him; the *French* in such a case advise a man to thred the needle *Nouer C'eguillette*, as much as to say, to piss through his wives wedding ring and not to spill a drop and then he shall be perfectly cured. Let him try it that pleaseth.

CHAP. III.

Signs that a woman is conceived with Child, and whether it be a Son or a Daughter.

Young women especially of their first Child, are so ignorant commonly, that they cannot tell whether they have conceived or not, and not one of twenty almost keeps a just account, else they would be better provided against the time of their lying in, and not so suddenly be surprised as many of them are.

Wherefore divers Physicians have laid down rules whereby to know when a woman hath conceived with Child, and these rules are drawn from almost all parts of the body. The rules are too general to be certainly proved in all women, yet some of them seldom fail in any.

First, if when the seed is cast into the womb, she feel the womb shut close, and a shivering or trembling to run through every part of her body, and that is by reason of the heat that draws inward to keep the conception, and so leaves the outward parts cold & chill.

Secondly

Secondly, The pleasure she takes at that time is extraordinary, and the mans seed comes not forth again, for the womb closely embraceth it, and will shut as fast as possibly may be.

Thirdly, The womb sinks down to cherish the seed, and so the belly grows flatter than it was before.

Fourthly, She finds pain that goes about her belly, chiefly about her Navel and lower belly, which some call the Water-course.

Fifthly, Her stomach becomes very weak, she hath no desire to eat her meat, but is troubled with sowr belchings.

Sixthly, Her monthly terms stop at some unseasonable time that she lookt not for.

Seventhly, She hath a preternathral desire to something not fit to eat nor drink, as some women with child have longed to bite off a piece of their Husbands Buttocks.

Eightly, Her Brests swell and grow round, and hard, and painful.

Ninthly, She hath no great desire to copulation, for some time she will be merry, or sad suddenly upon no manifest cause.

Tenthly, She so much loatheth her victuals, that let her but exercise her body a little in motion,

motion, and she will cast off what lieth upon her stomack.

Eleventhly, Her Nipples will look more red at the ends than they usually do.

Twelfthly, the veins of her breasts will swell and shew themselves very plain to be seen.

Thirteenthly, Likewise the veins about the eyes will be more apparent.

Fourteenthly, The womb pressing the right gut, it is painful for her to go to stool, she is weaker than she was & her visage discoloured.

These are the common rules that are laid down.

But if a womans courses be stopt, and the Veins under her lowest Eylid swell, and the colour be changed, and she hath not broken her rest by watching the night before; these signs seldom or never fail of Conception for the first two months.

If you keep her water three dayes close stopt in a glass, and then strain it through a fine linnen cloth, you will find live worms in the cloth.

Also a needle laid twenty four hours in her Urine, will be full of red spots if she have conceived, or otherwise it will be black or dark coloured.

To know whether the Infant conceived be male or female I refer you to *Hippocrates*, *A-*
pher-

pho. 48. for it is a very hard thing to discover.

1. If it be a boy she is better coloured, her right Breast will swell more, for males lye most on the right side, and her belly especially on that side lieth rounder and more tumified, and the Child will be first felt to move on that side, the woman is more cheerful and in better health, her pains are not so often nor so great, the right breast is harder and more plump, the nipple a more clear red, and the whole visage clear not swarthy.

2. If the marks before mentioned be more apparent on the left side it is a Girle that she goes with all.

3. If when she riseth from the place she sits on, she move her right foot first, and is more ready to lean on her right hand when she reposeth, all signifies a boy.

Lastly, Drop some drops of breast Milk into a Bason of water, if it swim on the top it is a Boy, if it sink in round drops judge the contrary.

CHAP,

CHAP. IV.

Of false Conception, and of the Mole or Moon Calf.

Many women themselves have thought that they had conceived with Child because their bellies were swoln so great, and their courses were staid and came not down according to natures custome; whereas this swelling of the belly more and more, and stopping of the Termes proceeded from nothing else but an ill shaped lump of flesh which grows greater every day in the womb, and is fed by the Terms that flow to it; and this is that Midwives call a Mole or Moon-Calf; and these are of two sorts, one the true, the other the false Mole.

The true Mole is a mishapen piece of flesh without figure or order, it is full of Veins and Vessels with discoloured veins or membranes of almost all colours, without any entrails or bones, or motion; it is bred in the wombs hollowness, and cleaves fast to the sides of it but takes no substance from it, sometimes it hath a skin to cover it and is empty within, sometimes it is long or round, and some women

men have cast forth three at a time like the Yard of a man: sometimes these Moles are without sense, sometimes they have an obscure feeling; sometimes they are bred with the Child, and then is the Child in great danger to be opprest by them; sometimes they are voided when the Child is delivered, or before or after. Widows have been known to have had these Moles formed in their wombs by their own seed and blood that flows thither. But ordinarily I think this comes not to pass, but it proceeds from a fault in the forming faculty, when the mans seed in Copulation is weak or defective and too little, so that it is overcome by the much quantity of the womans blood, the faculty begins to work but cannot perfect, and so onely Veins and Membranes are made but the Child is not made, yet this Mole is of so different kinds that it is not possible to set them down according to their several varieties; but doubtless a Mole is sooner formed if Men and Women ly together when they have their courses, and the blood is not fit for formation by reason of impurity, so that neither heat nor cold are the chief cause of this error, but the uncleanness of the matter that is not endued with a forming faculty; from corrupt seed or menstruous blood bad humours are in-

gendred

gendred and nature works in vain.

Some are called false Moles, and of those are four sorts, as their causes are; for either they proceed from wind and are called windy swellings, or from water flowing to the womb, and called watry swellings, or else diverse humours cause this swelling, and sometimes it is nothing but a bag full of blood. If the Child be conceived with a Mole, it draws the nourishment from the Child. Both sexes doubtless contribute to the making of most Moles, the seed of the Man being choakt with the blood of the woman, and wrapt both in a caule, Nature will make something of it though nothing to the purpose. If it be true that some widdows have had them, they were neither of the same shape nor substance, but voided will consume into water, and this can be supposed only of dead Moles, for living Moles that have some sense or feeling or true motion in them can never be produced but mans seed must be a part of their beginning; as for Maids they cannot breed any true Mole, because a true Mole must be made of the greatest part of the womans blood coming into the womb, but the vessels & passages in maids are too narrow, so that there is no flux of blood thither to make this Mole of, as it is in women

men that have had the use of man: but without dispute, the principal cause is womens carnally knowing their Husbands when their Terms are purging forth, from whence Moles, and Monsters, distorted, imperfect, ill qualified Childred are begotten. Let such as fear *God*, or love themselves, or their posterity beware of it.

The windy Mole proceeds from an overcold womb, Spleen and Liver, which breeds wind that lastneth in the hollow of the part. Sometimes the womb is weak and cannot transmute the blood for nourishment, but it turns to water which cannot be all sent forth, but part of it remains in the womb; also the womb ofttimes receives a great confluence of water from the spleen or from some parts nigh unto it.

The Mole made of many humors flowing to the womb, proceeds from the Whites, or ill purgations coming from the menstruous Veins. The fourth Mole is a skin full of blood with many white diaphanous vessels, if you cast it into the water, the skin coagulates like a clod of seed; and the blood runs away.

It is very hard to know a false conception from a true until four moneths be past, and then the motion of the body of the thing conceived

ceived will shew it; for if it be a living Child, that moves quick and lively; but the false conception falls from one side to another like a stone as the woman turns her self in her bed, if it stir at all it is but like a sponge, trembling and beating, and contracts and dilates it self like the beating of the pulse almost.

This false conception hath many signes whereby it personates and shews like a true Conception; for the Terms stop, their stomachs fail, they loath their meat, they vomit and belch sowrly, their breasts and belly swell, cunning Midwives and women themselves that have them are deceived, taking one for the other.

There are many other things bred in the womb sometimes besides these Moles; Two famous Physician of *Senon*, tell us of a woman that had a Child in her womb, that did not corrupt, nor stink, though it lay long dead there untill it was turned into a stone; cold, and heat, and driness might keep the child from corrupting, but there was also a petrifying humour mixt with the seed and blood, or it could never have been turned into a stone; there is but this single History that I ever read of this kind, and Authors say the mother lived twenty eight years after she was delivered of it; but it is no great wonder why it did

not

not stink nor corrupt in the womb, for many aged women live many years with a Mole in the body, yet it never stinks nor corrupts though they keep it in them till they dye.

As for Monsters of all sorts to be formed in the womb all nations can bring some examples; Worms, Toades, Mice, Serpents, *Gordonius* saith, are common in *Lumbardy*, and so are those they call *Soole kints* in the *Low Countries*, which are certainly caused by the heat of their stones and menstrual blood to work upon in women that have had company with men; and these are sometimes alive with the infant, and when the Child is brought forth these stay behind, and the woman is sometimes thought to be with Child again; as I knew one there my self, which was after her child-birth delivered of two like Serpents, and both run away into the Burg wall as the women supposed, but it was at least three moneths after she was delivered of a Child, and they came forth without any loss of blood, for there was no after burden. Again in time of Copulation, Imagination oftentimes also produceth Monstrous births, when women look too much on strange objects.

To distinguish then false conceptions from true, but if there be both true and false at once that is very hard to know.

False

False Conceptions cause the greatest pains in their Backs, and Groins, and Loyns, and Head; their Bellies swell sooner, they faint more, their Faces, and Feet, and Legs swell, their Bellies grow hard like a Dropsie, they have such pain in their Bellies that they cannot sleep because they carry such a dead weight within them; and though their Faces and breasts swell, they grow daily soft and lank, and no milk in their Breasts but what is like water, or very little; whereas women with Child about the fourth moneth have their Breasts swoln with milk. Some women look well with these false Conceptions, but most of them look pale, and wan, and ill favoured: If it be a boy that is conceived he will stir at the beginning of the third Moneth, and a Girle at the beginning of the third or fourth moneth, and so soon as the infant moves there is Milk bred in the Breasts as any one may prove that will. The Child that is alive moves to all sides, and upward and downward without any help, but oftenest to the right flanck. A false conception may have a motion from the expulsive faculty, but not from it self, and being not tied by ligaments as a living Child is, it tumbles to one side or other, and if she lye on her back and one press it down with his hand gently, there it
will

will stay and not remove up again of it self. If she go with a Mole nine months compleat her belly will swell more and more, but she will wax lean and wan, and never offer to be delivered. Yet a woman may go ten or eleven months with child before her time be perfect to bring forth, but this depends upon the time when the child was begotten, and some women ordinarily go longer or shorter before they come to bring forth.

Those that have Moles are usually barren, or their Privities are ulcerated, for it hurts the womb and the whole fabrick of their bodies.

The windy Mole will swell the belly like a Bladder, and it will sound like a Drum, but it is softer than the fleshy Mole or the watry, it grows sooner, and sooner disappears, and she will feel her self lighter when it abates, but sometimes it will heat the belly with such violence as if she were upon the rack.

The watry Mole is a fluctuation of water from one side to another, as the woman turns her self when she lieth, and then that side will be higher where the water falls, and the other side will sink down the more and grow flatter.

The Mole caused from many humours doth

not make the belly swell so much as the watry Mole doth, because the water comes more in quantity, and is clear, whereas the humours are reddish and stink when they come forth, like water wherein flesh hath been washed.

There is one observation more concerning false conceptions, that when they happen the Flowers stop presently and never come down, whereas they do sometimes the first two months in true conceptions, because they are superfluous in strong full fed persons before the child comes to want more nutriment, also the Navel of the woman doth not rise higher in false conceptions, but in true it doth.

Some women have their Terms well, and their wombs well disposed, yet their bellies have swoln and the cause not discerned till they were dead; for being opened; one or both corners of the womb have had little bags of water, or else clusters of kernels and strange flesh growing in them. Some women have also a piece of flesh hanging within the inward neck of the womb, fastned about a finger broad at the root, and growing dayly downward in form like a bell, and sometimes fills all the privy members orifice, and may be seen hanging forth, all these make the belly

swel

swell round, but are not properly Moles as they are before spoken of.

Amongst false conceptions all monstrous births may be reckoned, for a monster saith *Aristotle* is an error of nature failing of the end she works for, by some corrupted principle; sometimes this happens when the sex is imperfect, that you cannot know a boy from a girl; they call these *Hermaphrodites*: there is but one kind of Women *Hermaphrodites*, when a thing like a Yard stands in the place of the *Clitoris* above the top of the genital, and bears out in the bottom of the sharebone; sometimes in boys there is seen a small privy part of the woman above the root of the Yard, and in girls a Yard is seen at the *Lesk* or in the *Peritoneum*. But three ways a boy may be of doubtful sex. 1. When there is seen a womans member between the Cods and the Fundament. 2. When it is seen in the Cod, but no excrement coming forth by it. 3. When they piss through it. But Monsters most ordinarily falling out, are when the child born is of some strange feature, or like a dog, or any other creature, as the *Tartar* lately captivated by the *Germans* in their last war against the *Turks*; if the relation be true, he had a head and neck like a horse, some think he was begotten of a beast, a custom too frequent

quent amongst those miscreants. Some are monsters in magnitude, when one part, as the head, is too great for the body; or a Gyant or a Pigmy is brought forth. Sometimes in place, when the parts are displaced, as when the eyes stand in the forehead, or the ears behind in the poll; many such strange births have been in the world, and sometime children have been born with six fingers on a hand, and six toes, like those Gyants the Scripture speaks of, and others there are born with but one eye, or one hand, one ear, and the like.

CHAP. V.

Of the causes of Monstrous Conceptions.

WHat should be the causes of Monstrous Conceptions hath troubled many great Learned men. *Alcabitius* saith, if the Moon be in some Degrees when the child is conceived, it will be a Monster. Astrologers they seek the cause in the stars, but Ministers refer it to the just judgements of *God*, they do not condemn the Parent or the Child in such ca-

ses

ses, but take our blessed Saviours answer to his Disciples, who askt him, *who sinned the Parent or the Child, that he was born blind? our Saviour replyed, neither he nor his Parents, but that the Judgments of God might be made manifest in him.* In all such cases we must not exclude the Divine vengeance, nor his Instruments, the stars influence; yet all these errors of Nature as to the Instrumental causes, are either from the material or efficient cause of procreation.

The matter is the seed, which may fail three several wayes, either when it is too much, and then the members are larger, or more than they should be, or too little, and then there will be some part or the whole too little, or else the seed of both sexes is ill mixed, as of men or women with beasts; & certainly it is likely that no such creatures are born but by unnatural mixtures, yet *God* can punish the world with such grievous punishments, and that justly for our sins. *Aristotle* tells us that in *Africa* so many monsters are bred amongst beasts, because going far together to water, they that are of different kinds ingender there, and so dayly new Monsters are begotten: But the efficient cause of Monsters, is either from the forming faculty in the Seed, or else the strength of imagination joyned with it; add to these the menstruous blood and the disposition of the Matrix; sometimes the mother is frighted or conceives wonders, or longs strangely for things not to be had, and the child is markt accordingly by it. The unfitness of the matter hinders formation, for an agent cannot produce the effect where the patient is not fit to receive it. Imagination can do much, as a woman that lookt on a Blackmore brought forth a child like to a Blackmore; and one I knew, that seeing a boy with two thumbs on one hand, brought forth such another; but ordinarily the spirits and humours are disturbed by the passions of the mind, and so the forming faculty is hindered and overcome with too great plenty of humours that flow to the matrix, or the spirits are called off and gone another way. But the imagination is so strong in some persons with child, that they produce such real effects that can proceed from nothing else; as that woman, who brought forth a child all hairy like a Camel, because she usually said prayers kneeling before the image of St. *John* Baptist who was clothed with camels hair: How the imagination can work such wonders is hard to say, but there must be some strength of mind that can convey the species from the external senses to the formative faculty, for by

this

this means there is a consent between the faculties superior and interior. The Soul is all in all, and all in every part of the body, yet it works in several parts as occasions serves. The child in the Mothers womb hath a soul of its own, yet it is a part of the mother untill she be delivered, as a branch is part of a Tree while it grows there, and so the mothers imagination makes an impression upon the child, but it must be a strong imagination at that very time when the forming faculty is at work or else it will not do, but since the child takes part of the mothers life whilst he is in the womb, as the fruit doth of the tree, whatsoever moves the faculties of the mothers soul may do the like in the child. So the parts of the infant will be hairy where no hair should grow, or Strawberries or Mulberries, or the like be fashioned upon them, or have lips or parts divided or joined together according as the imagination transported by violent passions may sometimes be the cause of it.

The *Arabians* say, a strange imagination can do as much as the Heavens can to make plants and mettals in the earth.

The second cause is the heat or place of conception, which molds the matter quickly into sundry forms. But imagination holds the first place, and thence it is that children are so like their Parents.

CHAP. VI.

Of the resemblance or likeness of Children and Parents.

THere are according to Philosophers and Physicians, three forms or likenesses in every living creature.

First, Likeness of kind, as when a creature of the same kind is produced, a man from a man, a horse from a horse; and herein the likeness proceeds commonly from the matter; and because the female usually brings more matter than the male, more children are like the Mother than the Father. So a she-Goat with a Ram breed a Kid, but a he-Goat and a Sheep beget a Lamb.

Secondly, there is a likeness of sex, and the cause why the child is a boy or a girl is the heat of the seed, if the mans seed prevail in mixing above the womans it will be a boy, else a girl.

Thirdly, there is a likeness of forms and figures and other accidents, that the child by
them

them more resembles, the father or the mother, as these accidents, are found in it more like to either of the two; this, saith *Galen*, comes from the difference of parts and conformation of the members.

  Hence one is black, another white, one with a high forehead or a Roman nose, the other not. Sometimes the child is very like the father, sometimes the mother, and ofttimes like them both in many respects, sometimes like neither, but the grandfather or grandmother: and there are many examples where children have been like to those who have had no part in the work; but a strong fansie of the mother hath been the reason of it. Authors and Travellers say, that the *Chineses* children are like their Sires in many limbs and parts of their faces, as the forehead, nose, beard, and eyes. In some Countries where they have Wives in common, as a people called *Gamnate* have, Men make choice of their children by the likeness to themselves. There are also childrens marks, proper to some Families, that are visible upon their bodies, *Thyestes* had the likeness of a Crab, some of a star. The *Thebans* and *Spartans* a Lance: *Delemus* and his offspring had their thighs crooked and like to an anchor, and that lascivious strumpet *Julia*, Au-

gustine

gustus's daughter, had no children but resembled her self, for she was so cunning, that she would admit of none besides her husband till she had conceived.

Some are of that opinion, that all this proceeds from the strength of imagination, so *Empedocles*, so *Paracelsus* determine it, and the last thought the Plague to be infectious only to those that phansie made it so. But the *Arabians* ascribe so much power to imagination, that it can change the very works of nature, heal diseases, work wonders, command all kind of matter, and they impute as much or more to that, than Divines do to having Faith, to which nothing is impossible; but I cannot be altogether of their opinion.

Imagination is powerful in all living creatures, for by it *Jacob*'s Ewes conceived spotted, and grisled, the peeled rods being set before them when they were in conjunction.

Galen taught an *Æthiopian* to get a white child, setting a picture before him for his wife to look on.

Their opinions also are not wide, who say the cause of this likeness lieth much in the motion of the Seed and the forming faculty, this was *Aristotles*'s judgment. We deny not but both may be true, for imagination can do nothing

thing without it, and by the forming faculty Imagination works this similitude, yet so that they both concur to the business. The Soul lyeth in the Seed which makes its own house, for all confess a forming faculty, and this faculty must come from some substance that lyeth close in the seed, though it appear not in the first act for want of fit organs to work with. Three things are requisite to form a child.

1. Fruitful seed from both sexes wherein the Soul rests with its forming faculty.

2. The mothers blood to nourish it.

3. A good constitution of the matrix to work it to perfection; if any of these be wanting you must not expect a perfect child: But as for the marks, or likeness to the Parents, sometimes this vertue lyeth hid some ages in the seed, and appears not, and then the child comes to be like those from whom it was descended by many succeeding generations, for *H lin* had a white daughter by a Black, but that daughter had a black son born of her, the forming faculty still continuing in the seed when it hath been stirred up by new imagination.

Plants being grafted, experience shews will bear fruit of the nature of the graft, but the kernels

kernels of that fruit sowed will bring fruit like the stock it was grafted on. Graft an Apricock on a Pear stock you shall have Apricocks, but a stone of those Apricocks set grows a Pear stock. If the forming faculty be free, children will be like their Parents, but if it be overpowred or wrested by imagination, the form will follow the stronger faculty; if the mother long for figs, or roses, or such things, the child is sometimes markt with them. *Avicen* gives this reason for it, that the aery spirits that are nimble of themselves, are soon moved by the phansie, and these mingle with the nutrimental blood of the child and imprint this likeness from imagination. This is a deep speculation, but it may be compared and represented to our understanding by those equivocal generations made in the air of frogs, and flies and the like by the forming faculties of the Heavens, so are the forms imagination sends forth engraven on the light spirits, for the quick spirits receive all forms from the imagination, and the seed that passeth through all parts and is derived from the whole body retains the images of them all.

CHAP.

CHAP. VII.

Of the sympathy between the womb and other parts, and how it is wrought upon by them.

IT is strange to consider that the womb should discern between sweet and stinking scents, and to be so diversly affected with these smels that some have miscarryed by smelling the snuff of a Candle, insomuch that some have thought the womb to be a creature of a discerning quality, and it receives this judgement from every part of the body, it is delighted with sweet scents, and displeased with the contrary. Wise Men have been at a stand to give a reason for it. Some refer it to a hidden quality, but that is still the last refuge for ignorance. There are indeed many things in nature secret to us, of which we can give no certain reason, as for the Loadstone to draw Iron; we see it is so but we cannot say how it comes to pass. In fits of the Mother sweet smels are good, for they disperse the ill qualities and venenosities of the Air, and so by a peculiar quality strengthen the womb, by
draw-

drawing down the spirits, and humours, but the different way of applying them will do good or harm. For the sweetest things that are, as Musk, or Civet, will cause fits of the Mother, if you apply them to the womans nose, for the womb consents or dissents by sympathy and antipathy, and sweet things applied to the privities profit in such cases, and stinking things to the nose, as burnt leather, feathers, or the like. There is a great agreement between the womb and the brain, as *Hippocrates* proves by a smoke to try barrenness by, and there is the like between the womb and the Heart by Nerves and Arteries. Sweet scents are pleasing to all womens wombs, and ill savours offend, but not in all women alike, for where the Matrix is well disposed and not disaffected by reason of ill humours that it is charged with, those Women are much delighted with sweet smels, but it is not so with others who are unclean, for they cannot away with sweet smels, for no sooner do they begin to scent them, but they fall into those fits, for while the womb resents those sweet swels, the ill humours that lye hid in the womb, especially where the seed is corrupted, fly up with the spirits and carry the bad humours with them to the Heart, and to the brain, and so cause these stiflings of the womb. This

This is general for all sweet things, that the Matrix is pleased with them rightly applied; for apply any sweet thing to the Privities, the womb is quiet and well refresht by them, and so the humours are still, or else they move downward, but contrarily stinking things by Antipathy with the womb are thrust out by the spirits when we apply such stinks to the nose, for the spirits fly downwards, and often there is an abortion thereby.

The womb cannot smell scents no more than it can hear sounds or see objects, for scents belong to the nose which is the Organ of smelling, as colours to the eyes that are the instruments of seeing, & the ears of hearing, but the womb partakes with these scents by reason of a thin vapour or spirit that comes from any strong smell, for the womb is affected as our senses are, very suddenly as it feels exactly, wch is in some kind a general sense, and is common to every part of the body. our spirits are refresht with sweet vapours, not discerning them but as they are placed and strengthened by them. But how doth the womb chuse sweet smels and refuse the contrary if she cannot discern? I know not why it is so, unless the reason be, because of the impurity of those vapours that arise from stinking things, for all such things are noy-
some,

noyfome, and not well concocted, and defile the fpirts contained in the parts of Generation, and fo caufe faintings, and fwoundings; whereas fweet fmels are pleafant, and refrefh the fpirits. But why then doth *Ambergreece* and Musk caufe fuffocations being fo extreamly fweet fcented; and *Affafetida* and *Caftoreum*, two ftinking cure it? The Anfwer is, that all women are not fo affected, but onely they whofe wombs, as I faid, are charged with ill humours, and then quick fpirits arifing from fweet fmels prefently move the brain and the membranes of it; and fo the membranous womb is foon drawn into confent, the bad vapours that lay ftill before being ftirred and raifed by the Arteries, flee to the heart and the brain, and by fecret paffages caufe fuch fits, but noyfome fmels being raw and ill tempered, ftop the pores of the brain, and come not to the inward membranes to prevent them. Alfo Nature being offended with deftructive ill qualified fcents, raifeth up all her forces as againft an open enemy to oppofe them, and fo cafts out of the womb with the ill vapours the ill humours alfo from which thefe vapours rife, fo comes a crifis in acute difeafes, if Nature be ftrong fhe cafts them forth; and when a man takes a purge, Nature helps her felf againft the ill qualities of the

Medica-

Medicament, which she can no way conquer but by casting it forth, and so what humours were peccant are cast forth with it.

It was the judgment of *Hippocrates*, that womens wombs are the cause of all their diseases; for let the womb be offended, all the faculties Animal, Vital, and natural; all the parts, the Brain, Heart, Liver, Kidneys, Bladder, Entrails, and bones, especially the share-bone partake with it: but no part is so much of consent with the womb as the Breasts are. The agreement between the womb and the Brain comes from the Nerves and membranes of the marrow of the back, some see great pains in the hinder part of the head, some are frantick, others so silent they cannot speak, Some have dimness of sight, dulness of hearing, noyse in their ears, strange passions and Convulsions.

It agrees with the Heart by the Arteries of the Seed and lower belly, and if these be stopt or choked by a venemous air, the hearts natural heat is dissolved, & faintings, and swoondings, and intermission of pulse follow, with stopping of their breath, so that you cannot perceive them to breath unless you apply a clear looking-glass to their mouth, and if they breath at all there wilbe left a dewy vapor upon the Glass, if not they are dead; for some of these women draw in no more air than what comes in by the pores of the skin into the Arteries and so goes to the Heart; and such persons sometimes lye in such fits twenty four hours at least, and many of them have lain so long that their Friends have thought them to be dead and have caused them to be unhappily buried when they were alive, and would no doubt have revived when the fit had been over. I speak this for a warning to others, to beware what they do upon such occasions, and to give at least two or three dayes time before they put them into the ground; some have been taken alive out of their Coffins long after they were thought to be dead.

The womb and Liver agree by Veins running from the Liver to the womb, which is the cause of Jaundies, Dropsies, and Green-sickness, if the blood be naught that comes to it. And that the Kidnies by the Seed-veins consents with the womb, is manifest by the pains of the loins women suffer when they have their Courses; for the left Seed-Vein comes from the left emulgent or kidney-vein on the same side. So the womb, the bladder, and the right gut agree, for if the womb be inflamed, presently follows a desire to go to stool, and to make water, by reason of the nearness and communion these parts have one with

with the other, by the membranes of the *Peritonæum*, that tyed the womb and these parts together, and by common Vessels running betwixt, for from the same branch of the vein of the under belly run small Fibres to these three parts: but the consent of the womb with the breasts is most observable, the humours passing ordinarily from one to the other, whereby we may know the affections of the womb, and how to cure them, and of the state of the Child contained in it. *Lusitanus* tells us that he saw two women that voided monethly blood by their Nipples when their Courses were stopt. *Hippocrates* confirms this, affirming that women are in danger to run mad when blood comes forth at their Nipples. *Brassavolus* tells us of womens milk that came like blood; but it was raw unconcocted blood; and that might be, for Nurses Courses are alwayes stopt because the blood runs to their breasts to make Milk. By the colour of the nipples the state of the womb is perceived; if the Paps look pale or yellow that should look red, the womb is not well. Also if you will stop the Terms that run too much, set a great cupping glass under the Breasts, for that will turn the course of the blood backward.

Farther you may know the Child if it be a

Boy

Boy to be three moneths old, and if a Girle to be about four moneths old, if you find Milk in the Mothers breasts, for at those times the Child first moves, and then is there Milk found in the breasts of the Mother.

If the right breast swell and strut out the Boy is well, if it flag it is a sign of miscarriage, judge the same of the Girle by the left breast, when it is sunk, or round and hard, the first signifies abortion to be near, the other health and safety both of the Mother and the Child.

CHAP. VIII.

How the Child grows in the Womb, and one part after the other successively made.

MEn are of several minds concerning the time when each part is made; I think they are in the right, who maintain that the membranes are first made which wrap the Child, with the Navel-vessels, by which the Child is fastned to the Mothers womb, and draws nutriment from her, and all parts are made sooner or later, as dignity and necessity of the parts require, but this is thought to be the hardest piece of *Anatomy*, because it is seldome to be observed, because if women dye in child-bed they first miscarry and dye afterward. Some follow *Galen* herein, who never saw a woman Anatomized; others *Columbus*, some *Vesalius*, but few or none know the truth. The stones of a woman for generation of seed, are white, thick and well concocted, for I have seen one, and but one and that is more by one than many Men have seen. In the act of Copulation both eject their seed, which is united in the womb; and Boys or Girls are begotten as the seed is that prevails stronger or weaker, so the greater light puts out the lesser, the Sun the light of a Candle. Nature desires to beget its like in all things, a Man a Man-child, a woman one of her own sex; but we follow desire not nature when we wish the contrary. If the Horse or Mare trot, it were strange that the Filly should amble.

The seed of both persons being joyn'd, the Matrix presently shuts as close as may be, to keep in, and to fasten the seed by its native heat, and so womens bellies seem lank at their first conception. The first thing that works is the spirit of which the seed is full, this is stir'd up to action by heat of the womb, and though the seed seems to be homogeneous and all one substance, yet it consists of very different parts, some pure and some impure; the spirit then in the seed divides between these parts, and makes a separation of the earthy, cold, clammy, grosser parts, from the more aerial, pure, and noble parts. The impure are cast to the outside, to circle in and keep close the seed which is pure, and of the outside are the Membranes made, by which the seed inclosed is kept from danger of cold and other ill accidents; just as it is in Trees so it is here, the cold winter congeals the vital spirits of the Tree, but the Suns heat revives it in the Spring, and opens the pores of the Tree, and separates the clean from that which is unclean, making of the pure juyce flowers, of the impure and gross juyce leaves and bark.

The first thing Nature makes for the child, is the *Amnios* or inward skin that surrounds the Child in the womb, as the *Pia mater* doth the brain: next is the *Chorion* or outward skin made, which compasseth the Child, as the *dura mater* the brain; this is soon done by nature, for *God* and nature hate idleness, and no sooner are these two coats made, but presently the Navel-Vein is bred, piercing both these skins whilest they are exceeding tender; and conveighs a drop of blood from

the

the mothers womb-veins to the feed; of this one drop is formed the Childs Liver, from the Liver is bred the hollow Vein, and this Vein is the fountain of all other Veins of the body, so this being done, the feed hath blood sufficient to feed it and to form the rest of the parts by. It is a vain fancy that some hold, how that all the parts are formed together, others that the heart is first framed; it must receive a right construction what *Aristotle* saith, that the Heart lives first and dyeth last, for the Liver is made much before the Heart. Nor is that if it be well understood to be found fault with, that a Man lives succesively, first the life of a Plant, then of a Beast, and lastly of a Man. For first the Child grows, then it begins to move, last of all it becomes a reasonable Soul. Next to the hollow Vein of the Liver being made, are the arteries of the navel made, then the great Artery which is the Tree, and all the small Arteries are but branches coming from it; & last of all the Heart is framed, as *Columbus* proves upō very sufficient reason, for all the arteries are made before it, for the Body receives its life by Arteries, and the Navel arteries are bred from the Mothers arteries, and therefore are made next to the Veins, to give vital blood to the Seed, as the Liver feeds it with natural blood to build a frail house for poor

mor-

mortals. Next in order, so far as reason and *Anatomy* can guide us, the Liver sends blood to the Arteries to make the Heart, for the arteries are made of seed, but the heart and all fleshy parts are made of blood; last of all the brain, and then the Nerves to give feeling and motion are produced. If the most noble parts were first framed, as the *Peripateticks* suppose, then the brain and heart should be first made, which is not agreeing to reason and observation. As for the forming of the bones in order, I think *Aristotle* said true, that the whirl bones and the skull are first made. I confess all these things have been questioned by some, but I love not impertinent disputes, as it was the quality of the *Grecians*, who have made a large dispute, whether the Elephants Tusks be Horns or Teeth. *Hippocrates* divides the forming of the infant into four divisions: First the seed of both sexes mixed have not lost their own form, but resemble curdled milk covered with a film or cream: the next form is a rude draught of the parts, or a chaos like a lump of flesh. And next in order there is a more curious draught, wherein the three chief parts, the Brain, the Heart, and the Liver, may be seen together with the first three, and as it were the warp of all the seed parts, and this is called *Embrion*: But fourthly,

Book II. *The Midwives Book.* 137
fourthly, To perfect the whole work, all the parts are set in order and perfected, so that Nature hath nothing to do but to hasten to delivery, that this work of hers may be brought forth into the world. When the spirit in the seed begins to work, it parts the more noble from the base, and the pure from the impure, so that the thick, cold, clammy parts are kept out to cover the more thin and pure parts, and to defend and preserve them. Nature begins her conformation with the cold clammy parts of the seed, and makes skins and membranes of them to cover the rest, and stretcheth them out as need requires. Men have only two membranes, the outward or *Chorion* which is strong and nervous, and wraps the infant round, and this membrane is like a soft pillow for the Veins and Navel-arteries of the Child to lean upon, for it had been dangerous for the Childs Vessels coming from its Navel to pass far unguarded : but the inward Coat which is wonderful soft and thin, called the *Amnios* or Lamb-skin is loose on each side except it be at the cake, where it growes so fast to the skin that it cannot easily be parted; this skin receives the sweat and Urine, and from thence the Child is much helped, for it swims in these waters like as in a bath, and time is for delivery, it moistneth the orifice of
the

the Matrix, makes it glib and slippery, whereby the woman is more easily and more speedily delivered.

These two Coats grow so close together that they seem to be but one garment, and it is called the *Secundine* or after-burthen, because it comes forth after the Child is born, for the Child first breaks through it, & sometimes brings along with it a piece of the said Lambskin upon the face and head, which is called by Midwives the Caule, and strange reports they give of it.

Some think it ridiculous and fabulous, but as all extraordinary things signifie something more than is usual, so I am subject to believe that this Caule doth foreshew something notable which is like to befall them in the course of their lives.

But notwithstanding all that hath been said, some Anatomists do a little vary from it, for they maintain, that within the first seven days wherein the generative seed is mingled and curdled in the Mothers womb by the heats motion, many small fibres are bred, in which shortly the Liver and his principal Organs are formed first, and through these Organs the vital spirits coming to the seed in ten days makes all the distinction of parts, and through some small Veins in the *Secundine* the

blood

blood runs, and of that is the Navel made, and there appears at the same time three clods of seed or white lumps like curdled Milk, & these are the foundation of three principal parts, viz. the Brain, the Liver, and the Heart. But the Liver is conceit to be first made of a blood gathered by one branch of this Vein, for the Liver it self is nothing else but a lump of clotted blood full of Veins which serve to attract and to expell; but immediately before the Liver is made, there is a two-forked Vein formed through the navel, to suck away the grosser part of the blood that rests in the seed. In the other branch of this vein more veins are made for the spleen and lower belly, and all of them coming to one root meet in the upper part of the Liver in the hollow Vein, & from hence other Veins are sent out of the *Midriff* to the thighs below, & to the upper part of the back-bone; next this the heart is made with its veins, for these veins draw the hottest part of the blood & that which is most subtil, & so make the heart; within the membrane called the *Pericardium* or skin that covers the heart, the hollow Vein runs through the inward part of the right side of the heart carrying blood to it to feed it: from the same branch of this vein and the same part of the heart is there another vein that beats but faintly; therefore

fore called the still Vein, amongst the pulsative Veins, and this is provided to send the more pure blood by from the heart to the Lungs, they are covered with a double Coat as the Arteries are.

The Artery called *Aorta*, that conveighs the vital spirits through the whole body from the heart by the beating Veins or arteries, is bred in the hollow of the left Vein of the heart, and under this artery in the same hollow place of the heart is another Vein bred which is called the vein-artery, that brings the cold air from the Lungs to cool the heart, for the Lungs are made by many Veins that run from the hollow of the heart, and come thither to frame the Lungs; and they have their substance from a very thin subtil blood that is brought thither from the right hollow of the heart.

The breast is first framed by the great Veins of the Liver, and after that the outmost parts, the legs and arms.

But last of all the Brain is made in the third little skin I speak of, for the seed being full of vital spirits, the vital spirits draw much of the natural moisture, into one hollow place where the brain is made; and covered with a Coat which heat drieth and bakes into a skull.

The Veins come all from the Liver, Arteries

ries from the Heart, Nerves from the brain, of a soft gentle nature, yet not hollow as Veins are, but solid; the Brain retains and changes the vital spirits; from hence are the beginnings of sense and reason.

After the Nerves the pith of the back-bone is bred which cannot be called Marrow, for Marrow is a superfluous substance made of blood to moisten and strengthen the bones, but the pith of the back and brain are made of seed, not to serve other parts, but to be also parts of themselves, for sense and motion, that all the Nerves might grow originally from thence; also Bones, Gristles, Coats, and Membranes are bred from the seed, Veins for the Liver, Arteries for the Heart, Nerves for the Brain, besides all other pannicles and coverings the child is wrapped in. But all fleshy substance as the Heart it self, Liver, and Lungs, are made of the proper blood of the birth; this is all ended in eighteen days of the first month, and all that time it carrieth the name of seed, and afterwards is called the birth; and this birth so long as it is in the womb is fed with blood received through the Navel, and therefore when women are with child the courses cease; for after conception this blood is severed into three parts, the best and finest serves for the childs nourishment, the next
in

in pureness though not so pure as the first, riseth to the breasts to make milk, and the grossest part of the three stays in the womb and comes away with the birth and afterbirth.

But this is a long dispute how the child comes to be fed in the womb. *Alcmeon* thought the childs body being soft like a sponge did draw nourishment by all parts of its body, as a sponge sucks water, not only drinking from the mothers veins but from the womb also. *Hippocrates* as well as *Democritus* or *Epicurus* seems to say, that the child sucks both nourishment and breath at the mouth, from the mother when she breaths, for these two causes.

1. Because it could not suck so soon as it is born were it not used to it before.

2. There are excrements found in the Guts of a new born child; but all creatures that suck will do it presently by instinct of nature; as Chickins that never fed before, will presently pick up their food; and as for the excrements found in the Guts they are not excrements of the first concoction, for they think not, but are gross blood that came from the Vessels of the spleen to the Guts and are dried there; but how it is agreed by all since the truth is found out, that the child in the womb

is fed by its Navel, only they differ about the food it lives on, the *Peripateticks* say it is fed by menstrual blood which is the excrement of the last nutriment of the fleshy parts, which at certain times is purged forth by the womb in a moderate quantity, but primarily ordained for the generation and nutriment of the child.

But *Fernelius, Pliny, Columella,* and *Columbus* deny this, because such blood is impure, and will, where it falls, destroy Plants, and Trees, Dogs will run mad that eat it, and ofttimes hurts the women themselves, causing swimmings of the head, pains, swellings, and suffocations, this then were ill food for a tender infant.

But to answer all: If the woman be in good health, her monthly courses are no bad blood for quality though they hurt in quantity being more than she can concoct; and therefore she sends forth what is too much; but if her body be ill affected, the blood that stays in the womb is naught as well as that she voids by her terms; but when the courses are not duly voided but stay, in being stopt beyond their time of evacuation, then they cause those ill effects formerly mentioned, else not: but women have not these courses the greatest part of the time they are with child,

nor

nor yet when they give suck, for the most part; if the child be not fed with this blood what becomes of this blood when women are with child? certain it is it turns into milk, when time serves, to suckle the infant with. Yet *Hippocrates* was mistaken, who says, that the last part of the time the child lieth in the womb after it is quick, its fed partly by the mother milk; but this is certain that the infant in the womb is fed with pure blood conveyed in the Liver by the Navel-vein which is a branch of the great vein, and spreads to the small veins of the Liver. And here this blood is more refined, the thick, gross, crude part goes to the Spleen and Kidneys, and the gross excrement of it to the Guts, and that is it is found in the Guts as soon as they are born. The most pure part goes into the hollow vein, and from thence through the whole body by small branches; this blood hath a watry substance with it, as all blood hath, to make it run and keep it from clodding, and this water in men and women breaths forth by sweat, & so it doth in a child, and is contain'd in the Lamb-skin, as I told you. This watry substance that is joined with the blood, when the blood comes to the kidneys, parts from the blood, and is sent by the kidneys that make their separation, by the Ureters

Book III　*The Midwives Book.*

ters to the bladder, nor doth the infant, p_s as he lieth in the womb, by the Yard; but the Urine is carryed by the *Urachos*, a vessel to carry it, which is long and without blood, to the *Allantois*, or skin that is made to hold the childs water in, so long as it remains in the womb; this *Urachos* or passage goeth from the bottom of the bladder to the *Allantois*, and hath no muscle belongs unto it, that the child may void the Urine, when nature requires, but when the child is born it hath muscles at the root of the bladder, to shut and open that we may make it not a meer natural, but partly a mixed action, to follow our business, and make water, not alwayes but when we please; but this is not the course with the child continually, for the first month the childs Urine comes out through the passage of the Navel, but in the last month by the Yard, but it never goes to stool in the womb, because it takes no nutriment by the mouth. After forty five days, the child lives, but moves not, commonly he moves in double the time he was formed, and is born in thrice the time after he began to move. If the child be fully formed in forty days, he will move in ninety days, and be born in the ninth month, but he receives daily more food after the third and fourth month to the day of his birth. A child

L　　　　　　　　born

born in six months is not perfect and must die, but one born in seven months is perfect, but one born in the eighth month cannot live, because in the seventh month the child useth all its force to come out, and if it cannot, it must stay two months longer to recover the strength lost upon the former attempt that had made it too feeble to get forth in the eighth month; for if it come not forth at the seventh month it removes its station and changeth it self to some other place in the womb; these two motions have so weakened it, that it must stay behind a month longer, for if it come forth before, it is almost impossible for it to live. But Astrologers determine this business another way, for they affirm, that children born in the seventh month do live by reason of the compleating of the motion of the seven planets, allowing one month to each of them, beginning with *Saturn* thus; *Saturn, Jupiter, Mars, Sol, Venus, Mercury, Luna*. Now if the child come not forth at the seventh month, but stay till the eighth month, the Planets having ruled every one his month, *Saturn* begins to rule again, who is an enemy to conception in all his qualities, and so the child born in the eighth month will be born dead, or live a very short time; yet other Philosophers maintain, that

Saturn

Saturn is no enemy to conception, but ruling in the first month, by his influence and retentive faculty, the child is fixed in the womb; but as the celestial bodies have their influence upon the terrestial and upon all the elements, they cause all the changes here below, and are not changed themselves: for that the Heavens, and the fixed Stars, and the Planets are still the same they were in the first creation; and that the twelve Signs and Planets do rule over the bodies of men and women; and how that *Scorpio* which is the house of *Mars*, rules over the womb and makes it fruitful; and that *Leo* is a barren Sign, because Lions seldom bring forth young, and so is *Virgo* for they are no maids that conceive with child. But then why should not *Taurus* be a barren but a fruitful Sign, when Bulls never bring forth any. But not to trouble the reader with Astrological dreams. I think it is not the seven Planets that by this compleatment of seven make the child to live, but I should rather impute it to the perfection of the number seven; which is easily proved by Scripture to be the most perfect number; and will appear so to be by the Sabbath the seventh day of the week commanded for rest; also the Sabbatical or every seventh year, and the year of Jubilee seven times seven. So that *Hippocrates*

was

was out in three books, where he endeavours to prove that a child born in the eighth month cannot live; *Aristotle*, *Plutarch*, *Galen*, and others were of the same judgement. But to oppose them, the writers of *Spain*, *Egypt*, and of *Ninas* prove the contrary by divers examples: *Hippocrates* might be also misunderstood, whether he meant *Solar* months that consist of thirty one days a piece, or very near, being the time the Sun is passing through the *Zodiack*, or *Lunar* months, the time the moon is in any Sign of the twelve, and her stay there which is but twenty seven days, with some few hours and minutes; besides all this, the woman *Hippocrates* mentions, might not make her reckoning right; for, if you trust to womens account you can be at no certainty, scarce one of a hundred can tell you true. And as for *Saturn*, who is so much blamed for playing the ill Midwife in the eighth month, he is as much commended for his good office in the first month; but there is no man, or Planet that can alwayes have every mans good word; yet I am of opinion they do him wrong: but Astrologers may say what they please without reason, for they never prove any thing but one dream by another: *Aries* forsooth is not fruitful because it is the House of *Mars*, and is not *Scorpio* which

they

they praise for fructifying the house of *Mars* too? Every Planet is maintained by them to rule the several parts of mans body, and that by degrees according to their signs and several Houses they are in. I have found no Table concerning this business to have any truth in it, wherefore I have drawn forth one exactly which you may safely rely upon, if upon any Table at all, and by this Table you shall find that every Planet when he is in *Scorpio*, which signifies fruitfulness of the womb, rules those parts of the body which are under the same Sign: the two great Luminaries, I mean the *Sun* and *Moon*, excepted, which do it by reception; a clear proof that they have a great influence in framing the child in the womb, and that the two Luminaries in that work, mingle their influence one with the other.

The Table.

The first month Authors give to *Saturn* to retain the conception, for he, say they, fixes the seed. The Second month to *Jupiter*, and upon him they lay the foundation of encreasing, of sense and reason, but the true foundation is then laid, when the Seed of both man and woman are well mingled. *Mars* rules

rules the third month to give heat and motion to the infant. *Any Tooth good Barber.* The *Sun* governs the fourth month to give the child vital spirits; yet *Mars* gave it motion a month before without any spirits at all; I cannot understand there can be voluntary motion and no vital spirits. *Venus* in the fifth month adds beauty; the body we all know is fashioned in thirty or forty days, but beauty must not come till three months after. As for the sixth month that is *Mercuries* part, to distinguish the parts of the child, which *Venus* it seems could never do with all her beauty, as if the child were but a Chaos, and a rude mass till the sixth month, yet it was very beautiful a month before. As for the seventh and last month in the Planetary revolution, that is the *Moons* part, to make the child complete. Here is much ado to small purpose. It is no error I confess to impute much to the operation of the Planets. But they are much mistaken about the times that such and such Planets do work, for doubtless the Planets do not operate by succession as some would have it, so that when one rules, all the rest are idle and lie still, but they cooperate and work altogether, and that continually. Their motion causes mixation, for the motion of the Sun, saith *Potolomy*, of the *Earth*, saith *Copernicus pernicius*, distinguisheth night from day. The *Sun* gives heat to all things here below, the *Moon* moisture, and our life consists in heat and moisture. The *Sun* is the Sire of all living creatures, and is first active in the seed of both sexes, in the very middle of the seed, and so he enlivens and moves every part to its proper action. That which *Aristotle* speaks of the Heart, the *Microcosmical* Sun in man's production, is partly true both in and after conception, to frame vital spirits and cause motion & action. For as the earth is preserved by the element of water from being scorched and burnt up by the beams of the Sun, so the *Microcosmical* Sun, the Heart; but which is the *Moon*, the brain or the Liver is hard to say, adds moisture to this conception from first to last, I mean as long as the child lives, and thus the radical moisture is preserved. *Aristotle* thought the brain by its coldness tempered the heat of the heart, and for my part I think he said very true, I see no man give a sufficient reason to the contrary. There must yet be something to ballance the heat and moisture of the *Sun* and *Moon*, and that they say is *Saturn* by his coldness; for he fixeth them both in the work of conception, and the dry bones are his work, which are the Pillars and supports of this frail building. But be-

L 4   cause

cause there is no Generation, but first there must be corruption, for the corruption of one is the generation of another, whereby it comes to pass that there is not a total decay in the world: the beams of the *Sun* & *Moon* working upon the seed of both sexes fixed by *Saturn* are purified and concocted by the equal temperature of heat and moisture that the Planet *Jupiter* lets fall amongst them; but then comes *Mars* with his heat and dryness; and what is overplus in the conception, as there must needs be some superfluities, that *Mars* draws forth, and turns to excrements, and hardens into Coverings and Coats for the child by his calcining heat, what is bred by moisture and is not fixed by cold and dryness. *Mars* heats (still a fiery calcination) but *Venus* she tempers the heat of *Mars* by her moisture, for she is a cold moist Planet, and fitly added to abate the courage and violent heat of warlike *Mars*. So there is a great sympathy between *Mars* and *Venus*, and therefore surely the Poets speak so much of their conjunction; for they are eminent in this of mans generation.

You may by this find out the causes of sympathy and antipathy in natural things, and seeing all things are made up of such contrary qualities, what is generated must in time be corrupted, nothing is eternal in this world;

but

but a perpetual motion breeds mutation, and not man nor any thing else can continue in the same stay. *Mars* and *Venus* do here play their parts in mans production, for they are the nearest of the five Planets to the earth, but next to them is *Mercury*, of a changeable disposition, and applieth himself to the rest of the Planets with several aspects, and he causeth the desire of knowledge in man; sense and reason also some maintain to be the work of *Mercury* by his influence upon the child in the womb. It is not denied but a piercing acute humour proceeds from him, which is most likely to effect not alone the sensible but the rational part in man.

CHAP. IX.

Of the Posture the Child holdeth in the Womb, and after what fashion it lieth there.

HEre Physicians are at a stand and are never like to agree about it, not twie in twenty that can set their horses together; the speculation is very curious, insomuch that the Prophet *David* ascribes this knowledge as more peculiar to God, *Psalm* 139. *My reins are*
thine

thine, thou hast covered me in my mothers womb: I will give thanks unto thee for I am fearfully and wonderfully made, marvellous are thy works, and that my soul knoweth right well: my bones are not hid from thee, though I be made secretly and fashioned beneath in the earth; thine eyes did see my substance, yet being unperfect, and in thy Book were all my members written, which day by day were fashioned, when as yet there was none of them.

Yet Anatomists have narrowly enquired into this secret Cabinet of nature, and *Hippocrates* that great Physician tells us in his Book *De naturâ Pueri*, that the infant lieth in the womb with his head, his hands, and his knees bending downward, towards his feet: so that he is bended round together, his hands lying upon both his knees, the thumbs of his hands, & his eyes, meeting each with other, & so faith *Bartholinus* the younger of the two. Likewise *Columbus*'s opinion is, that the child lieth round in the womb with the right arm bended, and the fingers of the right hand lying under the ear of it, above the neck, the head bowed so low that the chin meets and toucheth the breast, and the left arm bowed lying above the breast and the face, and the right elbow bended serves to underprop the left arm lying upon it; the legs are lying upwards

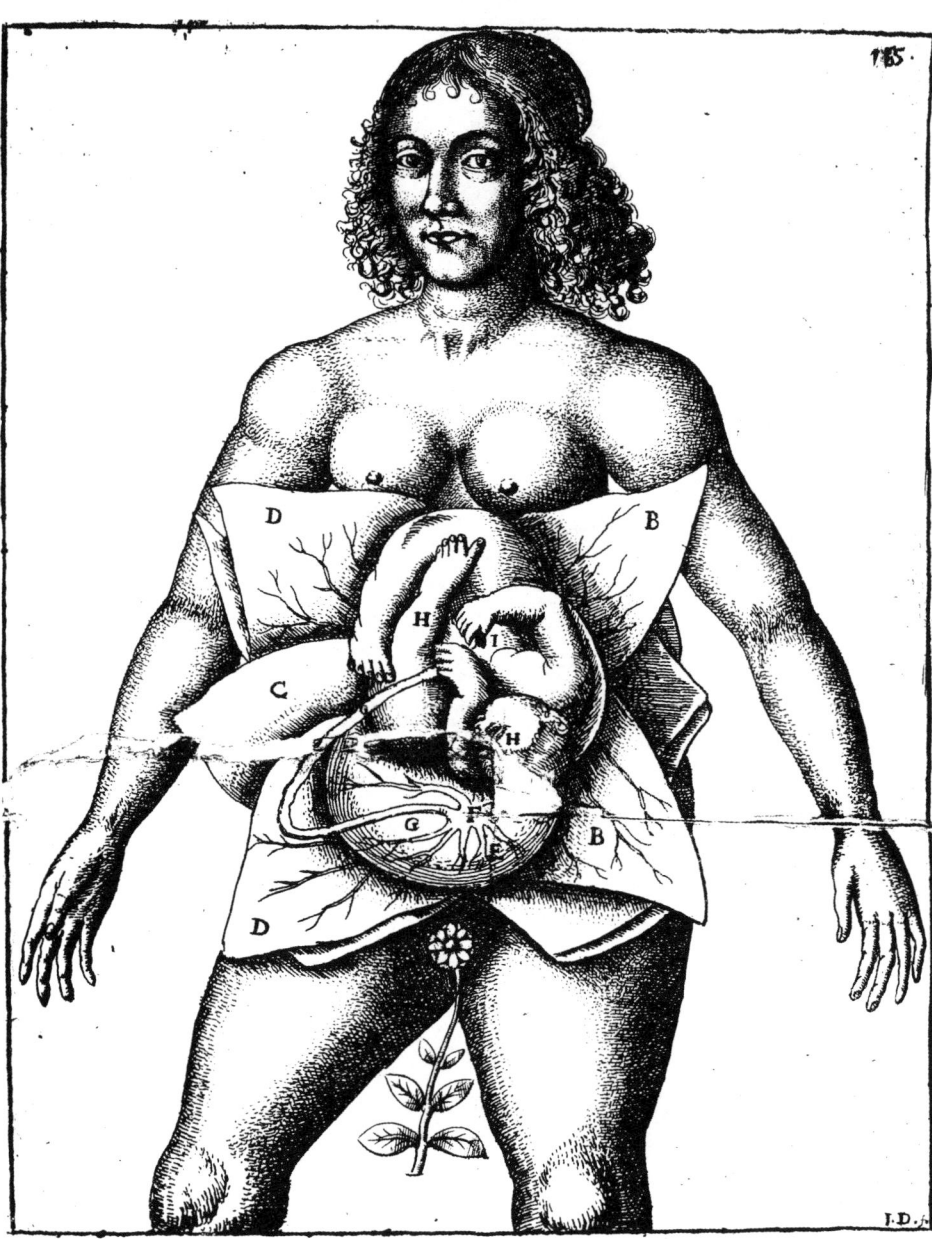

wards, and the right leg is lifted so high that the infants thigh toucheth its belly, the knees touch the Navel, and the heel toucheth the left buttock, and the foot is turned backward and hides the privy members; as for the left thigh, that toucheth the belly, and the left leg is lifted up to the breast; the stomach lyeth inwards. But the expert *Spigelius* hath the fashion of a child near the birth, whose figure I have here laid down, and I believe it is very proper; for, as well as I am able to judge by the figure, it is the very same with that of a child that I had once the chance to see when I was performing my office of *Midwifry*.

Here insert the Figure of the Child near its Birth.

This is a general observation, that the Male Child most commonly lyeth on the right side in the womb, and the Female on the left side; but *Hippocrates* layeth it down as the most universal way, to have his hands, knees, and head bending down toward the feet, his nose betwixt his knees, his hands upon both knees, and his face between them, each eye touching each thumb; but he is wrapt as he lieth in two mantles or garments, as I said,

for

for a boy hath no more; that which immediately covers him and lieth next to his skin, is called *Amnios* the skirt or Lamb-skin, it is wonderful soft and thin, and is loose on all sides, only it grows so fast to the Cake, that it can hardly be parted from it; the use of it farther is to receive the Childs sweat and Urine, which moisteneth the mouth of the Matrix also, and makes the birth more easie; but the outward coat called *Chorion*, is very strong and sinewy, and encloseth the child round about, and like a soft pillow or bed bears up all the veins and Arteries of the Navel, which would have been in danger, to have been carried so far, without some soft bolster to sustain them.

These coats growing fast together seem to be but one coat, or one to be the beginning of the other, and this altogether taken is called the after-burden or *Secundine*; for when the Child is grown strong enough to come out of the womb, and the time of his birth is at hand, he breaks through these coverings, and the coverings come forth after the child is born: yet sometimes a piece of the *Amnios* covers the childs face and head when he is born and women call it the caule, and hold it to be a Sign of some great happiness that will befall the child in the following part of his life;

life, but some think it is neither here nor there, one born without this caule may be as happy as he that is born with it. There belong to the child whilest it lieth in the womb some things that are proper for it, some to cloath it, and are only for that time that it lieth in that place, and afterwards of no known use, though some have tried to make use of them in Physick and Chirurgery, but commonly they cast it away. Some things again serve to nourish and feed it in the womb, and those are the Navel-vessels which are four in number, two arteries, one vein, and that vessel which is called *Urathos*, which carrieth away the childs water in the womb to that skin that is prepared to hold that water so long as the child staies in the womb and it is called *Allantois*. The vein I speak of comes from the Infants Liver, and when it is passed the navel, it brancheth into two branches; and these again divide and subdivide, the skin called *Chorion* supporting the branches of it, and these are joined to the Veins of the mothers womb, and serve to suck and to carry the mothers blood from thence to feed the infant with, whilest it stays there.

This Vein is for that end that the infant may be fed from the first time of conception untill it be born; and then its use is over as to

the

the first intention, when the child comes to feed it self, for then it hath no need to suck blood from the mother as it did before.

The Arteries are two on each side, and these spring from the branches of the great artery of the mother that comes from the small Guts and these serve to carry vital blood to feed the Infant with, when it is first well prepared and concocted by the mother.

The next part for servile use, is a Nervous production called *Urachos*, and it comes from the bottom of the bladder of the child to its Navel, and it serves, as the name also implies, to carry the childs Urine to the *Allantois* or skin that must retain it. But Anatomists are not all of one mind about it, for some say there is no such thing to be found in the afterburden of women, but in beasts it is. Let their ignorance or disputes be what they will to no purpose, I shall satisfie all by true experience, which cannot be contradicted; he that reads the *Anatomy* Lecture of *Montpelion* in *France*, *Bartholomew Cabrollus* a skilful Chirurgion professeth that he saw a maid whose Urine came forth at her Navel, the ordinary passage of her water being obstructed: and Dr. *John Fernelius* tells the same story, of a man who was thirty years old, who had a stopping in the neck of his bladder so that for

many

many months continually, his water came forth by his Navel, yet he found no hurt at all by it but was very well in health, and *Fernelius* faith, the reason was, becaufe his Navel-ftring was not well tied, and the paffage of the *Urachos* gave way, becaufe it was not well dried. And there is another example that *Vulchier Coiler* lays down of a *German* maid of *Noremberge*, fhe was thirty four years of age. Thefe diftempers are not frequent, becaufe fhe muft be a very unskilful Midwife that knows not how to tie and cut the Navel ftring, yet thefe accidents are fufficient in fuch a dark matter to prove that there is fuch a thing as a *Urachos* or Urine-carrier from the Navel in both fexes, men as well as women.

Thefe four veffels, as I faid, namely one Vein, two Arteries, and the *Urachos*, join together near the Navel, and they are tyed by a skin they have from the *Chorion* or outward coat of the *Secundine*, and fo they feem to be a Chord or Gut without any feeling, this is that that all People call the Navel-ftring, if woman or man doubt of the truth of this relation, let him only take the childs Navel-ftring when it is cut off, and untwift it, and open it and fo they shall be able to fatisfie themfelves. Thefe Veffels are fo joined for to ftrengthen
them

them that they will not be broken, nor yet are they entangled together; when the child is born into the world: then these Vessels as they hang without from the Navel serve for no other use but to be knit fast and to make a strong band to cover the Navel-hole. Yet experience hath found a way to make a Physical use of them, that what is spar'd from tying and to be cut off, may not be thrown away; as for the *Secundine* and the parts of it, the parts of it are held to be four. I shall shew you a little more concerning the description and use of them. The first part is that which is commonly called a Sugar-cake in Latine *Placenta*, and indeed it is very like a cake in the form of it; it is tied both to the Navel and to the strong outward, sinewy Coat of the Child in the womb called *Chorion*; and this is that which makes the greater part of the after-burden or Secundine; the flesh hereof is soft and of a red colour, much like the spleen or milt, tending somewhat to black; there are abundance of small Veins and Arteries in it, and it should be probable that the chief use it serves for, is to cloath and keep the infant in the womb. *Columbus* a very good Anatomist, yet was much deceived when he affirms the *Chorion* or strongest and outward membrane that wraps the Child in the womb to be no

skin

skin. It is undoubtedly known, that the *Chorion* and *Amnios* do compass the child round, above, beneath, and on all sides, but the *Allantois* that contains the childs Urine doth not so. *Columbus* he mistook this skin for the *Placenta* or cake, but *Hippocrates* gives this name Secundine as general to the whole; in that book he hath written of womens diseases: for the *Chorion* is a skin very white, and thick, light and slippery, and it is laced, and adorned, and branched with a great many small Veins and Arteries, and we must not think that it serves only for a covering of the child in the womb, for it serves farther to receive and to bind fast the roots of the Veins, and Arteries or Navel-Vessels which I spake of before.

The *Allantois* or skin to contain the childs Urine in the womb is denied by many that there is any such Vessel to be found in mans body, I must confess reason must help us to discern it, for we can hardly see it or find it. It is said that in *Holland* men are wont to be present at their wives labours as well as women, and that few of the women use stools, but they sit in their Husbands laps when they are delivered; and they say there is such a thing. *Galen* maintains, that there is as much reason and experience for it in men as in beasts

beasts, good women as well as my self have done, may look for it, and find it too if they please, a very fine, white, soft, exceeding thin skin, and it lieth just under the cake or *Placenta*, and there it is tied to the *Urachos* from which it takes in the Urine, and its office is to keep the Urine apart from the sweat, that the saltness of the Urine may not hurt the tender Infant, which it must needs do, were it not kept up in a place by its self. The *Amnios* is the last and inmost skin, and it is wonderful fine, soft, white, transparent, fed and interwoven with many Veins and Arteries; this skin not only infolds the Infant, but also holds the sweat that comes from it whilest it lieth in the womb.

BOOK

BOOK. III.

CHAP. I.

What it is that hinders Conception and may be the causes that some women are barren.

BArrenness, as I said, is either by Nature, and that may be when two persons are joined in marriage, that either both are deficient by reason of ill conformity of the generative parts, or but one of them; for if both be not perfect to all respects, as to that work of copulation, they shall never have any children, and such marriages are not lawful by the Laws of *God* or man, because that procreating and bearing children is one of the chief ends of marriage; but accidental barrenness may happen to them by reason of some curable infirmity, and when that is removed they may be as fruitful as others that are naturally so. Physicians and Midwives have tried many ways to discover when man and wife cannot fructifie, where the fault lieth, whether the hinderance be from the man or from his wife, or from both; the best experiment that ever I could find, was to take some small quantity of Barley, or any other Corn that will soon grow, and soak part of it in the mans Urine, and part in the womans Urine, for a whole day and a night; then take the Corn out of both their Urines and lay them apart upon some floor, or in parts where it may dry, and in every morning water them both with their own Urine, and so continue; that Corn that grows first is the most fruitful, and so is the person whose Urine was the cause of it; if one or neither part of these grains grow, they are one or both of them barren: almost all men and women desire to be fruitful naturally, and it is a kind of self-destroying not to be willing to leave some succession after us; nay it seems to be more general and to tend to the ruine of the world, which cannot be continued without fruitfulnels in copulation; Virginity

nity and single life in some cases, is preferred before Matrimony, because it is a singular blessing and gift of *God*, which all people are not capable of: But for men or women to mutilate themselves on purpose, or use destructive means to cause barrenness, besides the means prescribed of Prayer and fasting, I cannot think to be justifiable, though some persons have presumptuously ventured upon it. Let the Votaries of the *Roman* Church look to it, when they make vows of chastity, which the greatest part of them doubtless are never able to keep but by using unlawful means. I much doubt whether they pray and fast so much as they pretend to. The principal cause of barrenness in man or woman lieth in the generative parts, and if children be born defective it is not we that are Midwives can cure it, what Nature wants, Art can hardly make perfect. It is not my design so much to speak of unfruitfulness in men, but of women in relation to their Conception, and Child-bearing; and I conceive the chiefest cause of womens barrenness to be from the womb of them that is ill formed, or ill disposed, and not as naturally it should be in those that may have children. There are many infirmities that we women especially are made unfruitful by,

but

but *God* hath appointed several remedies for most accidents, that none need to despair of help: true it is that the Scripture relates of a woman that had an issue of blood twelve years and could find no cure, but had spent all upon Physicians, yet at last she was cured by touching the hem of *Christ's* Garment: it is probable *God* would not have her cured by man, that her faith might be confirmed by the surpassing vertue she found in *Christ*. But before I come to speak of this, I shall speak of the things that are most proper to follow in order, namely concerning delivery of women with child.

CHAP. II.

Of great pain and difficulty in Child-bearing, with the Signs, and causes, and cures.

I Have done with that part of *Anatomy*, that concerns principally us Midwives to know, that we may be able to help and give directions to such women as send for us in their extremities, and had we not some competent insight into the *Theory*, we could never know

how

how to proceed to practice, that we may be able to give a handsome account of what we come for.

The accidents and hazards that women lye under when they bring their Children into the world are not few, hard labour attends most of them, it was that curse that *God* laid upon our sex to bring forth in sorrow, that is the general cause and common to all as we descended from the same great Mother *Eve*, who first tasted the forbidden fruit; but the particular causes are diverse according to several ages, and constitutions, and conformations, or infirmities. For sometimes Maids are married very young at twelve or fourteen years of age, and prove so soon with Child, when the passage is very little dilated, but is very strait and narrow; in such a case the labour in Child-bearing must needs be great for the infant to find passage, and for the Mother to endure it; and it must of necessity be much greater if some diseases go along with it, which happens oft in those parts, as Pushes, and Pyles, and Aposthumes, that Nature can hardly give way for the Child to be born: Sometimes the Bladder or near parts are offended, and the womb is a sufferer by consent, and this will hinder delivery: And so if her body be bound that she cannot go to stool, the

belly

belly stopt with excrement will make the pain in travel the greater, because the womb hath not room to enlarge it self. So if women be too old as well as too young, or if they be weak by accident, or naturally of feeble constitutions, if they be fearful, & cannot well endure pain; be they too lean or too spare bodies, too gross or too fat, or if they be unruly & will not be governed, they will suffer the greater pain in Child-birth; and it is not without reason maintained also, that a Boy is sooner and easier brought forth than a Girle; the reasons are many, but they serve also for the whole time she goes with Child, for women are lustier that are with Child with Boys, and therefore they will be better able to run through with it: the weaker they are the greater the pain, because they are less able to endure it; and the strength of the Child is much, for it will sooner break forth, than when it is weak though it be of the same sex; if the Child be large, and the passage strait, as it is alwayes, though not alike in all, she must look for a great deal of pain when the time of delivery comes; but none more painful and dangerous than Monstrous births. Sometimes the Child doth not come at the time appointed by Nature, or it offers not it self in such a posture as that it may find a passage
forth,

Book III. *The Midwives Book.* 169

forth, as when the feet first present themselves to the neck of the womb, either both feet together, or else but one foot, and both hands upwards; or both knees together, or else more dangerous yet, lying all upon one side thwart the womb, or else backward or arselong; or two Children offer themselves at once with their feet first, or one foot and one head; the postures are so many and strange, that no woman Midwife, nor man whatsoever hath seen them all. We have an example in Scripture of two Children that *Judah* got incestuously upon his Daughter in Law *Tamar*, who offered themselves to the Birth at the same time, Gen. 38, 26. *And it came to pass in the time of her travel, that behold Twins were in her womb, and when she travelled, one of them put forth his hand, & the Midwife took and bound upon his hand a scarlet thred, saying, this came out first; and it came to pass, that as he drew his hand again back, his brother came out, and she said, how hast thou broken forth? this breach be upon thee, therefore his name was called Pharez. And after him came his brother that had the Scarlet thred upon his hand, and his name was called Zerah.* We do not read but that she was safely delivered of them both, and neither Mother nor Child died in the Birth. But we find an example that will serve to our purpose

pose concerning hard labor, and that of *Rachel*, a good woman, wife to the Patriark *Jacob*, Gen. 35. 17, 18. *Rachel travelled, and she had hard labor, and when she was in travel the Midwife said to her, fear not, thou shalt have this Son also, but her soul was departing, for she died*, &c. A single birth, and a Boy, which is easier labour as I said, than of a Girle, and a young woman who had born one child before; yet Child-bearing is so dangerous that the pain must needs be great, and if any feel but a little pain it is commonly harlots who are so used to it that they make little reckoning of it, and are wont to fare better at present than vertuous persons do, but they will one day give an account for it if they continue impenitent, and be condemned to a torment of hell which far surpasses all pains in Child birth, yet these doubtless are the greatest of all pains women usually undergo upon Earth.

There are many more causes of great pains in travel than have been yet spoken of; for if a woman miscarry before the due time of Child birth, if she come in three, or four, or five Moneths after she hath conceived, the womb at that time is close shut by the course of nature, and must be forced to open, which, if the Child come at the just time it should come

come, opens it self, but Abortion makes the woman that she ofttimes never can conceive again, for she can hardly ever retain the mans Seed any more, there is such a weakness caused in the retentive faculty, or else she will hardly ever conceive again. And I have heard some women complain that have miscarryed, of the great pains they have endured at such a time, and to profess that they have found less pain in bearing ten Children than when they have miscarryed with one.

But there is yet something worse than all this, when a Child comes to be dead in the womb, and is of full age to be born; for then it cannot help the woman because it stirs not, nor can it be turned that it may be brought forth but with great difficulty; and if the woman have been long sick her self, the infant cannot be strong in her womb, if she have by some accident had her courses come down much, after she is conceived with Child, or had some extraordinary flux, or looseness, and if the Child do not stir, as a living and healthful Child will; these are signes of imbecillity.

Moreover the *Secundine* which covers the Child in the womb, of which I gave you the description before, that it is the Membranes, and

and Coats, *Chorion* and *Amnios*; and these are ofttimes so strong that they will not break to make passage for the Child to come forth, & it may cause hard labour; also if the *Secundine* be too thin and weak so that it cleaves asunder before the child be turned, or fitted to come to the birth, for by this means all the moisture and humours run forth of the womb and leave the after-birth dry, and the Birth can hardly pass because the womb is not slippery wanting due moisture. Cold also shuts the womb closer, and heat causeth the woman to faint, if either of them exceed, so that she must be kept in a due temper or her delivery will not be so easy as it might be otherwise. Besides these, Diet is to be taken into consideration; for sower and binding things will straiten the Orifice of the Matrix; as Quinces, and Chesnuts, and Services, and Medlars, and Pears, all these and such like cause dolour by contracting the womb; sweet scents cause hard delivery, because they draw the matrix upward; too much hunger or thirst, weariness, or watching extraordinarily, and to use cold baths after the fifth moneth, or astringent mineral baths of Alum, Salts, or Iron, or of vegetables that bind much, will produce the like painful effects. The woman may be assured also by the pains she feels before travel,

if

if they be above the Navel and in the back only, and not below as they should be in time of delivery, that all is not so well as not to put her to more than ordinary pain: the signes of easie Birth are contrary to these; for then the pains bear downwards and not upwards and so they are not so violent, if she have usually been delivered with ease; if the woman have cold fainting sweats, and she swoon away, and her Pulse beat out of measure, there is much danger, but if she be strong and lusty, and the Child tumbles and strives much to come forth, and the pains fall to the bottom of the belly there is no fear; but know this, all women are most in danger to miscarry in the first, and second moneth after they have conceived, for then the ligaments and all parts of it are weak and easily spoiled and torn in sunder, and about the end of her going with Child, the Child is heavy and the womb begins to open, and so causeth danger of abortion; but in about four, five, or six moneths there is least danger in taking Physick, or letting blood if the women be oppressed with it, for then she will not easily miscarry. I told you before, that women are all ready to be brought a bed at seven moneths end, for that number of seven is the perfection of all numbers; *Pythagoras* saith, that

that seven is the knot that binds Mans life, and *Hippocrates, lib. de Principiis*, saith, that the time of all men is determined by seven, every climatericall or seven years breeding a new alteration in the body of Man: Children cast their Teeth at seven, and Maids courses begin to flow at fourteen. Seven times seven is of great danger to Mans life; and the great Climaterical which few escape is seventimes nine, which makes sixty three. But the signes of miscarriage in Childbirth are; if the Child be faln lower toward the wombs mouth and so out of its true place; also if the woman have blackish courses, chiefly if she be far gone with child, she is in danger to lose the Child; many women have their Terms in the first moneths, but they are but watry, pale coloured, not fitting for the nourishment of the infant, and they are also superfluous, so that nature at first sends them out as being useful neither for nutriment for the Mother nor the Child. I said before, that the breasts will shew danger, and of Twins which is most likely to suffer, if the right breast flag she will miscarry of a Boy, if the left of a Girle, and the head shaking as with a Palsie, the body trembling, the face flushing with red, the eyes pain'd inwardly, if the body be afflicted with wind, there is fear of miscariage in child birth, but if she travel when she is sick of a sharp Feaver, or some such dangerous disease, seldom doth either Mother or the child escape death: but the ordinary causes of Abortion are, when the womb is too weak, or corrupted by phlegmatick, slippery, slimy, or watry humours, so that it cannot retain the Child, the pains of inflammation and Imposthumes hinder delivery, extream Costiveness of the body by straining to go to stool forceth the child downwards, and the dung staying in the right gut, when the woman is bound, oppresseth the child; if she fall into a *Tenesmus* which is a great desire to go to stool and can do nothing, *Hippocrates* saith, Abortion is like to follow: Piles and Hemorrhoids cause pain and miscarriage, fat women have slippery wombs, and lean women have as dry and want nourishment for the child, neither are fit for child-bearing. Bleeding is bad for childing women, unless there be great need; purging, especially in the first, or second, or about the last months, and vomiting is far worse; too much fasting starves the child, too much eating and drinking will stifle it; great heats or baths, or stoves, force the child to press for a more free air, and great cold is not good for it, all immoderate exercises, passions, desires, longings, falls, strokes, and all violent

running

running, leaping, coughing, lifting and such like will bring on this misfortune.

There being then so many causes, and accidents whereby women usually fall into such mishaps, 'twill be profitable for women with child to observe some good rules beforehand, that when her time of delivery is at hand, she may more easily undergo it, and not so soon miscarry. But as there are diverse causes of miscarriage, so the times are diverse that we are to provide for, either before or after conception. And before she be conceived with child, let her use means both by diet and physick to strengthen her womb, and to further conception : Drink wine that is first well boyled with the mother of Tyme, for it is a pretious thing. If the womb be too windy, eat ten Juniper berries every morning, if too moist, the woman must exercise, or sweat in a Stove, or Hot-house, or else take half a dram of *Galingal* and as much Cinnamon mingled in powder and drink it in Muskadel every morning, but if she use moderate labour, perhaps she may have no need of this: but the most frequent cause of barrenness in young lusty women that are of a cholerick complexion, is driness of the Matrix ; and this is easily known by their great desire of copulation. It is to be corrected by cooling drinks, and e-
mulsions

mulsions made of barley-water, blanched Almonds, white poppy seeds, Cucumbers, Citrons, Melons, and Gourds, and to drink frequently of this; all violent exercise, drinking of wine, or strong waters must be forborn. The Oyl of Nightshade is good to annoint the Reins; some report, that the seeds of Mandrakes are very useful to cool and purge a hot and foul womb, such diseases are common to salt complexions, and the dose of half a dram of Mandrake seed bruised and drunk at once in a cup of white wine, cannot be dangerous, for though the leaves be cold, yet the seeds have a vital spirit in them to beget their like; cold begets nothing, but heat is an active quality for production. There are many conjectures concerning those Mandrakes that *Reuben* found, and that *Rachel* so much desired because she was then barren, *Gen.* 30. it may be she knew that they were fit to cure her barrenness. I grant that sometimes *God* is the cause of barrenness, who shuts up the womb, and will not suffer some women to conceive; we have multitudes of examples in Scripture for it, *Rachel* doubtless was not barren of her self, and she was angry with *Jacob*, that she said unto him, *Give me Children or else I die*, but he acknowledgeth *God* to be the chief cause of it, *And he said unto her, Am I God, who hath withheld the fruit of the womb from thee?* And again he makes the barren women to keep house and be a joyful mother of Children.

Prayer is then the chief remedy of their barrenness, not neglecting such natural means, to further conception and to remove impediments that *God* hath appointed, and those means are chiefly, either by a well ordering of the body and mind, or else when need requires by taking of Physick. The good order of the body consists in seasonable moderate eating and drinking of wholsome meats and drinks, moderate exercise, for idleness is a great enemy to conception, and that may be the reason that so many City Dames have so few children, &if they have any, they are commonly sickly and short lived; it is not so with Country women who are always working, they usually have many children, and they are lusty and strong, for moderate labour raiseth natural heat, revives the spirits, helps digestion, opens the pores, and wasts excrements, comforts all the parts, and strengtheneth the senses and spirits, helps nature in all her faculties, and that is the way to have strong and many children. As for working too much, it wasts and destroys nature, but I think few women are guilty of this fault. Moderate rest refresheth nature, as well as moderate work, but there is a large difference between moderate rest and extreme idleness, which dulls both mind and body, and hastens old age; and therefore *Lycurgus* commanded all the *Spartans* to work at least four hours in a day. If women will be fair let them work, as it is with the body so it is with the mind, the mind must alwayes be intent upon something that is good, yet this also admits of some relaxation and rest, or else we are never able to endure; but above all we must take heed of discontent, for that wonderfully hinders conception, whereas content of mind dilates the Heart and Arteries and distributes the vital blood and spirits through the body, which exceedingly recreates nature in all her operations. Much might be said in Divinity against discontent, sullenness, and murmuring, which many women, especially, are too much guilty of; for it troubles the imagination, which should be pure in the act of conception; it stirs up ill affections and draws away vital heat from the Circumference to the Center, consuming the vital spirits; Discontent hinders People from what they desire, denies *God*'s Providence, and shews that our spirits are too much fastened to the World; yet sometimes the best woman of us all cannot

not avoid it. But it is the Physical part that I pretend to. And therefore let such as desire to have children, look to it that their courses come down orderly, and be well coloured, for then there is no fear but such women will be easie to conceive, but they must be sparing in the act of Copulation, else one act will destroy another; like *Penelopes* web, what she spun in the day, she unreathed at night; too frequent use makes the womb slippery, and therefore whores have but few children, and some honest women conceive presently when their Husbands return after a long absence; women will soonest conceive two or three dayes after their Terms be staid; she must avoid all meats and drinks that hinder conception, as drinking of sweet Wine the *Hollanders* call Stum, that keeps women from conceiving, or eating Ivy berries, wearing Saphyre, or Emerald stones about them; but a Laodstone carryed causeth concord and fruitfulness, and so doth the heart of a male Quale; for a man, of a female for a woman; to eat *Eringo* root, or *Ctyrions*; take *Castorium* half a dram in Malmsey, spread a plaister of *Lsbdanum* and lay to the womb; take a scruple of *Galingal* in White Wine every morning, or a dram of Fox or Boars stones in Sheeps Milk, or a dram of a Bulls pisle; eat the brains of Sparrows and Pidgeons, and the flesh too if you please.

But to leave this which is concerning means before women have conceived, that they may more easily prove with child, and retain it their full time, and be afterwards in due time happily delivered of it.

I come in the next place to shew what the woman must do that is gone with child; and first let her drink every morning a good draught of Sage Ale, for though Sage do provoke the courses yet it will not do so here, but it strengthens the womb; many things by sundry qualities they abound with, will cause contrary effects; so *Cinnamon* a great binder for a loosness, will stop the courses when they flow too much, and make them come down when they are stopt. I have proved that *Aurum Potabile* will stay the bloody flux, yet if a body be full of ill humours, it wil purge sufficiently.

Garden Tansie Ale made and drank like Sage Ale is good if the woman fear to miscarry; if you bruise the Tansie and sprinkle it with Muskadel and apply it to her Navel, it is more effectual than a toast of bread that some dip in the said wine and apply the same way. Let women that are in the said danger alwayes keep the sirrup of this Tansie by them

them, it is made with the juice of the herb, clarified and boiled up with a double weight of sugar, give a spoonful or two to the labouring woman, it may save many a womans life, and her childs. Let her abstain from all binding diet, let her boyl Mallows when she comes near the time of her delivery, or Holyhocks in fair spring water, and with Honey, or Sugar enough to sweeten it, and add half a spoonful of white salt, for a Glister. Let her eat meats and drink such things as nourish well, but take heed of surfeiting or excess, and let her keep her body loose, roasted Apples eat with Sugar in the morning will do it, or let her take a bolus of *Cassia Fistula*, called Pudding pipe, about an hour or less before dinner, there is no danger in it and it opens gently, she may make a Glister with Chicken or tender flesh broth, adding course Sugar or Honey, and half a spoonful of white salt, or let her boyl *Mercury* in her broth to make a suppository with Castle-sope or Lard.

The Eagle stone, I have seen abundance of them every day to be sold in *Hamburgh*, and they are to be had in *London*; but they are of four kinds, the best is brought from *Africa*, and is taken out of an Eagles nest, for the Eagle some write, cannot lay her eggs if she want these stones by her, it hath the name from

hence

hence, and it is called from the likeness it hath with it, a stone with child: it is but a small stone with another stone that shakes and sounds within it, it is but of a small body and easily beaten to powder; some say there is a male Eagle stone and this is a female, I think there is both male and female in stones and Plants. There is a second and that is called the male Eagle stone, and it comes from *A-rabia*, it is as hard as a gall, of a dark red colour, and hard to be powdered; the third is brought from *Cyprus*, not unlike that of *Africa*, but it is much bigger. The fourth brought from a place called *Taphimsius*, is so denominated also, it is round and white, and another stone within it, it is found in Rivers, this is held to be the worst, but in some respects very good, and the best of all the four as it is used for some occasions: but herein must we needs admire the works of *God*, for I have proved it to be true, that this stone hanged about a womans neck, and so as touch her skin, when she is with child, will preserve her safe from Abortion, and will cause her to be safe delivered when the time comes; but since the fall of our first Parents it is hard to find the vertues and secret qualities of the creatures. But when I give these and the like rules, I know poor women are not able to provide

provide in such cases, but their rich neighbours should do it for them; for I do not question but that all women will be glad to eat and drink well, and to take all things that may do them good if they knew but what, and can procure them.

A Bath for a woman great with child, and near her time to be delivered, is very good for her to sit in, and it may be thus made: Holyhocks leaves and roots two handfuls; Betony, Mallows, of each one handful; Mugwort, Marjeromo, Mints, Camomille, of each half a handful; Linseed, Pursly, Pursly bruised two handfuls; put all in Bags together, and boil all in well-water sufficient for the woman to sit up to the Navel in; when it is warm to sit in, hold one bag to her Navel, and let her sit upon another, after this done, warm this Ointment following and anoint her back, her belly, and secrets. Take Oil of sweet Almonds, of Lillies, of Violets of each half an ounce, Ducks greafe, and Hens greafe, of each 3 drams, Wax a little to make the Ointment; you may add if you please to this Ointment in compounding it Holyhock rubra, Fenugreekseed, Butter, of each a quarter of an ounce, Quince kernels, Gum tra ganth, of each an ounce; stamp the seeds, slice the roots, boil till in Rain water, take out the mucilage and

mix

mix it with the foresaid Oyles, then let the pounded Gum traganth, and hens grease boil so long till their mucilage come to a Salve. Use this annoynting every day for five or six weeks before she lye in. But before I come to her time of delivery, I shall speak a word of one frequent cause of womens miscarriage, and that is their longings, and sometimes of their unnatural and unreasonable desires after they have conceived with Child. You must know, that to exceed in the things not natural as Philosopers call eating and drinking, fullness, emptiness, sleep and watchings, exercise and rest, and too great intention of the mind, may hasten the birth, and cause abortion, Those women that use moderation in the foresaid things, are not so often longing for what they can not easily attain to. Nay sometimes you have Ladies at Court, and Citizens Wives, and Country women too will long to eat sand and dirt; but their Children seldome live long that are begun thus. That some women with child will desire to steal things from others, this is no small argument that the Child she goes withal will be a Thief; wherefore she must take care to give it good education, and to bring it up in the fear of *God* When nature is thus perverted in what she defires, she is forced to leave the conception be-

cause

cause she cannot attain what she looks for. This may be prevented by a decoction of vine leaves frequently taken; it may be provided by preparing a decoction strong of it at time of the year, and to boil that into a sirrup, to use when need requires, for it is said to be very proper for this distemper, though I cannot call it a disease.

There is another cause not far unlike in the effects to womens longings, and that is suddain fears, for many a woman brings forth a Child with a hare lip, being suddenly frighted when she conceived by the starting of a Hare, or by longing after a piece of a Hare; *Miraldus* thought so, and many women cannot deny it to be true; but he was a notable conceited old Philosopher, and he bethought himself how he might find out a remedy to do poor women good, and it is this, which is easily proved; let a woman slit her smock like her husbands shirt, and that he saith upon his knowledge will do it.

BOOK,

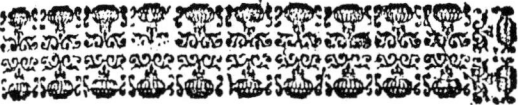

BOOK. IV.

CHAP. I.

Rules for Women that are come to their Labour.

ALl Women, Midwives especially should be well seen against this time of necessity, and all things provided that may cause them to be easily delivered, and Childbed linnen at hand, having first invoked the Divine assistance by whom we live and move and have our being.

When the Patient feels her Throws coming she should walk easily in her Chamber, and then again lye down, keep her self warm, rest her self and then stir again, till she feels the waters coming down and the womb to open;

pen; let her not lye long a bed, yet she may lye sometimes and sleep to strengthen her, and to abate pain; the Child will be the stronger.

Sometimes the Child is dead in the womb before, and you may know it to be dead, when the Breasts suddenly hang down slack, Nature makes no Milk of provision for them, for there is no reason she should.

Secondly, she is cold all the belly over, chiefly the Navel.

Thirdly, Her water is thick, aud hath a stinking substance that falls to the bottom.

Fourthly, The Child moves not though you wet your hand in warm water and rub it over her belly, which is a true trial, and it will stir if it be alive.

Fifthly, She dreams of dead people, and is frightned with it.

Sixthly, Her breath smels filthily.

Seventhly, She longs to eat strange things unfit for to eat.

Eightly, She looks ill favouredly, and sorrowfully.

Ninethly, The Child falls to the side she lyeth on like a lump of lead: But Garden Tansey or the Eagle stone will bring the Child to its right place if it be weak onely; but if it be dead there is no way to help that but to hasten

hasten delivery as fast as may be, for it is a misery beyond expression for a woman to go with a dead child in her womb; as for two Twins to be born that grow together and one of them dead, the living Child cannot long endure. *Virgil* tells us of *Mezentius* a Tyrant,

> *Dead bodies to the living he did place,*
> *Joyning them hand to hand and face to face.*

Tenthly, Corrupt stinking humours run from the womb, chiefly if she have had some ill disease.

Eleventhly, Her eyes look hollow, and her nose strangely, her lips wan and pale.

Twelfthly, Her breath stinks if the Child have been dead two or three dayes.

The more of these signs appear at once the more certainty of the death of the Child. Wherefore presently use medicines to expel it forth, or Manual and Chirurgical operations with all care to save the Mothers life, for she is in great danger of death also. The signs of greater danger to her are.

1. If she swoond in labor, or be in a trance and memory be gone.
2. If she be extream weak.
3. If she will not answer when you call, or very hardly.

4. If she hath Convulsion fits or shrinking together in travel.

5. If she loath meat.

6. If her pulse beat high and quick.

But if none of these signes appear, there is not so great danger; wherefore presently hasten by medicaments to provoke the expulsive faculty to cast it forth, but the physick must be stronger than for a live Child, for a dead Child makes no way, wanting motion, but a living Child doth.

The vertue of the Eagle stone in such cases some commend, but I fear it is but a fansie of *Miraldus*, for I never saw it tried.

There must be no delay at such times especially to drive the dead Child forth before it be corrupted, for then the Mother can scarcely escape, Nature is sometimes strong and able to cast forth a dead Birth, without helps, but then the danger is the more when help wants.

The causes that some Children dye in the womb are.

1. Want of nutriment.

2. Corrupt diet.

3. Gluttony and surfeiting, that choke the Infant.

4. The Cups are sometimes broken by strokes, sudden fears, much sneezing, coughing, violent

motion, extream joy, sorrow, or trouble of mind; or by medicaments that corrode, or bitter drinks the infant loaths, or things that provoke the courses, or by acute diseases, or lasty by hard labor or difficulty in bearing of Children. These following Medicaments will, *God* willing, cause her to be delivered of the dead Child, and her self escape death by them; make her sneeze with powder of Pepper and white Hellebore snuft up into her nostrils, drink a dram of Basil powdered, with white wine, it makes the delivery easy, *&c.*

But if it fall out that these medicaments prevail not, as sometimes they do not, that disease is beyond the power of medicine or ordinary Midwifry, then we must come to chirurgery, and the method how to perform it is thus.

1. Lay the woman along upright, the middle of her body lying highest, and let sufficient help keep her down, that when the Child is drawn forth she rise not with it.

2. The midwife must first annoint her hands with Oyl of white Lillies, Butter, or Ducks grease, then holding down her fingers let her shut her hand and thrust it up into the womb to feel how the Child lyeth, for sometimes it may be drawn forth with the hand, but

but if it cannot be done so, then use Chirurgeons Instruments, having first found with your hand the posture of the Child.

1. If the head come forward, fasten a hook to one eye of it, or under the chin, or to the roof of the mouth, or upon one of the shoulders, which of these you find best, and then draw the Child out gently that you do the woman no hurt.

2. If the feet come first fasten the hook upon the bone above the privy parts, called *os pubis*, or by some rib or back bones, or breast bones, then draw it not forth, but hold the Instrument in your left hand, and then fasten another hook upon some other part of the Child right against the first, and draw gently both together that the Child may come equally, moving it from one side to another until you have drawn it forth altogether; but often guide it with your fore-finger well annointed; if it stick or stop any where, take higher hold still with your hooks upon the dead child.

3. If but one arm come forth and you cannot well put it back again, the passage being too narrow, or for some other reason, then tye it with a linnen cloth that it slip not up again, and draw it down gently till the whole arm come forth, and then cut it off with a
sharp

sharp knife from the body, do so also if both hands appear together, or one leg, or both; if you cannot easily put them back or take them forth with the body; as you cut the arms from the shoulders, so you must cut the legs from the thighs, your instruments being very sharp for quick dispatch; when some parts are cut off from the body, then turn the rest to draw it out the better.

4. If the childs head be swollen with watry humours, that it be too great, to come forth at so narrow a passage, then put in your hand, holding a sharp incision knife between your fingers, and so cut open the head, that the humours contained in it may come forth and the head abate; but if it be too great of it self and not by disease, you must divide the skull and take it out by pieces with instruments for that purpose; if when the head is come out the breast be too large to follow, then cut that asunder also, and bring it forth in pieces, and so must you do with the whole body, or any parts that are swollen too great.

5. If the child come sidelong, then annoint your hand and her secrets, and turn the child to the best posture you can; the womb and all the Privities must also be perfumed with such things as may dilate the place and
make

make it slippery; there are many medicaments prescribed in this book will be very proper for it, but when all fails you must cut the child asunder and draw it out by pieces.

6. If the womb be diseased or hurt so that it be ulcerated, whereby the parts are made dryer and narrower, it must be dilated by oyls, unguents, baths and fumes, such you will find set down to help delivery for a living child, and you must use them for a child that is dead.

You must observe in this work, that if by violent drawing forth the child, the Privy parts and Genitals of the mother be so torn that her Urine and excrements come out against her will, which often happens in such cases, the cure will be the same as for the Palsie, and wounds of these parts, with a general evacuation of her body; also make a Bath of all these herbs and roots following, or as many as you can get, *viz.* of the decoction of *Bay-leaves*, *Sage*, *Betony*, *Brank*, or some *Hogs-Fennel*, *Origanum*, *Penni-Royal*, *Tanicle*, *Tormentil*, *Plantane*, *Rupture-wort*, *Mugwort*, *Mouseeare*, *Lady-Mantle*, *St. Johnswort*, *Cammomile* flowers, *Oaken* leaves, *Camphire-roots*. The woman must sit in this Bath, and presently after her bathing, she must annoint

noint her Privities and Fundament with this following Unguent.

Take Oyl of worms, of Foxes, and of the Lillies of the Vallies, each alike, boyl a young blind Puppey in them, so long that his flesh part from the bones; then press forth all strongly, and add to the straining, *Styrax, Calamint, Benzoin, Opopanax, Frankincense, Mastick*, of each one dram, a little *Aqua-Vitæ*, a little *wax*; mix them and make of them an Ointment; then let her drink often of this Potion following.

Take Pennyroyal, Balm, Motherwort, Mousear, Ladies Mantle, of each one handful, Mace one dram, boyl all in a Pottle of the best wine, strain it and drink a little draught morning and evening, or boil nothing but Ladies Mantle in her broth; drink a pint of it every morning fasting; or if her stomach will not bear it, take but four or five Ounces at a draught.

The *Cesarian* Birth is the drawing forth of the child either dead or alive, by cutting open the Mothers womb, it was so called because *Julius Cæsar*, the first *Roman* Emperor was so brought into the world. Physicians and Chirurgeons say it may be safely done without killing the Mother, by cutting in the *Abdomen* to take out the child; but I shall wish no man to do it whilest the Mother is alive; but if the Mother dye in child-bearing, and the child be alive, then you must keep the womans Mouth and Privities open that the child may receive air to breath, or it will be presently stifled, then turn the woman on her left side, and there cut her open and take out the Infant. This is also a *Cesarian* Birth, but it is not like that which is used whilest the Mother is alive. It is used three ways.

1. The Mother living and the Child dead.
2. The Child living and the Mother dead.
3. When both are living.

Mathias Cornax relates of a woman that carried a dead Child in her womb four years, it was cut out of the belly and womb, and the Mother lived and conceived with child again; she fainted not when her belly and womb were cut, and they grew well again without stitching; but she had hard labour the second child, and the Chirurgeon offered to cut her again, but the women would not suffer it, so she fainted, but the Chirurgeon delivered her of a second boy, but this last was dead.

Roderigo de Carstro saith, that a child cannot live in the womb when the Mother is dead,

dead, if it be not presently taken forth so soon as her breath is gone, or vital spirits last, because when the Mothers life and motion cease, the childs must needs cease that depends upon it; but it is an error, for the child hath a Soul and life of its own, and may live a while without the Mother; but the Midwife must keep the womb open that it be not stifled till the Chirurgeon cuts it out; you shall feel the Child leap when the Mother is dead.

Charles Stephen shews how to cut out a dead Child. And *Francis Rufet* saith, a live Child may be cut out of the womb & both child & Mother do well; it is possible and sometimes necessary to be done, and it stands by reason, for women receive sometimes wounds in the *Peritoneum* and the Muscles of the lower belly, more dangerous than the *Cesarian* cut, and yet escape well enough.

A Child may be sometimes very weak, yet not dead, take heed you do not force delivery in such occasions till you be sure it is time, for children may be sick and faint in their Mothers bellies. But to prevent danger, burn half a pint of white-wine adding no Spice to it, but half an ounce of Cinnamon and drink it off: if your Travel and throws come upon you, be sure it is dead; but if it be but sick and weak, it will refresh it and strengthen it.

If the Child be dead in the womb, the juyce of Garden Tansey annointed on the secrets, or an oyl made in Summer with the herbs before it run to flower, and boil'd in oyl till the juyce be wasted, and set in the Sun a moneth before you boil it, is an especial oyl for Midwives.

The Eagle-stone held near the privy parts will draw forth the Child, as the Loadstone draws Iron, but be sure so soon as the Child, and afterburthen are come away, that you hold the stone no longer, for fear of danger.

Any of these herbs half a dram in powder drunk in white-wine will do much, *viz* of Bettony, or Sage, or Penny-Royal, Fetherfew or Centory, Ivy-berries and leaves, or drink a strong decoction of Master-wort, or of Hysop in hot water, it soon will bring the dead Child forth; because the afterbirth is corrupted in such cases and comes forth by pieces, it is fit to drink of the same drink till all be come away, or the roots of Polipody stamped and warm'd laid to the soles of her feet presently works the effect.

The same things almost all are proper when the Child is living and comes to be born, but if her Travel be long, the Midwife must refresh her with some Chickens broth of the Yolk of a potched Egg, with a little bread,

or

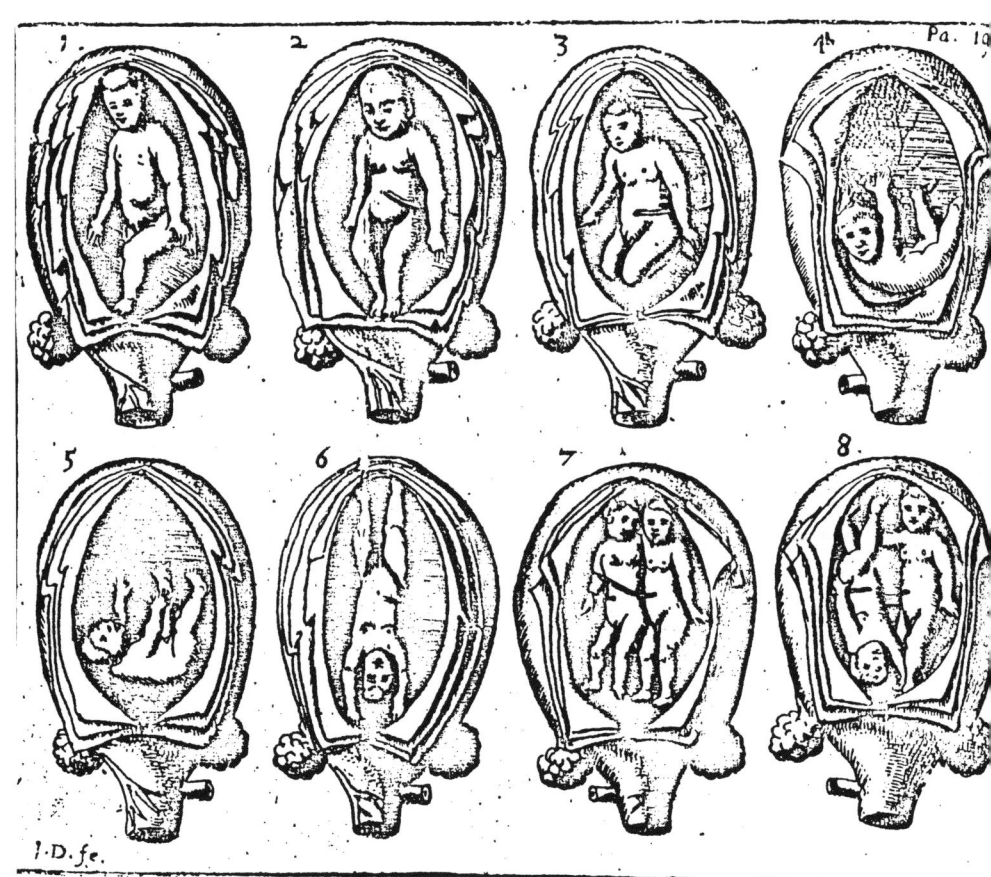

or some wine, or strong water, but moderately taken, and withal to cheer her up with good words, & stroaking down her belly above her Navel gently with her hand, for that makes the Child move downwards: She must bid her hold in her breath as much as she can, for that will cause more force to bring out the Child.

Place here the Picture of all sorts of postures of Children.

Take notice that all women do not keep the same posture in their delivery; some lye in their beds, being very weak, some sit in a stool or chair, or rest upon the side of the bed, held by other women that come to the Labor.

If the Woman that lyeth in be very fat, fleshly, or gross, let her ly groveling on the place, for that opens the womb, and thrusts it downwards. The Midwife must annoint her hands with Oyl of Lillies, and the Womans Secrets, or with Oyl of Almonds, and so with her hands handle and unloose the parts, and observe how the Child lyeth, and stirreth, and so help as time and occasion direct. But above all take heed you force not the birth till the time be come, and the Child come forward and appears ready to come forth.

Now the danger were much to force delivery, because when the woman hath laboured sore, if she rest not a while, she will not be able presently to endure it, her strength being spent before.

Also when you see the after-burthen, then be sure the Birth is at hand; but if the coats be so strong that they will not break to make way for the Child to come forth, the Midwife must gently and prudently break and rend it with her nails, if she can raise it, she may cut a piece of it with a knife or pair of Scissers, but beware of the infant.

Then follows presently a flux of humours and the Child after that, but if all the humours that should make the place slippery chance to run forth by this means before the child come, the parts within and without must be annointed with Oyl of Almonds or Lillies, and a whole Egg Yelk and white beaten, and poured into the privy passage to to make it glib, instead of the waters that are run forth too soon.

If the child have a great head and stick by the way, the Midwife must annoint the place with Oyl as before, and enlarge the part as much as may be; the like must be done when Twins offer themselves; if the head coms first,

the

the birth is natural, but if it come any other way, the Midwife must do what she can to bring it to this posture.

Sometimes the infant comes with the legs forwards, and both arms downwards close to the sides, this way the Midwife may endeavour to take it forth if it continue the same posture, by annointing and gently handling the place; but it is safer if she can, to turn the Legs upward again by the Belly, that the head may first come down by the back of the womb for that is the natural way.

If the child come forth with both legs and feet first, and the Childs hands both litted above the head, this is the worst for danger of all the rest; she must strive to turn the Child, and if she cannot she must try to bring the hands down to the sides, and to keep the legs close that it may come forth, or else to bind the feet as they come out with some linnen Cloath, and tenderly to help delivery, but it will be hard to it.

Sometimes the Child will come forth with one foot, and the other lifted upward. Then let the woman in Child-bed be laid upright on her back, & hold up her thighs and belly, that her head be lower than her body; then let the Midwife with her hand gently put back the leg that is come forth into the womb again,

and

and bid the labouring woman to stir and move her self, that by her stirring the birth may offer it self the head downward, and if so, you may then set her in a Chair as she was at first that she may have a natural delivery, but if this cannot be done, then the Midwife with her hand must discreetly bring forth that leg that is not yet come forth; but beware she put not the Childs hands that lye close down by its sides out of their place; if the side of the child come towards the passage, she must turn the child to its natural posture, but if it come the feet forward and the legs abroad, she must joyn the legs and feet together, taking care that she remove not the hands from the place they should hang down close by the side.

If the infant with one or both the knees first strive to come forth, she must put them back that both feet may first come down to the passage.

If the child come headlong with one hand thrust out, then she must put the Child back with her hand upon the shoulders, that the hand may goe to its natural place; if this will not prevail, lay the woman upright with her thighs and belly upwards that it may pass forth as it should do.

If both hands come out first, she must thrust
the

the Child back by the shoulders as formerly, till the hands hang down by the sides of the Child.

If it would come forth arsewards, the buttocks first, she must return it back with her hands till the legs and feet may present themselves, or the head first if it be possible, which is most natural.

If the infant present both hands and both feet together to come forth so all at once, she must take the Child carefully by the head and put the legs upward to take it forth.

If the shoulders come first, she must put it back by the shoulders that the head may come first.

If it come the breast forward, the legs and hands lying behind, she must take it by the feet or by the head as she finds it to be most easy, putting the other part upward that it may come forth right.

If a Woman have two Children at once that come together headlong, she must take forth one after the other, but beware the other retreat not back in the mean time; so also must she receive them both that come together with the feet forward, taking them out one after the other.

If they come one with his feet, the other with the head forward at the same time, she
must

must receive that first which is most likely, and next the passage, and that which cometh with the feet first, if she can, receive last, taking heed that they do not hurt one the other.

But let this general rule be observed, still to annoint the passage with Ducks grease, or Oyle of Lillies, or sweet Almonds, or such things as may smooth the passage and ease womans labour, and likewise when she toucheth any part of the infant, this will help much if there should be any aposthume in the place.

Particular helps to delivery, are to lay the woman first all along on her back, her head a little raised with a Pillow, and a pillow under her back; and another pillow larger than the other, to raise her buttocks and rump; lay her thighs and knees wide open asunder, her legs must be bowed backwards toward her buttocks and drawn upwards, her heels and soles of her feet must be fixed against a board to that purpose laid cross her bed. Some woman must have a swathe-band above a foot broad four double, this must be put under her Reins, and two women standing on each side of her must hold it up straight, and these two persons must lift up the swathe-band equally, just when her throws come, or else they may do her hurt; and two more of the standers by must

must lay hold on the upper part of her shoulders, that she may with more ease force the child forth. The woman must hold her breath in and strive to be delivered, and the Midwife must stroke down the birth from above the Navel easily with her hand, for that will, as I said before, make the Infant move downwards.

CHAP. II.

To know the fit time when the Child is ready to be born.

I Shall desire all Midwives to take heed how they give any thing inwardly to hasten the Birth, unless they are sure the Birth is at hand, many a child hath been lost for want of this knowledge, and the mother put to more pain than she would have been. Let not therefore the child be forced out, unless there fall down an extreme flux of blood, for in such cases it is best to save the Mothers life to drive forth the Child, but there is great skill and care to be used, or the woman were as good be set upon the Rack. It is hard to know when the true time of her travel is near, because many
women

women have great pains many weeks before the time of delivery comes. But I think the heat of their Reins is the cause of these pains, but you may know whether the heat of their reins be the cause of it or not, for if their legs swell their reins are too hot, and the cure will be to annoint their backs, to cool the reins with Oyl of Poppies, water Lillies, or Violets: women whose reins are hot have alwaies hard labour. A strong decoction of Plantane leaves and roots in water, then strained and clarified with the white of an egg, boil'd then to a sirrup with its weight in Sugar is excellent, take a spoonful or two when you please, or drink often the water and sirrups of Violets and water Lillies.

But if the birth be at hand, you shall know when the skins *Amnios* and *Allantois* which as I told you serve to hold the sweat and urine of the child in the womb, and by the means of which skins the infant is also supported in the Matrix, do break by the violent motion of the child, so that these excrements fall down to the neck of the womb, Midwives call it the water, and when that runs forth then the Birth is near; this is the truest sign that is, for when those skins are broken, the Infant can no longer stay there than a naked man in a heap of snow.

These

These waters make the parts slippery and the birth easie, if the child come presently with them, but if it stay longer till the parts grow dry it will be hard, therefore Midwives do ill to rend these skins open with their nails to make way for the water to come, nature will make it come forth only when she needs it and not before; but if the water break away long before the birth, it is safe to give medicaments to drive the birth after the water. But there are other signs of the birth approaching, let the Midwife look well on the womans belly, for if the upper part of it be sunk and hollow, and the lower part big and full, it is certain the child is sunk down; again, if the womans Throws be quick and strong, coming from the reins downward all along the belly and not staying at the Navel but falling still lower to the groins, and inwardly to the bottom of the belly, where lieth the inmost neck of the womb, this is another sure sign.

Then let the Midwife, her hand annointed with fresh butter or with oyl of sweet Almonds, put up her hand, and if she feel the inward neck of the womb open, or any substance to push forward, the child is coming; but if the skin break and the waters come down, that is the last and surest sign, as I said,

when

when the waters preeede and the child doth not follow presently in some reasonable time, these things following hasten and ease delivery.

Featherfew or Mugwort boil'd in white wine, let her drink a draught of the decoction, the sirrups of either may be made in summer with their juice clarified and boyled to a sirrup with twice as much Sugar, a spoonful at a time to be taken; or drink a dram of the powder of Cinnamon in wine or the distill'd water of Mugwort, Betony, Dittander, Pennyroyal, or Featherfew.

Tansie bruised and applyed, or the Oyl of it, as I said, will do it, but the Eagle stone held to the secrets, draws out both Child and *Secundine*, hold it to no longer for it will draw forth Womb and all; *Miraldus* tells of many more pretty ways.

But for more assurance take this powder made of Dittany, of Crete, Penni-royal, Roundbirthwort, of each ten grains, Cinnamon and Saffron of each twelve grains; beat them to fine powder, and let her drink it in wine, or some fit liquor, in the decoction or distill'd waters of red Pease, Penniroyal, Parsly, &c.

Outward means is good applied to the secrets; take Agrimony leaves and roots, but
after

after cast it away lest it draw forth the Matrix; Henbane, Polypody, or Bistort roots are commended for the same use. But let all hot and violent remedies be avoided, for many times they bring the woman into a dangerous Feaver.

Also too much fasting, or too much eating breed peril to women in travel, a woman that is with child cannot so well digest her meat as they can that are not with child; Midwives therefore must ask how long it was since that the woman did eat, and what and how much, that vpon occasion she may give her something to strengthen her in her labour if need be, as warm broth, or a potched egg; and if her delivery be long in doing, give her an ounce of Cinnamon water to comfort her, or else a dram of *Confectio Alkermes* at twice in two spoonfuls of Claret wine, but give her but one of these three things, for you may soon cast her into a feaver by too much hot administrations, and that may stop her purgations, and breed many mischiefs.

CHAP. III.

What must be done after the woman is delivered.

IT will be profitable when a woman hath had sore travel, to wrap her back with a sheep-skin newly flead off, and let her ly in it, and to lay a Hare-skin, rub'd over with Hares blood newly prepared, to her belly; let these things be worn two hours in winter, and but one hour in Summer, for these will close up the parts too much dilated by the childs birth, and will expel all ill melancholly blood from those parts.

This being done, swathe the woman with a Napkin about nine inches broad; but annoint her belly with Oyl of St. *Johns wort*, and then raise up the womb with a linnen cloth many times folded, cover her flanks, with a little pillow about a quarter of a Yard long, then swathe her, beginning a little above the hanches, rather higher than lower, winding it even; lay warm cloths to her breasts, forbearing those that repulse the milk till longer time, and the body be setled, lest repercussives should do her hurt, let then her blood be first setled ten or twelve hours, and
that

that the blood which was cast upon the lungs by violent labour may return to its own place; but you may ease the pains of her breasts and comfort them, laying a linnen cloth doubled and not warm'd, dipt in Oil of St. *Johns wort* and of Roses, with the yolk and white of an egg beat together, of each an ounce, with an ounce of Rose-water, and as much of Plantain-water. Let her not sleep till about four hours after she is delivered, but first give her some nourishing broth or Cawdle to comfort her; let her eat no flesh till two dayes at least be over, for she may not use a full diet after so great loss of blood suddenly, as she grows stronger she may begin with meats of easie digestion, as Chickens, or Pullets: she may drink small wines with a little Saffron, Mace and Cloves infused, equal parts, all tied in a piece of linnen, and let them lie in the wine so close stopt, she may drink a small draught of it at dinner and supper for the whole month, and besides her ordinary food she may if she will take nourishing broths and Aleberries, with bread, butter, and Sugar. Let her drink her Beer or Ale with a tost, she may drink a decoction of Liquorish, Raisins of the Sun and a little Cinnamon : if the child be a boy she must lye in thirty dayes, if a girl forty daies, and remember that it is the time of her purification that her husband must abstain from her.

CHAP. IV.

When and how to cut off the Childs navel-string, and what is the Consequent thereof.

THe Navel-string is twisted that it might be the stronger, and that the blood by that delay might be better prepared: had the Vein in the Navel, or the Arteries, or *Urachos* that carryes the piss being single, the different postures of the child in the womb, or the difference of the womans standing, sitting, or lying, might press a single vessel, and stop the passage of the blood in the Vein, spirit in the Arteries, or water in the *Urachos*, but the twisting hath prevented that.

The cutting of the Navel-string helps much, for it keeps the blood and spirits in, after the Child is born. A Midwives skill is seen much if she can perform this rightly.

The time to do it is so soon as ever the Child is born, whether he bring a part of the
Secundine

Secundine out with him or not, for sometimes the infant brings a piece of the Coat *Amnios* upon his head, and that they name the caule: I know no wonders this Caule will work, but if you find this Caule on the childs head you shall miss it in the after-birth, if it be in the after-birth it will not be on his head. The reason why some Children bring it with them on their head into the world is weakness, and it signifies a short life, and proves seldome otherwise: But if it come with it or without it, so soon as it is come forth, consider whether the Child be strong or weak, for by the Navel-string the Mother gives both vital and natural blood to the Child; wherefore if the Child be weak, you must gently put back part of the vital and natural blood into the childs body by the Navel, for that will refresh a weak child; if the child be strong you need not do it. Many children seem to be born dead that recover by this meanes, as very weak children often do; but you must crush out six or seven drops of blood out of the navel-string, I mean that part which is cut off, & give it the child by the mouth to drink.

But in what place this string must be cut, Midwives and Physicians can scarce agree. *Elias lib. 4. c. 3.* saith, it must be cut four fingers breadth from the body, but what is this,

this, Midwives fingers are not equal, I suppose he means four inches, for that was the opinion of the Antients; *Miraldus* was critical in this point, and from him some errors were begotten about it in late writers, and Midwives. Hence it is, if *Spigelius* speak truth, that Midwives cut the Females Navel-string shorter than they doe the Males, for Boys privy parts must be longer than womens, but if Females are cut short they say it will make them modest, and their secrets narrower. *Spigelius* and others laugh at this conceit, for if Midwives by cutting their Navel-strings can make their secrets wider, all women that have hard labour have good reason to complain of their Midwives for cutting their Navel-string so short. *Miraldus* bids cut the navel-string long in both sexes, for that the Instruments of Generation in both follow this proportion, if womens Navel-strings be cut too short, it will hinder their Childbearing. *Taisner* an excellent Astrologer was of this mind. If Nature framed the child by the Navel-string in the womb, there is no small use of it afterward: *Miraldus* saith, that if a childs Navel-string be cut off and let fall to touch the ground, that child shall never hold its water sleeping nor waking. Also if you carry a piece of a Childs Navel-string about you, you

may,

may, saith *Miraldus*, wear it for a foil in a Ring, you shall never be troubled with convulsion fits, nor the Falling sickness. I have known all this tried, but he saith farther that it will defend those that carry it from Devils and Witch-crafts, and one may try this if they please.

If the Child be very weak when it is born, put back gently the natural blood by the Navel vein, and the vital by the Navel arteries and you shall see the child almost dead before, to revive like one awak'd out of sleep; if the child seem full of life and spirits, then stop the navel-string near the Navel that no blood nor vital spirits go back, and that will keep the child strong as it is; having done this bind the Navel-string with a strong ligature, and cut it not off too near to the string, least it unloose; you need not fear to bind the Navel-string very hard, because it feels not, and that piece of the Navel-string you leave on will fall off in a very few days; for the whole course of Nature is soon changed in the Child, and another way ordain'd to feed it. It is no matter what you cut it off with, so it be sharp to do it neatly. The reason of so many nodes or knots in the childs Navel-string is, that the blood and vital spirits might not come in too fast to choke the child,

child, Nature is a careful Nurse; but Midwives say, these knots in number signifie so many Children, the reddish boys, the whitish Girls, and the long distance between knot and knot, long time between child and child; but all false, for all women almost have equal knots, and more knots with their last Children than with the first.

When the Navel-string is cut off, apply a little Cotten or lint to the place to keep it warm, least the cold get in, and that it will do, if it be not hard enough bound, and if it do you cannot think of a greater mischief for the Child; when part of the Navel-string left is fallen off, Midwives use to burn a rag to tinder and to apply to the place, a little powder of *Bolearmoniack* were better, because it drieth; Beasts can lick the Navel-string round enough to keep out the air, but the curse lyeth heavier on women for our Grand-Mothers first sin, than it doth upon beasts.

CHAP.

CHAP. V.

What is best to bring away the Secundine, *or after-burden.*

WOmen are in as great danger if not more, after the young is born, but Beasts are not; the Caule or inward chamber of the womb the child did lye in, stayeth ofttimes long after the child is born, wch should presently follow it, & when it so happens, if it begins especially to corrupt as it will soon do, it causeth grievous pains and ofttimes death, wherefore make hast to drive it forth, but be sure the means you use be very gentle, for the woman is now grown weak and her womb is quick of feeling but the *Secundine* is dead, let the quick then cast forth the dead.

Midwives long nails may do mischief, I grant delays are dangerous, for if it be retain'd till it corrupt, it will cause Feavers, Imposthumes, Convulsions, and such like; know this, that what brings away the birth, will also do good to cast forth the after-birth; then comfort the woman, let her snuff up a little white *Hellebore* in powder to make her sneese;

but

but put the woman to as little trouble as you can, for she hath endured pain enough already.

The herb *Vervain* boil'd in wine, or a sirrup made with the clarified juice, as I told you, of Tansie, Featherfew, and mugwort do the same but hardly so forcibly; *Alexanders* boiled in wine, and the wine drunk is excellent, Sweet-Cecely, Angelica roots, or Master-wort doe the same so used.

The smoke of Mary-Gold Flowers taken in by a Tunnel at the secrets, will easily bring forth the *Secundine* though the Midwife have let go her hold. Mugwort boil'd soft in water & applied like a Poultess to the Navel, brings birth, and after birth away, but then remove it least it bring the womb after all.

Women suffer great pains in Child-birth, because the womb that hath many Nerves and Sinews, by which the body feels, is strait till time of delivery, and then it is stretched, which causeth great pain; and some women have more pain in bearing than others have, because some womens passages are narrower, and their wombs more full of Nerves as *Anatomy* will shew; and some think the reason of the great soreness of some women is, because the share-bone and *os sacrum*, or holy-bone

bone do part or give way in hard travel; it was that excellent Anatomist Doctor *Reads* opinion, and I believe it to be true; for nature strives to the utmost in such times. *Crook*, and *Columbus* deny this, but the bones are joyned with Cartilages, and Ligaments, which being wet with much moisture may give way though the bones open not, but in all labour, the Nerves that carrry feeling through the whole body, are then stretcht and cause soreness till they have rest and be settled again.

CHAP. VI.

Of the great pains and throws some Women suffer after they are delivered.

Sometimes a woman delivered shall for two of three days after, and now and then longer, feel such bitter pains in her belly and above the Groin as if she should be delivered again; these pains are not in the body and bottom of the womb, but in the Vessels and Ligatures by which the womb hangs,

and

and so it passeth to the sides and belly. The causes are, the cold air that is got in by her sore travel in child-birth, or sharp or clotted blood sticking in the womb and pricking for expulsion; these pains make the woman weak and very troublesome, wherefore you must strive to abate them.

Some women are so hardy, that to hinder this, they will drink cold water so soon as they are delivered; if the woman be cholerick she may do it with a crust of tosted bread, otherwise it is dangerous.

CHAP. VII.

Of the Chollick some women are afflicted within the time of their travel.

Some women have the Chollick at the time they should bring forth a child, which hinders the delivery, and the pains surpass the pain of their travel, you can scarce distinguish one of these pains from the other, but whilst the chollick lasts the birth comes not forward at all, the causes of this disease are, great crudities, and indigestious of the stomach.

Let

Let her take Cinnamon water one ounce, with two ounces of Oyl of sweet Almonds newly drawn; if this do it not, then give her a Glister against wind, or use fomentations against wind, both are good in this cases. More remedies there are against wind, for Child-bed Women, but these may suffice.

CHAP. VIII.

Of Womens Miscarriage or Abortment with the Signs thereof.

THere are abundance of causes whereby women are driven to abort, or miscarry, and I have spoken somewhat of this before; I shall add a little more to it, the better to know the signs, causes, and remedies against it; it is the bringing forth an untimely birth or fruit before it be ripe, if it happen in seven daies after conception it is but an effluxion, but if in fourteen daies after it is an untimely birth; sometimes an untimely birth may be alive, but it is very seldom that it continues, the elder and stronger it is the more hopes for life; some women have such large wombs, or flippery, & full of slimy humours that the Seed cannot be contain'd but slips away; sometimes it is an imposthumation causing pain, that hinders retention, but this is rather effluxion than abortment. But sometimes the Cups or Veins whereby the conception is tied to the womb, through which also nourishment passeth to it, as we said before, are stopt with viscous ill humours, and so swollen with wind, or inflamed that the Cups break and the fruit is lost for want of food; this happens commonly in the second or third month; so *Hippocrates* tells us, that this is the certain cause, if the woman that miscarries be of a good state of body, not too fat nor too lean. Sometimes the right Gut or the womb may have an Ulcer, or Piles, or the Bladder or Ureters swollen with the Stone or Strangury, and the pains thereof may break the Cups; or if she have a *Tenasmus*, great provocation to stool and can do nothing, she brings forth her birth by straining downward, and that before she should. Also great coughs make the woman feeble and consumptive, and the child consumes within her, great bleeding at the nose, or any great loss of blood, or too great flux of her courses after conception cause miscarriage, if they flow in in the third month, else not. Also opening of

a vein

a vein may cause it if the woman want blood, but such as are sanguine may let blood after the fourth month and before the seventh month, but it is good to see there be cause for it, else not. Violent purging before the fourth month, or after the seventh causes abortment. But gentle purging between the fourth and the seventh month are safe. Violent fluxing, or vomiting make women strain too much, especially lean folks, and may perish the child and break the Cups. If the woman hunger much for want of food, Nature hath nothing to spare to keep the child alive; it is the same thing with Beasts, and Plants, that want nutriment, and too much will choak it. Sharp diseases or Pestilential Feavers, Imposthumes in the breast, Palsies, falling-sicknes kill the child, and sometimes the child is sick in the womb. Also change of weather may cause miscarriage, saith *Hippocrates*, when the winter is hot and moist, and the Spring cold and dry that follows it, the women that conceive in that Spring will easily abort, and if they do not, they will suffer hard labour in child-birth, and the child will be weak and short liv'd; the reason may be because the body is opened and made more tender by the foregoing heat and moist weather, and then the succeeding cold makes it

more

more dangerous. Great labour, as dancing, leaping, falls or bruises, great passions suddenly coming not lookt for, may make a woman miscarry; let all women beware of it for it is more painful than a true delivery, because one is natural and the other against nature, nature helps the one but not the other. Signs of Abortment I have spoken of in part, but commonly about the third and fourth month womens bodies that will swell and puff up with hardness and stiffness, stitches and windiness running about her, yet she feels no more weight in her body, this is a sign of miscarriage if it be not prevented.

There is nothing better after conception, to prevent abortment than good natural food moderately taken, and to use all things with moderation, to avoid violent passions, as care, and anger, joy, fear, or whatsoever may too much stir the blood; use not Phlebotomy without great cause, nor yet violent purgatives.

If the Matrix be too much dilated, use things that contract and fasten, as Baths prepared, Unguents, Ointments, Fumes, Odours, Plaisters. Some remedies are specifical against miscarriage, and if the woman be in danger she may use them, and that in divers ways that she may take them; as thus, take red Coral

ral in powder two drams, shavings of Ivory one dram and a half, Mastick half a dram, and one Nutmeg in powder, give half a dram in a rear egg, &c.

A Powder to hinder Abortion.

Take Bistort-roots one scruple, Kermes berries, Plantane, and Purslain seeds, of each one dram, Coriander prepared two scruples, Sugar all their weight, take every day one scruple with a little Maligo Wine if the body be not costive.

For an Ague.

Sometimes women with Child fall into an Ague, then take Barley meal, juice of Sloes, and of Housleek a sufficient quantity, and with Vinegar make a *Cataplasme*, and lay it upon a double cloth, and lay it often upon the womans belly, and this will preserve the child from it.

For the minds.

Some are much troubled with wind that will cause them to miscarry, then take Cummin seed and boyl it in water, give her four
spoonfuls

spoonful of it twice a week with a dram of *Methridate*.

Against sudden frights.

Take Mastick, Frankincence, of each one dram, Dragons blood, Myrtles, Bolearmoniak, Hermes berries, of each half a scruple, make them into powder and give half a dram at once with White Wine or Chicken broth.

To strengthen the Child in the Womb.

Take two pound of the crumbs of the inward part of white Bread, Cammomile flowers one handful, Mastick two drams, Cloves half a dram; bruise them and mingle them well with some Maligo Wine and two ounces of rose Vinegar, boil them to a Pultise and lay it on a double Cloth to the *Os pubis*.

Purgations may not be used unless the belly be bound, and then a gentle Glister, or some *Manna* or *Cassia* about half an ounce is safe to give by Potion.

Slipperiness of the womb is cured by an injection made of Pomegranate pills boil'd in Oyl of Lillies. Or take Mastick, Myrtle, *Gal-*
lia

Book IV. *The Midwives Book,* 227
lis *moscala* of each half a dram, mix them with Goose-greafe, and Sheeps-Wool, and sew them in a linnen cloth and make a paftry and tye a ftring to it to pull it out again when you have put it up into the place.

To ftrengthen the Matrix.

Take four ounces of the Oyl of Nuts, Barrows-greafe one ounce and half, Cyprefs-nuts, Maftich of each one dram and half, boyl them all about five hours, and with this annoint her belly, womb, and reins of her back.

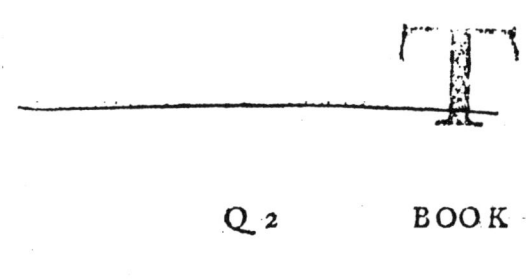

BOOK. V.

CHAP. I.

How women after Child-birth must be governed.

THere is great differences in Womens constitutions and education; you may kill one with that which will preserve the other; tender women that are bred delicately must not be governed after the same manner that hardy Country women must, for one is commonly weak stomach'd, but the other is strong, if you should give the weak woman presently after delivery strong broth, or Eggs, or milk, it will cast her into a Feaver, but the other that is strong will bear it, but tender women must be tenderly fed, and nothing given them that is of hard digestion nor yet

what

what they have no mind to, provided that what she desires be not offensive; but for the first week she lies in, let her have boil'd and not roast, Jellies, and Juice of Veal, or Capon, but no mutton broth for that may make her Feaverish, let her drink barley water, or boyl one dram of Cinnamon in a pint of water, dissolving two ounces of fine Sugar in it, if she will drink wine, mingle twice as much water or two third parts with it, but let it be white wine in the morning, and Claret in the after-noon; she may sometimes drink Almond-milk, but beware of crudities.

Some women when they lie in are still sleeping, some cannot sleep; if she cannot sleep let her drink barley water well boyled not straining it at all, but let her forbear it after the first week, lest it nourish too much, and stop the Liver.

Baths for Child-bed Women.

For the first week let her Womb and Privities be bathed with a decoction of *Chervil*, a good handful boiled in a good quantity of water, adding to it after it is boiled one ounce of Honey of Roses, this will draw away the purgations, and cleanse and heal the parts; and it will take away all inflammations.

For the second week boil Province Roses, put in Bays, Wine, and water, and with this decoction bath her secrets.

Keep her not too hot, for that weakens nature, and dissolves her strength, nor too cold, for cold getting in will cause torments, hurt the Nerves, and make the womb swell. Let her diet be hot; and eat but little at once; some Nurses perswade them to eat apace because they have lost much blood, but they are simple that say so, for the blood voided doth not weaken but unburden nature, for if it had not come away, long diseases, or death would have succeeded; some say Oat-meal Caudles are good for them, but oat-meal makes people troubled with the green sickness by its binding quality, boyling will never make a binding thing to purge ill humours as they say it doth Child-bed Women, but purging things by boyling may sometimes be made to bind.

Let her for three daies keep the room dark, for her eyes are weak and light offends them; let all great noises be forborn, and all unquietness, remembering to be praising *God* for her safe delivery.

First then, so soon as she is laid, give her a draught of white wine burnt, with a dram of *Sperma cety* melted in it.

Viv. is

Vervain is an herb that fortifies the womb, it is fit to gather in *May* and *June*; you may dry it in the *Sun*, and keep it to boil with her meat, and drinks; you shall profit more in two daies with it than in two weeks without it.

If the woman be Feaverish, boil Plantane leaves and roots with it, and if she be not, yet they will do well together, for the heat of the one is tempered by the coldness of the other. But if her purgations stop, for Plantane take Mother of tyme.

If her purgations be clotted, and smell filthily, or the after-burden be not quite come away, boyl Featherfew, Mugwort, Pennyroyal, Mother of time in white wine sweetened with Sugar, let her drink that; new laid eggs and Sugar Penides are best for her to eat often of moderately, and boyl Cinnamon in all her meats and drinks. Let her talk little, nor stir much, especially if she be weak, for six or seven dayes after she is delivered; a decoction of Mallows with a little red Sugar is a good Glister if she be too costive. *Crato* prescribes Coleworts, and *Chrysippus* makes them to be a universal remedy for all diseases, but they are too windy for women in Childbed.

After the first week if she be near clean of her

her purgations, she may use Comfry and knot-grass in broths to close the womb that hath been so much opened, you may use a little purging with them. Therefore put in some Polypody, of the Oak that is best, leaves and roots both being bruised, the quantities are almost at your discretion.

Sometimes pains encrease after delivery, *Hippocrates* saith, women are most subject to them after the birth of their first child; some Physicians think it is by reason of the thinness and sharpness, others from the thickness and sliminess of the blood, but if you use the former directions, these pains may be prevented. What I said of *Vervain* before is a good remedy, or else boil an egg soft, and mingle the yelk with a spoonful of water of Cinnamon and let her drink it; also a fume of the powder of bay-berries cast on a chafing dish of coals received at her secrets, is a great help. And for present ease boyl an equal quantity of tar and barrows grease together; when it boyls put in a little pidgeons dung to it, spread it on a linnen cloth and lay it hot to her reins: she may drink half a dram of Bay-berries in powder in a quarter of a pint of Muskadel; you may see by this that cold and wind cause these pains.

For

For Excoriation of the Privities.

Annoint them with Oyl of sweet Almonds, or Oyl of St. *John's-wort*, which is better.

Against the Piles or Hemorrhoids.

Take Polypody bruised and boyl it with your drinks or meats.

Let her be let blood in the *Saphena* vein.

Cut a great hole in an onion, fill the hole with Oyl, roast it and stamp it and lay it warm to the Fundament.

Also take snails without or with shells, I mean either kind, and bruise them with some Oyl, warm it and lay it to the place; Sows or wood-lice called Hog-lice so bruised with Oyl are as effectual.

The Menstrual blood stopt.

We read *Levit.* 12. that a woman delivered of a Boy, must continue in her purification thirty three dayes, and for a girl sixty six days. *Hippocrates de Natura pueri*, saith, a woman must continue purging her blood forth so long as the child was forming in the womb that is thirty dayes for a Male and forty two dayes for a Female; *Hippocrates* rules may be calculated chiefly for his own Country of *Greece,* and the *Levitical* Law most concerns the feed of *Abraham*; but this is to be observed though not so precisely to a day by all women after delivery, for women that give their own children suck, have their purgations not so long as those that do not. It is not good for a woman presently to suckle her child because those unclean purgations cannot make good milk, the first milk is naught, for even the first Milk of a Cow is salt and brackish and will turn to curds and whey.

You shall know if a woman be well cleansed by her health, for if she be not, she cannot be well and lusty. I shewed you before what herbs will bring her purgations down. She may if she please take every morning two or three spoonfuls of Briony water to be had at the Apothecaries; or a dram of the powder of Gentian roots every morning in a cup of Wine; the roots of Birth-work are as good, or take twelve Peony seeds powdered in a little *Carduus* posset drink to sweat, and if it cures not do it again three hours after.

Against

Against the too great running down of the Menstrualblood.

This disease seldom troubles women after delivery, if it should, Comfrey, and Knotgrass are good remedies; or else take Shepherds-pouch boyled in drink and powdered, or bramble leaves, a dram of either every morning in a little wine, or a decoction made of the same.

Women when they ly in use to be costive because they keep their bed, and some foolish Nurses are so bold as to purge them with *Sena* before nature be setled, whereby many sad accidents have followed, but neither loosning broths, nor Prune broths, nor bak'd Apples are then good, but rather gentle Glisters and suppositories taken twice a week will prevent mischief and make the breasts abound with good milk.

CHAP.

CHAP. II.

Of looseness of the Womb.

THis may proceed from sundry causes, as when great fluxes of humours take the ligaments and relax them; falls or great burdens carried in the womb will unloosen them; or chiefly when women travel before their time, they overstrein themselves because the passage is then shut, but unskilful Midwives often make it so, when they thrust in their hand to pull forth the *Secundine*, they tear part of the womb away with it, for the *Secundine* is fastened to its bottom; sometimes they cause the woman to cast out the *Secundine* by strong vomit, or by holding Bay salt in her mouth. All causes, except those that come from strong defluxions which must first be removed, will be cured by the same remedies.

Take Nuts of *Cypress*, and Galls, and flowers of Pomegranates, and Roch Allum two ounces of each, Province Roses four ounces, Scarlet Grains, Rinds of Pomegranates, and Cassia Rinds of each three ounces, waters of Myrtles, of Sloes, an ounce and half, Smiths water & wine of each 4 ounces and a half, then boil

boil two little bags, each a quarter of a yard long, in the said waters in a new pot, then hold the womans head and Reins low, and apply these bags first one and then the other upon the *os pubis*, and chafe her often. Let her take in the morning a little *Mastick* in an egg or some Plantan seed; but if the disease be long confirmed, then make a Pessary half round and half oval of a thick Cork with a great hole in the middle for her Terms and ill vapours to come out by, tye a pack threed to the end of it to pull it out by, cover it over with white wax that it may not be offensive, dip it in sallet Oyl to make it go in, it must be strait that it may not quickly fall out, when she doth her need let her hold it with her hand, take it not away till her purgations be over; the thickness of the Cork makes the Matrix mount higher; if she be in Child-bed, the Midwife or Nurse must not suffer the woman to strain, but must keep her with her hand or finger to keep back the Matrix, laying her head low and her Reins high with a pillow under her hips.

Women that are troubled with this disease must not lace themselves too strait for that thrusts down the womb, makes the woman got-bellied, makes her carry her Child upon her hips, hinders it from lying as it should in

the

the womb, and though the womans waft may be made flender by it, her belly is as great and ill favoured. But fomtimes there happens a relaxation of the skin that covers the right gut, when the head of the child, when the woman begins to travel, falls downward and draws it low; lacing Childing women too hard is a frequent caufe of it alfo, for this makes fo much wind fly to thofe parts, that fome are deceived and think it is the head of the child, and the women can hardly ftand or go; let her then be kept foluble and eat Annis, & Coriander feed to difpell wind, a fume of Sage, Agrimony, Balm, Motherwort, wormwood, Rue, Marjoram, a little Time, and Cammomile, pick out the ftalks, cut the herbs fmall, mingled, put them into a maple platter, put hot cinders upon them and another handful of herbs upon them, cover the platter clofe with a cloth, and let her take the fume beneath.

The womb falls out of its place when the ligaments by which it is bound to other parts of the body are by any means relaxed; it is bound with four ligaments, two broad membraces and above, that fpring from the *Peritoneum*, and two round hollow nervous productions below; alfo it is tied to the great veffels by veins and Arteries, and to the back

by

by Sinews, but the Bottom of the womb is not tied, the ligaments being onely upon the sides of it; sometimes it falls forward quite out of the Privities, but whether it can ascend and go upward is doubted by some; Physicians say it will if sweet things be held to the nose, if to the secrets it will fall downward; if stinking things be put to them it flyes from them, it may be discerned by their breathing and by some meats the womb greedily accepts. But *Galen* saith, it is very little that the womb can go upward, it cannot reach the stomach the ligaments are so strong that tye it down, and the falling of it down is onely by reason of moisture that relax the ligaments, but that will not make it ascend; and though it be enlarged in conception, that is not presently but by degrees, nor are the ligaments always much relaxed in Childbearing; but what is that if it be not, the womb that may sometimes be felt to move above the womans navel as round as a Ball, that round ball is the womans stones together with that blind Vessel *Fallopius* found out, like to the great end of a Trumpet, and is therefore called *Fallopius* his Trumpet: the stones they hang, and the body of the Trumpet is like a pipe that is loose and moving, and when they are full swoln with vapours and corrupt seed, they stir to and fro,

fro, and come up to the navel ; and *Riolanus* faith, this Trumpet and the stones make this great round Ball. Whafoever fills them with corrupt feed and venemous windy vapours cauſeth this moving, and from thence ſuffocation of the womb ; when theſe poyſonous vapours are freely carried by the Nerves, veins, and arteries to all the principal parts, the Brain, the Heart, the Liver, and the reſt, it is not extream dangerous, yet it may turn to the ſtrangling of the womb if means be not uſed, ſuch as are good againſt ſuffocations of the womb, when they ſeem to be ſtrangled, but of that afterwards. Sometimes it falls as low as the middle of the thighs, and ſometimes near the knees, when the ligaments are looſe, it falls by its own weight, when the Terms are ſtopt, and the Veins and arteries are full that go to the womb ; it is drawn on one ſide, if there be a Mole on one ſide. the Liver veins too full on the right ſide, or the ſpleen on the left, are the cauſe of it. But how it comes to be looſe is queſtioned. *Hppocrates* faith, great heat, or cold of the feet or loyns, violent cauſes external, leaping or dancing may do it, for theſe moiſten and ſoke the ligaments, if the woman take cold after ſhe is delivered and the Terms flow. *Pſaterus* aſcribes it to the looſening of the fibrous neck

from

the adjacent parts by the weight of the Matrix falling down, but then the ligatures must be loose or broken; but when a woman is so in a dropsie, it is the salt water that causeth it and that drieth more than it moisteneth. The signs to know it are, that the womb is only fallen down, if there be a little swelling within or without the privities, like a skin stretched, but if the swelling be like a Goose egg, and a hole at the bottom, there is then a great pain in the *Os sacrum*, the bottom of the belly, the loyns and secrets to which the womb is tied, because the ligaments are relaxed or broken, but the pain will abate soon and the woman can hardly go, sometimes the vessels breaking blood comes forth, the woman falls into Convulsions and a Feaver, and cannot void her excrements by stool nor Urine; at first it may be easily helpt, but hardly afterwards, yet it is not mortal, though it be filthy and troublesome, if it come with a Feaver or convulsion it is mortal in women with child, if the ligaments be corroded the danger is the more. The cure is, thrust it up gently before the air change it or it swell and inflame, first administer a gentle Glister to void the excrements, then lay the woman on her back, her head downwards, her legs abroad and thighs lifted up and with your hand thrust it in gent-

ly, remove the humours with a decoction of Mallows, Marsh-mallows, Cammomileflowers, Bay berries, Linseed, and Fenugreek, and annoint it with Oil of Lillies and Hens-grease; if it be inflamed, stay a while before you put it up; you may fright it in with a hot Iron presented near it as if you would burn it, sprinkle on it the powder of Mastick, Frankincense, and the like; when it is put up, let her ly stretcht out with her legs, and one leg upon the other for eight or ten dayes, and a Pessaty with a Sponge or Cork dipt in astringent wine, with powder of Dragons-blood, Bole, or the ointment called the *Caunlesses* at the Apothecaries; apply a large cupping glass to the Navel or breasts, or both kidneys; use astringent Plaisters to her back, & fomentations, baths, & injections; if evil humors cause it to fall out, purge them first away because they sob the ligaments, and then use drying drinks of *Guaicum, China, Forta*, use Pessaries and ligaments, as for the Rupture to keep it in its place, of which see *Francis Rauseti*; you may use circles or balls in place of Pessaries, made of Betony roots cut round, or of Virgins wax, with white Rosin and Turpentine when they are dried, if it gangrene cut it off, or bind it fast that it may fall off it self. *Rausei* shews when you may ty it or cut
it

it off without danger: her diet must be drying and astringent, and astringent red wine to drink. If it encline to either side, apply Cupping Glasses to the other side, and the Midwife may annoint her finger with the oyl of sweet Almonds, and by degrees draw it to its place.

CHAP. III.

Of Feavers after Child-bearing.

THis disease frequently follows when she is not well purged of her burden or the purgations are corrupt that stay behind, about the third or fourth day they will be Feaverish also by the turning of the blood from the womb to the breasts to make milk, but this lasts not long, nor is it any danger: but you may mistake a putrid Feaver for a Feaver that comes from the milk; for the humours may be inflamed from her labour in travel, and corrupt, though they appear not presently to be so, the next day after she is delivered, but from thence you must reckon the beginning of the Feaver; it is probable then that this Feaver comes from some other cause, especially if her purggings be stopt, it may proceed from ill humours gathered in her body whilst she went with child, and are only stirred by her labour, if she be not well purged after travel, the blood and ill humours retreat to the Liver by the great veins and cause a putrid Feaver, but if they flow too much the Feaver may come long after. A feaver from milk will come on the fourth day with pains in the shoulders and the back, and the terms may flow well; if she kept an ill diet when she was big with child, the Feaver comes from ill humours if it come not from milk, if it do it will end about eight or ten dayes after; but if it come from stoppage of purgations, if she have not a loosness it is very dangerous; if black and ill savouring matter purge by the womb it is safe. But if the Feaver come from ill humours and the body be Cacochymical it is worse, for that shews the ill humours are many, which nature cannot send forth by the after-purgings, and the woman is weak already by her travel. Good diet and gentle sweating cure a Milk-Feaver, but there must be purging and many remedies used for the other, as bleeding in the foot, cupping of the thighs to provoke the after-purgations; but if the time of after-purging be over, if she be strong then open a vein in the Arm.

If

It is dangerous to purge the woman after the seventh day as some do, when she hath a Pleurisie, because of her weakness after travel, and because purges hinder the after-flux; but you may if the flux of blood cease, if need be, give a gentle purge with *Cassia* or *Manna*, sirrup of roses or *Sena* or *Rhubarb*. Too cold and sharp things are naught; take heed of cold drink, or too much drink; let her diet by degrees increase from thin to thicker.

If the Feaver came from too much milk or terms stopt, open a vein in her foot, then purge away the gross humours with sirrup of Maidenhair, Endive of each one ounce, waters of Succory and Fennel an ounce and half a piece.

Sharp and putrified humours must be purged away with proper medicaments, as water of Succory, and violets, of each two ounces, sirrup of the same of each one ounce; cooling Glisters are good here; if there be need you may purge stronger, but this is not usual. I shall give you one example; take two drams of *Rhubarb* in powder, *Diagridium* four grains, let them infuse all night in Succory and Annifeed water, two ounces and half of each, and one ounce of Borrage flower water, warm them gently in the morning, and strain them well through a linnen cloth add to the strained liquor one ounce of sirrup of Succory, Cinnamon water two spoonfuls, drink it warm.

Then after you have well purged away the ill humours you may gently sweat her to open the passages of the body and womb, you will find examples of them in the Treatise of the Courses stopt.

CHAP. IV.

Of the looseness of the belly in child-bed Women.

THis may be thought a small matter in respect of other infirmities, yet this is one of the most dangerous distempers and hardest to help in child-bed women, for stop the flux & you will stop her purgations; if you stop it not she will perish by weakness, nothing almost is safely given. Physicians are at a stand in such a case, but it is good be wary and moderate in what is done, and it may be helpt God willing. It is not safe to stop it presently, and if it continue it may cause a *Tenesmus* or a *dysentery*, if it come from ill diet let her

mend

mend that, and strengthen her stomach outwardly if yet it continue, use inward remedies that corroborate the stomach yet hurt not the womb, as Barley water, Honey and sirrup of roses, cleansing Glisters are good and to temper sharp cholerick humours. But the best way is, to observe what loosenes of the belly she is molested with, for if it be that they call *Diarrhœa*, that will only discharge her body of ill humours, therefore do nothing in that case but let her take strengthening food, for when nature hath eased her self sufficiently she will stay both the looseness of the belly and her purgations from the womb, and so no ill accidents will come; but if the flux be *Lienteria* that the food comes away with the stools undigested, annoint her belly with Oil of Mastick and of Myrtles, and give her some sirrup of dried Roses, *pulp* of *Tamarinds*, or some torrified *Rhubarb*, to purge the belly and not hurt the womb: But if it rise to a *Dysentery* called the bloody flux, then so soon as her Terms are purged away, try to stay it.

1. By purging, as take half a dram of bark of yellow *Mirobolani*, & of rosted *Rubarb* as much, finely powdered, sirup of Roses, or of Quinces one ounce, *pulp* of *Cassia* or of *Tamarinds* with Sugar half an ounce, Plantane or Oak-

en water four ounces, let her drink this at once.

2. *Abstersives* are good, as of whey, or barley water, or Glisters of Mallows, Mellilot, Wheat-bran and Oyl of sweet Almonds.

3. *Narcoticks* to ease great pains, *Philnium Romanum* two scruples, Rose-water two ounces, *Maligo* wine one ounce, give it when she goes to sleep, this is excellent.

In this case astringents are to be used but not in the former distempers, here they profit, there they are dangerous.

Of Womens vomiting in Child-Bed.

Women both before they fall in labour, and at the time of their travel, and also afterwards will sometimes fall to vomiting, and it may proceed from ill diet or raw humors, or from weakness of their stomach, or consent of the womb when the after flux is stopt, and sometimes they will vomit blood, for the blood that is stopped below, runs back to the great veins and liver, and being much and sharp finds a way into the stomach, and so comes forth at the mouth. It is ill after childbirth, especially the food being vomited there will be nothing to make milk for the child, and sometimes in hard labour a Vein is broken

broken and this may cause a dropsie; if ill diet cause vomit, rectifie that; if ill humours, stop it not presently but purge gently; it blood come, pull back by rubbing, or cupping, or bleeding, opening a Vein in the foot, harm, or ankle, and urging the after flux. Sometimes the woman is costive, then give her a *suppository*, with Castle sope or Honey, and then stay four or five days till you may give a Glister with *Manna* or *Cassia*. If her Urine run away against her will, bath her parts with a decoction of Betony, Bays, Sage, Rosemary, *Origanum*, *Stœchas*, and Penni-royal; for her vomiting give her three spoonfuls of Cinnamon water, one ounce and half of juice of Quinces, about a spoonful at a time. The leaves of Rosemary dried and brought into powder, and so drank about a scruple or half a dram at a time in a cup of wine will stay vomiting; preserve or Marmalade of Quinces, or Medlars eaten, or Pears or sowr Apples do strengthen the stomach, juice of Barberries, or of Pomegranates or sowr Cherries with Mint water.

There are many topical applications to be made to the pit of the stomach, which being laid on and so continued prevail much, as thus; take the crum of the inside of a white loaf, and tost it and steep it in good *Maligo* Wine, and

and strew it lightly over with the powder of Cloves and Nutmegs, or sirrup of Roses, *Rhubarb,* or *pulp* of *Tamarinds,* and astringents, of Roses, Plantane, Coral, Tormentil, if the Terms flow not at all the belly must be kept loose, but vomiting is so perillous that it ought to be stopt, alwaies provided it be done no sooner than it is needful aud with good provisoes.

CHAP. V.

Of Womens diseases in general.

WHosoever rightly considers it will presently find, that the Female sex are subject to more diseases by odds than the Male kind are, and therefore it is reason that great care should be had for the cure of that sex that is the weaker and most subject to infirmities in some respects above the other.

The Female sex then that it may be more nearly provided for wheresoever it is deficient must be considered under three several considerations, that is, as maids, as wives, as widows, and their several distempers that befall them almost commonly respect either the womb

womb or their breasts or both, and many of these diseases and distempers are common to all the Female sex, I mean they sometimes happen to them in any of the foresaid three estates of life, but Virgins, or Maids diseases that are more peculiar to them, though not essential, because many of them are incident to the rest, the causes may be the same; they are that wich is called the white Feaver, or green Sickness, fits of the Mother, strangling of the Womb, Rage of the Matrix, extreme Melancholly, Falling-sickness, Hedd-ach, beating of the arteries in the back and sides, great palpitations of the heart, Hypochondriacal diseases from the Spleen, stoppings of the Liver, and ill affections of the stomach by consent from the womb. But that I may make as perfect an enumeration as may be of all diseases incident to our sex, & give you some of the best remedies that are prescribed by the most Authentick authors, or what I my self have proved by long experience.

Know then that there are some diseases that happen about the secrets of women, as when the mouth of the Matrix is too narrow, or too great, when there is a Yard in the womb like a mans Yard, when the secrets are full of Pimples or very rugged, when there are swellings or small excrescenses in the

the Womb, or else Warts in the neck of it, or the Piles or Chaps, Ulcers, or Fistulaes, or Cancers, or Gangreens, and Sphacelus, or Mortification: all these and more that may be reduced to these heads, are found in the entrance or mouth of the womb.

2. As to the womb it self, it is frequently offended with ill distempers, being either too hot, or too cold, too dry, or too moist, and of these are many more compounded, as too hot and too dry, too moist and too cold; these are all to be cured by their contraries, cold by heat, moist by driers.

Or the womb is sometimes ill shaped and strange things are found in it, some women have two wombs, and some again have none at all. Again the vessels of the womb sometimes will open preternaturally, and blood run forth in abundance, sometimes the womb swells and grows bigger than it should be: It may be troubled with a Dropsie, with swelling of its veins from too much blood, also it may be inflamed, displaced, broken, and it may fall out of the body.

It may be rotten, or else cancerated, and sometimes womens stones and vessels for generation are diseased.

Further the womb may be troubled with an itch, it may be weak or painful, or suffer by sympathy

sympathy and antipathy from sweet or stinking smells.

Moreover the terms sometimes flow too soon, sometimes too late, they are too many or too few, or are quite stopt that they flow not at all. Sometimes they fall by drops, and again sometimes they overflow; sometimes they cause pain, sometimes they are of a evil colour and not according to nature; sometimes they are voided not by the womb but some other way; sometimes strange things are sent forth by the womb; and sometimes they are troubled with flux of seed or the whites.

As for women with child they are subject to miscarry, to hard labour, to disorderly births of their children; sometimes the child is dead in the womb; sometimes alive, but must be taken forth by cutting or the woman cannot be delivered; sometimes she is troubled with false conceptions, with ill formations of the child, with superfetations, another child begot before she is delivered of her first; with monsters or Moles, and many more such like infirmities.

And as for women in child-bed, sometimes the *Secundine* or after-birth will not follow, their purgations are too few or too many, they are in great pains in their belly, their privities are rended by hard delivelivery as far as their Fundament, also they are inflamed many times and ulcerated and cannot go to stool but their fundament will fall forth. They have swoonding and epileptick fits, watching and dotings; their whole body swels, especially their belly, legs and feet: they are subject to hot sharp Feavers and acute diseases, to vomiting and costiveness, to fluxes, to incontinence of Urine, that they cannot hold their water.

As for their breasts that hold the greatest consent with the womb of all the parts of the body, they are sometimes exceeding great or swelled with milk, or increased in number, more breasts than there should be by nature; sometimes the breasts are inflamed and trouble with an *Erisipelas*, or hard swellings, or *Scirrhus*, or full of kernels, or tumors called the Kings evil, or strange things may be bred in the breasts; besides this some breasts are diseased with Ulcers, and Fustulaes or Cankers, and some have no nipples, or are chopt or Ulcerated, and sometimes women have breasts will breed no milk to suckle the child with.

To speak then particularly to all these diseases that belong to our sex might be thought to be over tedious; however I shall so handle the matter, that I may not troubled the Reader

der with impertinences, that I shall apply my self to what is most needful for the knowledge and cure of them all; but because many diseases may be refered to the chief in that kind, and the remedies that will cure one may be sufficient to cure the rest, the judicious Reader may, according as he shall have occasion, make a more special application.

For it is in vain for any one to make use of what is written if they have no Judgement in the things they use, in such cases it will be best for them to ask counsel of others first, till they may attain to some farther insight themselves, and then no doubt but when they shall meet with sufficient remedies to cure the greatest distempers, they will be able to make use of the same without farther direction in the cure of those diseases that are lesse; not that I intend to omit any thing that is material in the whole, but that I may not trouble the Reader with needless repetitions of the same things, as too many authours doe, which breeds tediousness, and can give little or no satisfaction at all.

CHAP.

CHAP. VI.

Of the Green-sickness, some call it Leucophlegmatia, *or* Cachexia, *an ill habit or white Feaver.*

Though both wives and widows are sometimes troubled with this disease, yet it is more common to maids of ripe years when they are in love and desirous to keep company with a man.

It comes from obstruction of the vessels of the womb, when the humours corrupt the whole mass of blood and over cool it, running back into the great veins. For so soon as Maids are ripe, their courses begin to flow, Nature sending the menstrual blood from the Liver to the veins about the womb, but those veins and vessels being very narrow, and not yet open, if the blood be stopt, in that it cannot break forth, it will corrupt, and runs back again by the passages of the hollow vein and great Artery, to the Liver, the heart and the Midriff, and stops the whole body, which may be easily known, for their faces will look green and pale, and wan; they have trembling of the heart, pains of the head, short breathing

breathing, the arteries in the back, the neck, and the Temples will beat very thick; and though not alwayes, yet sometimes they will fall into a Feaver by reason of these corrupt humours, but it is alwayes almost attended with disgust and loathing of good nutriment, and longing after hurtful things.

The whole Body especially the Belly, legs, and thighs swelling with abundance of naughty humours, the Hypocondriacal parts are extended by reason of the menstrual blood runing back to the greater vessels, and they are much given to vomit; but all these signs are not found in all persons alike; but they are common to most, and in some you shall find all these meet. The cause is the Terms stopt, and from thence ill humours abound, for when the natural channel is stopt, the blood must needs return to the great vessels whence it came and choak them up, and so spoil the making of blood, nothing but raw and corrupt humors are bred which can never turn to good nutriment, or be ever perfectly joyned to the parts of the body; the blood is flegmatick slimy stuff, and sometimes it is bred from corrupt meats and drink that maids will long after as well as Childing women; they will be alwayes eating Oatmeal, scrapings of the wall, earth, or ashes, or

S   chalky

chalk, and will drink Vinegar; they are strangly affected with an inordinate desire to eat what is not fit for food, whereupon their natural heat is choaked, and their blood turns to water, their body grows loose and spongy, and they grow lazy, and idle, and will hardly stir; their pulse beats little and faint, as the vapours fly to several parts so they are ill affected by them; the heart faints, the head is dried and pained, and the animal actions are hurt when melancholy is mixed with the humours in too great proportion.

Sometimes this white Feaver turns to a Dropsie, or the liver grows hard like a stone that it can make no blood; some fall dead suddenly when the heart is choaked by ill vapours and humours flying to it; if the stomach be affected the danger is the greater, but if onely the womb be out of frame the remedy is much more easy.

The best time of the year to cure Maids and those that are sick of the green sickness is the spring, and the way of cure is, to heat the cold humours, and make the thick gross blood thin, and this cannot be all performed by one work, to draw away and to correct the whole mass of humours at once; wherefore you must purge gently and often, mingling things that heat and attenuate, as well

as

as purgatives to carry the ill humours forth.

But first it will be good to give a Glister, and next to open a Vein in the foot or ancle.

Moreover your physick must vary according to the parts of the body that are most stopt, and where the humors float.

If they lye above the stomach and mesentery, then vomit, if you find the Person fitted for vomit; likewise the Spleen, or liver, or womb must be respected in their several kinds with Physick accordingly; and to save you the labour of much reading, and me of writing too often of the same thing, under several heads, you may find what is to be done almost in all respects, where I write of the stopping of the Terms, and by this rule I wish the Reader to apply the rest when he stands in need, which he can never well do, as I said, till he have some judgement in it, and then it will become familiar to him.

But in this Disease principally for the cure respect the Liver, the Spleen, and the Mesentery, or Midriff, for these are certainly obstructed and must be opened; and above all be sure to keep a sparing diet and of a thin substance.

Secondly, Let blood in the arm first, though the courses be stopt, and after that in the foot.

If the disease be of long standing, you shall do well to give a gentle Purge.

First of all to purge the humours; as

Take powdered Rhubarb two drams, Chicory and Anniseed-water three ounces apiece; Infuse the Rhubarb all night, then let them boyl one walm onely, and then strain it forth, and in the strained liquor, dissolve sirrup of Damask Roses one ounce and a half, *Diacassia* half an ounce, Cinnamon-water half an ounce, five grains of *Diagridium*, let her drink it in the morning.

Next after this use opening decoction of Succory and Madder, and Liquorish roots of each half an handful, Anniseeds and Fennel seeds two drams apiece, a handful of Harts-tongue Leaves, Borrage Flowers and pale Roses of each half a handful, one ounce of the roots of Sassafras, stoned Raisins one ounce and a half, and half a dram of Cinnamon.

Boyl all these in Fountain water to a third part onely wasted, and then sweeten it with sirrup of Lemmons, she may drink it when she pleaseth.

An Electuary made of the rob or pulp of Elder-berries boyl'd to a just substance four ounces with one ounce of bay berries dried and powdered, two Nutmegs, and one dram of burnt-hartshorn, half a scruple of Amber, and four scruples of *species Diarrhoda*, mingled all with sirrup of Succory one ounce and half, is excellent.

And finally, it will not be from the purpose, but very useful, to anoint the womb and Liver with such Oyntments, as will open their obstructions, made with Oyl of Spike, and bitter Almonds, of each two ounces; and juyces of Rue and Mugwort half as much, and Vinegar a fourth part; waste the watery part of these by boiling: then add Spikenard, Camels Hay, Roots of Asarum, of each one dram; Cypress half a dram, Wax, sufficient to make an Unguent.

To provoke the Termes.

And that is effected with one ounce of the Five opening Roots, and with Madder, Elecampane, Orris Roots, Eryngo, dried Citron Pills, and *Sarsa*, of each half an ounce; Germander, Mugwort, Agrimony, of each a handful; two small handfuls of Savin, an ounce of wilde Saffron seeds, two ounces of Senna; Agarick and Mechoachan, of each half an ounce; two Pugils of Stœchas Flowers;

of Galingal, Annifeeds, and Fennel, of each two drams: Boil all this to a Pint and half, sweeten it for your Pallat, and add to it a spoonful of Cinnamon water.

Quercetans Pills of *Tartar*, and *Gum Ammoniacum* are commended; Take of each half a dram, Spike a scruple, three drops of Cinnamon, Extract of wormwood half a scruple; take a scruple, or twenty grain weight in pills an hour before Meat: Conserve of Marigold Flowers is very good. Some, after good preparatives, use Steel powder to much effect; giving first a vomit, if need require. This Medicament is good for all stoppings; but, if the Liver be stopt, let the Steel be finely powdered. Take prepared steel two ounces, Agarick, Species Diacrocuma, and Darrhodon of each a dram; two drams of Carthamus seed; Cloves one dram, Carrot seed, and red Dock Roots of each one dram and a half.

If the woman vomit, stop it not: but I approve not so well of steel taken in substance, as by infusion; I am sure it must needs be the safest way. Take steel (in powder) three ounces; three pints of white wine, and half an ounce of Cinnamon, let all stand in the sun eight dayes, stopt close in a Glass; and every day stir them well: the Dose is six or eight ounces for twenty daies together, four hours before dinner.

Steel is best used in the Spring and in the Fall: but alwaies you must purge the body, and exercise both before and after the use of it; and you must change the form of your Medicaments, or the Patient will loath, and grow weary of it: Sweating and bathing are good. Either Baths (by Nature, or Art) made with Mugwort, Calamints, Nifs, Danewort, Rosemary, Sage, Bays, Elecampane, Mercury, Briony Roots, Ivy: When the Obstructions are opened, and the body purged, you shall see all the former symptomes flie away: But let the diet be meats of good digestion, and good nourishment; The air must be temperately hot; all crude raw things must be avoided: as green fruit, Lettice, Milk, watry Fish: Wine is good drink: Sage and Cinnamon are good Sawce: put Fennel seed into your bread, and let it be well leavened: Sleep moderately: Marriage is a Soveraign Cure for those that cannot abstain. Maids must not be suffered to eat Oatmeal, or ashes, or such ill trumpery, though they desire them never so much; for they will breed and increase the disease: but Child-bearing women, if they cannot be perswaded, must have what they long for, or they will miscarry cairy. Exercise, I say, is alwayes good to keep maids from this disease, and to cure it when it is come: For idleness causeth crudities; but motion makes heat, and helps to distribute the Nutriment through the body; Yet moderation must be used; for it will weaken faint people if it be too much.

First, therefore onely rub and chafe the body, then by degrees, keep them from sleeping too much; then increasing the labour, after that the body hath been well cleansed by purging.

Hippocrates commends marriage, as the chiefest remedy for Virgins sick of this disease, if they once conceive; that is their cure: or as saith *Johannes Langius*, for this disease never comes till they are fit for Copulation, and then commonly it hasteneth; and it is cured by opening of Obstructions, and heating the womb; which nothing can so soon, and well perform, as the Venereal acts, to make the courses come down; but yet it is very dangerous, when these people are grown weak with this disease, and their bodies are full of corrupt humours; therefore they must purge them away before they marry: for I have known some that have been so far from being cured, that they died by it; perhaps sooner than they would have done otherwise: It may

may be good sometimes, when the disease is new, and the blood plentiful, to open a vein, when the courses are stopt; and are not changed into some corrupt humour, you may then bleed freely; this was the right judgment of *Hippocrates:* but when the passages are stopt, and the whole body is chilled with raw slimy humours, there is no time to bleed then; for that wil augment the disease.

And because we are now upon this remedy of marriage, for the cure of this infirmity; though I touch'd it before, I shall a little further discusse the matter: Whether all maids have that sign of their Maiden-head, which by *Moses*'s Law (*Deut.*22..) was so much to be taken notice of, and *Physicians* call *Hymen*, which signifies a *Membrane*, some do absolutely deny, that there is any such *Membrane*, or skin; and maintain also, that if any maid have it, it is only the closeness of the womb, a disease in the Organ, and not common to all: And some of the best *Anatomists* maintain the contrary; affirming that there is a *skin* in all, or should be, that is wrinkled with Caruncles, like Myrtle-berries, or a rose half blown: and this makes the difference between maids and wives: but it is broken at the first encounter with man, and it makes a great alteration; it is painful, and bleeds when it is broken: but what it is, is not certainly known. Some think it is a nervous *Membrane* interwoven with small veins, that bleed, at the first opening of the Matrix by copulation: Some think they are four Caruncles fastened together with small *Membranes*: Some observe a Circle that is fleshy about the Nimphe, with little dark veins; so that the *skin* is rather fleshy than nervous. Doubtless there is a main difference between Virgins and Wives, as to this very thing, though *Anatomists* agree not about it; because, though all have it, yet there may be causes whereby it may be broken before marriage, as I instanced formerly: and sometimes it is broken by the Midwives.

Leo Africanus writes that the *African* custome was, whilest the wedding dinner was preparing, to shut the married Pair into a room by themselves; and there was some old woman appointed to stand at the Door to take the bloody sheet from the Bridegroom, to shew it to the Guests; and if no blood appeared, the Bride was sent home to her friends with disgrace, and the Guests dismissed without their dinner. But the sign of bleeding perhaps is not so generally sure; it is not so much n maids that are elderly, as when they are very young; bleeding is an undoubted ed token of Virginity: But young wenches (that are lascivious) may lose this, by unchast actions, though they never knew man; which is not much inferior, if not worse than the act it self.

Amongst those signs of Maidenhead preserved, is the straightness of the privy passage; which differs according to several ages, Habit of body, and such like circumstances: But it can be no infallible sign, because unchast women will (by astringent medicaments) so contract the parts, that they will seem to be maids again; as she did, who being married, used a bath of *Comfrey* roots.

Some judge (but falsely) that if a maid have milk in her breasts, she hath lost her Maidenhead: There can be no milk, say they, till she hath conceived with child. Maids want both the cause, and the end, for which nature sends milk; namely to provide food for the child to be born: If a maids courses stop, they corrupt, and turn not to milk. The Breasts have a natural quality to make milk; but they do it not, unless convenient matter be sent to make it of; and that is not done, but for the foresaid end.

Hippocrates, Galen, & there followers say, that maids may have milk in their brests: True it is, that it is a certain sign of a living child in
the

the womb, when there is milk in the Breasts; and of a mole or false conception, when there is no milk: But that milk that maids sometimes have in their breasts, is only a watry humour, when their courses are stopt, and cannot get forth of the womb; then the Breasts by their faculty make whey, but cannot make milk, without there be first carnal copulation: it is white as milk is, but not so white, nor so thick: neither comes it to the breasts by the same veins that that blood that makes Milk comes into them by; for this breeds in the veins of maids from the superfluous nutriment of their breasts. But to enlarge a little more concerning that distinction of *Maids* from *Wives*, by the straitness of the *Orifice* of the womb: There are three diseases in this part of the secrets; either the mouth is too strait, or too wide, or sometimes there hangs forth the Yard of a woman. The Privity is too strait when there is not room for the Fore-man to enter; Such persons seldom child, and are delivered with great danger and difficulty: and if this come from ill conformation, that nature hath made them so, it will be hard to cure them by any thing but copulation, and bringing forth of Children, to enlarge the place: yet sometimes this straitness comes from the use of astringent Medicaments

caments, when whores defire to appear to be maids; fometimes the paffage is fo clofe fhut up on the outfide, that nothing can come forth but water and the courfes, and sometimes neither of them; becaufe they are attracted not bored nor pierced by nature. This difeafe is threefold; it is either in the mouth, neck, or middle body of the womb; it is never good for copulation, conception, or for the courfes to be voided by: I remember I faw a woman that had the Orifice of the matrix fo little, that nothing but the Urine and her courfes could pafs through; yet fhe conceived with child, no man can fuppofe how fhe received the mans feed, but by attraction of the Matrix: the midwives (when fhe was to be delivered) difcovered the difficulty; and a Chirurgeon made the Orifice wider, and fhe was by that means happily brought a bed of a Son: The cleft may be alfo clofe ftopt, by reafon of fome wound or Ulcer cured in that part. I faw a woman which by the French difeafe, had been much eaten off, yet when it was healed, it grew clofe together, that there was no paffage left, but for her Urine to come forth by: either proud flefh, in foul difeafes, or elfe fome membrane, by evil conformation may ftop the paffage: if it be in the mouth of the fecrets, it is vifible, but if in the neck it

lieth

lieth concealed; Unless it be when the courses are flowing, or Copulation is used, it is not painful: and maids are supposed to be with child; for the belly tumifies, and the body is discoloured. The Terms cannot well come forth of the neck, or the Veins of the womb, if there be an Ulcer or inflammation, you may know almost whence it came; but if a membrane stop it, the place is white: if the flesh be red, and you touch it, the touch will discover it; for a membrane is harder than the Flesh: the hazards are great for childing women.

CHAP. VII.

Of the Straitness of the womb.

Sometimes there are superfluous Excrescences, that fill up the Privites, and are like a tail: I spoke something before of a *Clitoris*; but these are not that: for a *Clitoris*, if it be rubbed, increases pleasure in copulation; but these fleshy excrescences are painful to be touched, and hinder copulation: you may safely cut them off, if you can come at them, because they are redundant.

There are a kind of wings in a womans secrets, much like to the comb of a cock for colour and shape; it swells like a Yard sometimes (in lust it is full of spirits) and is hard and Nervous at the top of it; sometimes it is no less than the Yard of a man, and some women by it have been suspected to be men; it proceeds from much nutriment, and frequent handling of the part that is loose. To cure it you must first discuss, and dry it with easie astringents; then you may go on to Causticks, that are not dangerous; as burnt Allum, or Egyptiac: if these cure it not, then you may at last cut it off; or tie it with a horse hair, or piece of Silk, till it fall off; but cut it not at first for fear of pain and inflammation: The way to cut it off is taught by *Ætius*, to cut it neatly between both the wings, causing as little pain as possible may be; and after that, foment the place with an astringent Decoction of wine with Pomegranate Flowers, Cypress nuts, Bay Berries, Roses and Myrtles.

Some call this disease *Tentigo*, when the *Clitoris* grows bigger by odds than it should be; it is a nervous piece of flesh, which is lapt in by the lips of the Privitie, and it riseth in the act of Copulation; it hangs below the Privy parts, outwardly, like a *Gooses Neck*

Neck in bigness; and it comes from a great Flux of humours to the part, being loose, and often handled: The way to cure it, is to purge superfluous humours forth, and to draw blood, and use a spare diet, and very cooling, and to discuss with the leaves of Mastich tree, or of the Olive: You may take away the excrescence by Sope, being boiled with Roman Vitriol; and last of all, add a little Opium, make some Troches, and sprinkle the powder upon the superfluous part; and after that cut it off, or cure it by ligature as I said before.

There is another fleshy substance, that sometimes fills up the privy parts, coming from the mouth of the womb, and hangs oftentimes out, like a Tail; it may be easier taken away than the former, by the same means of cutting or binding with a thread, or silk dipt in sublimate water.

There are many other *infirmities* that stop up the secrets of the womb, of which I shall briefly speak; but the straitness of the neck of the womb it self is not so usual, as too much wideness is; you may know when it is too strait, by the stopping of the Courses, and a weighty pain bearing down: It proceeds partly from ill conformation by nature, and partly from Diseases; sometimes it is so shut up

outwardly

outwardly, that neither the courses can come forth, nor the mans Yard enter in; that it is not possible for her to be with child: if the straitness be in the inward Orifice, the courses run back again for want of passage, and hinder conception. It may happen when the caule lieth to that, and presseth upon the neck of the womb; the stone in the bladder, or swelling in the straight Gut, may cause it also; if the parts cling together naturally, either soft red flesh, or a white hard skin causes this straitness as I said: But the straitness of the womb it self, and its vessels are sometimes natural by ill conformation; and such women will miscarry in the fourth or fifth month, because the womb that naturally stretcheth, as the child grows in bigness, & will after the woman is delivered, shrink as small as it was before, in some women will not be extended. But if the straitness be in the vessels or neck of the womb, Conception is hindered, because the terms cannot flow; gross humours, especially when the womb is cold and weak, stop the mouths of the veins and arteries.

Inflammations, or Swellings, or Scars, or Schirrhus, or the like, may be the causes; sometimes thick Flegm abounds, if there were a wound or the after-burden were forcibly pulled out.

T   If

If the terms be stopt, from an old obstruction of grown humors, the cure is hard; a Schirrhus, or humour that shuts up the vessels, cannot be cured; what is to be cured, must first be done by general evacuations of purging and bleeding; then use means to provoke the terms: if the straitness come from diseases, first cure them.

Sometimes the Secrets of women are full of pushes, and scurf, with itching and pain, wheals rising in the neck of the womb: They are of two sorts; some are gentle, but most commonly they are venemous, and come from the foul disease, and will impart it unto men: They proceed from burnt, sharp, cholerick, malignant humours, hard to be cured; Sirrup of Fumitory is very good in such cases: it is also profitable to wash the parts with wine and Salt-Peter.

Draw blood, if it abound, first in the arm then in the ancle: but first if it be the disease, drink the decoction of *Sarsa* and *Guaicum* for it: Avoid sharp sowr meats; it is good to purge with *Confectio Hamech*, or *Fumitory* Pills. You may see the cause of this great itching, and scurf, if you search with *Speculum Matricis*, an instrument Chirurgeons use. Sometimes Tubercles grow in the neck of the womb, with heat and pain; you may see them

them them, for they are a kind of swelling wrinkles, like the wrinkles you see when you close your Fist, but they are much larger; and when they swell they make these Tubercles: they are usual in the secrets, or Fundament, and come from the same malignant causes with the former; and some are more enflamed, and painful, than others are: The swellings are hard, proceeding from thick burnt humours; Powder of egg-shels burnt is good to strew upon them to dry them up, if they be new, and there be no inflammation; but if they be old and dry, they must first be softened. These wrinkled skins, when they are many, resemble a bunch of Grapes: Cure the Pox first, for usually that is the cause, and then they will vanish of themselves.

If Medicaments prevail not, some old authors bid us to use an actual Cautery, and to burn them away. Likewise Warts in the secrets are bred by a gross dreggy ill humour, and is of kind with the forementioned; Nature sends it forth to the outward skin, and there it becomes Warts: if they be hard or blew, and painful, you may know what they are, the Pox is in them, and hard to be got out, and they lie where medicines can scarce be applied to them to remain: if you apply sharp Topicals, use a defensative of

Bole and Vinegar, that you hurt not the parts; and so you may touch them with *Aqua fortis*, or *Spirit* of Vitriol, or of Brimstone. There are several sorts of these *Excrescences*; there are those that are called *Myrmeciæ*, leave an Ulcer; if you cut them off *Thymi*, & *Clavi* will grow again, but *Acrocordanes* leave no root, if they be once cut away.

The powder of *Mulberries* is good to cure Warts and swellings upon the privities of men; and I recommend it to women in the same cases: Sometimes women have the piles of the womb, like those in the Fundament; they proceed from gross blood, that staies about the ends of these veins, in the neck of the womb. Women that are thus troubled, look pale, and are very faint and weary: this may come from too long flowing of the courses, and grow thick, and cannot get forth; they are painful, and bleed disorderly; you may see them, by the help of *Speculum Matricis*, and touch them: The cure is by revulsion of the humour, by letting blood in the arm or heel; and by gentle applications if the pains be great: if nature open them and they bleed moderately, you may give way to nature; but if they run violently, open a vein in the arm two or three times: Purge with Rhubarb, Tamarinds, and Mirobolans

bolans mingled: and ufe Topicals to ftay the blood. The blind Piles bleed not at all: they are cured by letting young women bleed freely; and by foftening the parts with emollient Fomentations, to open the veins, and to difpel the humour, made with mallows, Marſhmallows, Cammomile, Melilot, Malius, Linſeed, Fenugreek: Anoint where the pain is, with butter, *Populeon* and *Opium*; if the pain be gone, and they bleed not, ufe Driers, of Bole, Cerufs, Allum, burnt Lead, waſh'd; if the veins fwell with blood rub them with Fig leaves, or with Horfe Leeches applied draw blood from them.

This difeafe of the Piles of the womb differs from the flowing of the courfes, becaufe this is with great pain; and moreover the courfes run from the veins of the womb, and the neck of it; but the Piles are caufed when the blood runs too much to the veins that force the fecrets; and either ſtops there, or comes forth fometimes by them: but fome fay they differ from the courfes, namely, by their great pain; but that they make the body lean, if they laſt long, and the blood comes not forth fo orderly, nor at certain periods, and fet times, as the courfes ufe to do: Sometimes the womb hath Ulcers bred there, fome are cleaner, and fome again are fordid

T 3 and

and malignant, all hard to be cured. They proceed generally from a virulent Gonorrhœa, or the Pox; but they may rise from inflammation, by abundance of sharp corroding humors, from abortion, or hard labour, or sharp medicines, or when the after-birth is pulled out by force, and rends the womb.

The pain of Ulcers is biting, and increased by sharp injections of Wine or Honey and Water: All Ulcers are hard to heal there, because of the sensibility, and moistness of the part: and a light Excoriation, or rawness, will not easily be healed; but eating Ulcers never are cured there almost but by Death. Ulcers by Venery, if they be cured, you must first cure the Pox.

All Ulcers in the secrets of Wombs may be cured, if they be not Cankered: and the way to cure them is by Purging and bleeding, to cleanse and carry away, and divert the ill Humours and moisture from the Womb: if there be great pain, abait that with Mucilage of Fleabane, and whites of Eggs; or, an Emulsion of Poppey Seeds. Warm Injections into the Womb will help forward the Cure, made of Barley, Lentils, Beanes, Lupines, of each one Ounce; and two drams of *Orris* Roots; and of Horehound, Wormwood, and a little Centry, of each half a handful, boil all in

Whey

Whey, strain it, and put some Honey of Roses, or Hydromel to it. Turpentine washed and with Liquorish swallowed is good: Drink Sheeps milk sweetened with Sugar. Fumes made with Frankincence, Myrrh, Mastich, *Storax Calamita*, Juniper Gum, received by a Tunnel do good; if there be a jealousie of the Pox, add a little Cinnabar; but Pessaries with Opium must not be held in above half an hour, for it will hurt the Nervous part of the womb: a scruple of the Pills of *Bdelium*, taken thrice a week, may be profitable. Vulnerary Potions drunk, and astringent powders cast upon the Ulcers must not be neglected.

Sometimes there are long Ulcers in the neck of the womb, like to those that eat the skin, and are seen upon some mens hands and feet in Winter; sometimes they are bleeding, and sometimes very dry, and have hard lips; much labour and sharp humours to the parts may cause them: when they are new they are easier cured; use a good moistening diet: if sharp humours cause them, purge them forth; and anoint the Ulcers with Oil of Linseed and Roses, mingle them in a Leaden Mortar with juice of Plantane, and the Yolk of an egg; when they are hard anoint them with deers Marrow, Turpentine, wax, and oil of Lillies

Lillies; when they are malignant they are cured, as Fistulaes are; if they itch, or cause pain, make an unguent of *Populeum* and *Diapompholix*, of either one ounce; Camphire & Sugar of Lead of each a scruple: when there is a great itching of the womb it is somewhat like the rage of it, then eat Sallets of cooling herbs, Purslain and Lettice, with a few Spearmints & oil and vinegar, or take conserve of Mints, and of Water-Lilly-Flowers, of each an ounce, Lettice candied six drams, *Agnus Castus* seeds one dram and a half, Coral one dram, Rue seeds half a dram, Camphire a scruple, with sirrup of Purslain, make an Electuary; annoint the Reins and secrets with *Galen*'s cold ointment, with a little Camphire.

As for the womb, it is soon ulcerated, because the parts are soft, and easily corroded, and hard to be healed: and these ulcers are of many kinds; hollow, crooked or strait; if the sharp humors be retained, it makes furrows and divides the parts; which growing hard with a callous cannot join again; thus it degenerates into a Fistula; it may be without pain, with hard Lips, and an ill matter may be pressed forth of it: sometimes it corrodes the bladder, and then the water passeth forth by the Fistula, and sometimes to the Fundament, and the Dung is voided by it:

An old Fistula is harder to cure than a new; and a crooked than a streight. General remedies and a good Diet may do much; and so leave the rest to nature to evacuate the excrements: but use a palliative cure by often Sweating, and purging twice a year; and by Injections and Corroboratives, laying on a Plaister of *Diapalma*: After general meanes, if it be not past hopes, Vulnerary Decoctions may help, made with Centaury, Bettony, Agrimony, Ladies mantle, and roots of male Fern. Topicks are useful, first dilating the Orifice with Gentian Roots, or with a Sponge; then make soft the Callous with Turpentine, wax, Deers Marrow, and Oyl of Lillies; then consume the Callous, which may be effected: For a new narrow Fistula use Black Hellebore, Egyptiac, or Vigo's powder, carried to it with a Pencil, or *Aqua Falopii*; or take Rose, and Plantane water, of each six ounces; put to it Sublimate half a scruple, set it on the Embers in a Glass; but if the Fistula be toward the womb, beware of violent means: if it be foul, and a hard Callous withall, a Potential Caustick may do good, but a Horrion is best; all these are safe in the outward part of the Neck of the womb, but in the inward there is greater danger.

A Cancer in the womb is seldome seen, nor can

can it be ever cured: but that which is in the Neck of the womb I shall instance in; which is either with an Ulcer, or without an Ulcer.

First, It comes without an Ulcer; but when long Applications are used to them, hard schirrhus Tumours, which spring from burnt black humours, and Terms, that flow to those parts, chang to an Ulcerated Cancer.

Secondly, It may be in the part not Ulcerated a long time, and not be known, because it is without pain; but at length there will be a pain felt in the Loins, and bottom of the belly: the swelling looks blew, and loathsome; when it becomes Ulcerated it is worse, and a thin black stinking matter comes from it. If much blood flow from it, that is dangerous; there will be a soft Feaver, red cheeks and loathing, by reason of the vapours that rise from it: Mild Remedies are not felt, and strong meanes make it worse; it growes harder daily: keep it from being Ulcerated, and you may live long with it. Prepare and Purge Melancholly, from whence it proceeds: Use no sharp biting applications at first, but onely Diapompholyx, or juice of nightshade, Plantane, or Purslane. Give every day three or four Grains of a Powder made of Oriental Bezoar

Bezoar stone, Saphyrs and Emeralds, of each one dram, in waters of Scabius, or Carduus; take also juice of Nightshade six ounces, burnt Lead washt, and Tutty, of each two drams, Camphire half a dram, put Cray-fish powder to them, and stir them well in a leaden Mortar.

An Injection made with a Decoction of Cray-fish is held to be very good; and, make a Cataplasm, and a Fomentation with milk, Saffron, water Lillies, Mallowes, Marshmallowes, Coriander, Dill, and Fleabane seed. Arsenick and Antimony may be good in some remote parts, but are dangerous here.

There was a Noble woman who had a Cancer Ulcerated upon her Face, and sought for help from all Countries; at last a Barber cut a Chicken in the midst, and often applyed that, and it drew forth the Ulciome, and the Lady was cured.

The womb is very soon corrupted by the many ill humours that flow thither, and it will quickly Gangreen, and the parts mortifie, the natural heat being extinguished; by reason of some preceding Ulcer, the neck of the womb will feel an unusual heat, and a Feaver runs through the body; the part is discoloured, and neither beats nor feels any thing;

thing; prick it, or cut it, it ſtinks: The Party that hath it faints and decayes; wherefore ſtrengthen the heart with cordials, and the principal parts, leaſt the Spirits be infected; cut off the dead fleſh: ſtop the corruption by ſcrarifying it, if you can come at it, then waſh the part with a decoction of wormwood, and Lupines, and Egyptiac; apply Epithems to the heart; it is worſe when it goes to the womb, than when it comes outward. Some have had their womb fall out and yet recovered as to life; wch was before endangered.

The Neck of the womb is onely ſubject to Ulcers: yet ſometimes the ſubſtance of the womb hath been Ulcerated, and rotted away. A dead child in the womb may cauſe an Ulcer; but all theſe Ulcers and Rottenneſs are to be dealt withal as I have ſhewed before: Sometimes there may be a Rupture of the womb; I never ſaw but one, and that was exceeding rare, it happens ſo ſeldome.

The womb is ſo fenced by the adjacent parts, that it is ſeldom wounded, unleſs the Chirurgeon chance to do it, in cutting the *Child* forth of the womb. There is more pain in the neck of the womb, than in the bottom of it: but this cutting may be cured by Injections and Gliſters for the womb, made with Decoctions of round Birthwort, Cypreſs

Nuts

Nuts, boiled in Steel water, and Astringent Wine, and a little Honyed water, and Agrimony, Mugwort, Plantane, Roses, Camels Hay, Horehound; If the pain be great use Anodynes, or Pessaries, made with a wax candle dipt in Vulnerary Oyntments ; as, take Turpentine, Goose Grease, wax and Butter, of each a dram ; Bulls Grease, Deers Marrow, Honey, Oyl of Roses, of each two drams.

I have refer'd all the foresaid Diseases to a natural, or Accidental straitness of the mouth, or neck, or Middle of the womb ; all of them being a hinderance to Copulation, and making compression upon the parts.

CHAP. VIII.

Of the Largeness of the womb

THe opposite to straitness of the womb is the largeness of the Orifice; and sometimes more Cuts than nature makes; which may proceed from Copulation, or bearing of Children.

By the largeness of the Orifice women are often barren, and sometimes the womb falls
out,

out, as *Hippocrates* saith : Nor do men desire to keep company with such women.

The cure after Child-birth is with Astringent Fomentations, and Bathes of Allum water; binding things of Bole, Dragons blood, Comfrey Roots, Pomegranat Flowers, Mastick, Allum, Galls, of each half a dram; powder all, and make a Pessary to thrust into the Orifice, dipt in this Mixture, made fit with steel'd water.

Hard Labour doth sometimes cleave the Privy parts as low as the Fundament ; whereby the rent is made so wide, that it goeth from one to the other hole; a long piece of Allum (put into the cleft) may do good to help it : but if there be many passages in the secret parts, it comes from an error in nature, there being a passage open from the womb to the straight gut.

There are some diseases whereby Physicians are much deceived, thinking the cause to lye in the womb when it doth not; for womens stones, and Vessels of procreation, may be sorely distempered, and their womb be no wayes affected with it.

Gasper Bauhin, and *John Scenkius*, tell us of a Maid whose belly was swoln, as though she had been with child ; but when she died, she desired to be opened, to let the World know

know her innocency, and it did so appear; for her stones were swelled as big as a white penny Loafe, they were blew, and spungy, and full of water.

 The womb is sometimes subject to great paines, besides what proceed from the former Diseases, for there is that which is called the Cholick of the womb; it is usual to women with child, as the Inflammation of the womb is, it binds the belly and stops the veins; all women are subject to it, either from sharp humours, or from clotted blood, that sticks to the hollow of the womb; Drinking of cold drink may cause it: sometimes it comes from retention, and corruption of the seed, that is cured as fits of the Mother; If it come from ill humours that lye there, purge them forth; if from windy vapours, that rise from the heat of ill humours, these must be discussed; give a Glister of Maligo wine, and Nut oyl, of each three ounces, Aquavitæ one ounce, oyl of Juniper and Rue distiled, of each two drams, apply it warm: lay on a plaister to the Navel, of *Tacamahac*, and Gum *Caranna*,

CHAP. IX.

Of the Termes.

THe Monthly courses of women are called *Termes*; in Latin *Menstrua*: *quasi Monstrua*, for it is a Monstrous thing, that no creature but a women hath them; or else *Menstrua* because they should flow every Moneth: and they are named Flowers because Fruit follows; and so would theirs if they came down orderly: they are then a sign that such people are capable of Children; it preserves health to have them naturally, but if they be stopt there must be danger; when the woman is conceived, then they stop: they begin commonly at fourteen years old, and stop at fifty, or in some at sixty years old; they are of no ill quality naturally, but are onely superfluous moisture and blood the Female sex abounds withal; for when they stop, the Child in the womb is supplied by them. The Termes run longer two or three dayes with some women than with others, for they differ as women do, according to plenty, or less plenty of good diet, and labour, or idleness, or the like,

Hippocrates saith, They should bleed in all
but

but two pints at most, or a pint and a half; the colour of the blood and substance differs, according to divers tempers; it should not be too thick nor too thin, without any ill scent, and of a red or reddish colour: and the veins of the womb are the passages, which are double from the Spermatick and Hypogastrick double branch on both sides, to send forth superfluous menstrual blood from all parts of the body; some say this blood is venomous, and will poison plants it falls upon, discolour a fair looking glass by the breath of her that hath her courses, and comes but near to breath upon the Glass; that Ivory will be obscured by it: It hath strong qualities indeed, when it is mixed with ill humours. But were the blood venomous it self, it could not remain a full month in the womans body, and not hurt her; nor yet the Infant, after conception, for then it flows not forth, but serves for the childs nutriment.

We read of a child but five years old, that had her monthly purgations: and *John Fernelius* writes, of one that was but eight years old that had them; but certainly it must be a sign of a lascivious disposition, and of a short life.

Some womens courses stop not only by conception, but from other causes, that have

V come-

come again very well seven or eight months after; but if the terms fail, there is either want of blood, or the blood is stopt: but some refer the causes of stopping the courses to four heads. *viz.*

    1. Corruption of the blood.
    2. The Womb ill disposed.
    3. An ill habit of the body.
    4. An ill Custome of the faculties of the Body.

    1. If the Womb be diseased, as it is subject to many, the Terms will increase or diminish, wherefore the womb must be first healed.

    2. If the blood be corrupt, it will be too thick, or too thin, by reason of ill humours and ill diet.

    3. If the body be ill disposed, it sends not blood as it should do: some laborious Country Women become so hot and dry like Men, that they have hardly any courses at all; as the *Indian* women have none: but they are barren, if they abound with no more blood than will nourish their body: Blood is wanting either because it is not made, or not dispersed where it should, but turned to other uses: Old age, cold constitutions, diseased bodies, will not make blood; also often bleeding of
the

the great vessels, and much loss of blood, or from Issues to make diversions, the womb is not supplied with it. Nature spends the blood in Nurses that give suck for an other end; and fat women wear it on their backs: sadness and fear not only wast, but cool and corrupt the blood.

4. The weakness of the woman hinders the courses; and so long as she continues weak, she will have none.

But all these things must be judged of by the relation of the party, whether the whole body be diseased, or the defect be in the womb or vessels, or the mouth of the womb turned aside: If the cause be from heat that her courses are stopt, her Pulses are swift and strong, she is very thirsty, and her head aketh, and such like signs of heat: If from cold, the woman is drowsie and sleepy, her Pulse beats slow, and she is not thirsty, the Veins are ill coloured; if the woman be fat or lean that will discover the inward cause of it.

The usual cause of obstruction of the courses is thick slimy humours; or from thick gross melancholly blood, proceeding from a cold distemper of the Spleen and Liver, by drinking cold Water, or eating gross Food.

The *Roman* women drank snow water, and that was the reason (said *Galen*) that they had few or no courses; but in such cases they could not be very fruitful: It will seem strange, that some women are so hot of constitution, that they have conceived, yet never had their courses at all.

Courses stopt in maids, are not the same as they are in women, for the effects are very different; Maids, they presently fall into the Green sickness by it, the blood going to and fro all the body over, and is corrupted: but in women, it runs to the womb commonly, and causes them to vomit, and to loath their meat, or to desire unnatural things: You shall know a woman with child, when her courses are stopt, from a maid that hath hers stopt; for the one looks wan and pale, the other lively and well: the one is sad, the other merry: the womans pains daily decrease, and the others increase. This obstruction causeth not only barrenness, but strange distempers, Suffocations, Swellings, Imposthumes, Coffing, Dropsies, difficulty of breathings, urine supprest, Costiveness, Heaviness, Megrims, Vertigoes, Head ach, and many more fearful distempers.

Hippocrates tells us, that when the terms are long stopt, the Womb is diseased, with humours

mours, imposthumes, ulcers, barrenness, Leucophlegmacy, vomiting of blood, heart-ach and head-ach, if the symptomes be great there is danger of death.

The best way to move the courses in weak women is to forbear Physick, and to feed them high with nourishing meats and drinks; this is where the Woman is lean; her Liver weak, and blood is wanting; but if blood abound, then give a gentle purge, or Glister: then open a vein to draw down the blood to the womb; open a vein in the foot, or ancle, one day, one leg, and another day the other, four or five daies before the time the courses should come down; use Frictions and binding of the parts below; but Issues, and opening of the Emrods do hurt, and draw from the womb: you may first loosen the belly with *Hiera Picra*, or Pills *de tribus*. For Phlegmatick bodies use the Decoction of *Guaicum*, or *Sarsa* and *Sassafras*; and *Dittany* fifteen drops, without sweating: purge with Agarick, Mechoachan, Turbith, and Scamony; or drink wine of their infusions: if the stomach be foul, give a vomit, lest it get into the Reins.

Things that provoke the terms are hot and thin: take Sirrup of Mugwort, and of the Fierwort of each one ounce and a half; Oximel simple, one ounce; Water of Motherwort and Mugwort, of each two ounces; Pennyroyal and Nip, of each one ounce, sweeten it with a spoonful or two of Cinnamon water, make a Julip to drink of thrice. Pessaries are not fit for maids, but Fumes may be used; if she be no maid bruise Mercury, with Centaury Flowers put in a bag for a pessary; begin with the mildest remedies: If it be from a Humour provoke not the Terms, but cure the swelling. Some say that the blood going to other parts cause the Terms to stop; but that is contrary, for the blood goes to other parts because the Terms are stopt.

Authors agree not what veins must be opened to move the Terms; *Galen* thinks the Ancle Vein, and most men conclude the same because it opens obstructions, and brings down the blood; open the ancle twice or thrice rather than the arm once: but in other diseases of the womb it is best to open a vein in the arm; as when the Terms a re too many, or drop, or the womb is inflamed.

The *Saphena* is opened by putting the foot into warm water, few terms flowing, if the blood be but little there is no harm: Diseases grow when they are stopt by thick blood, as the Cancer, Schirrhus, and Erisipelas, when the time is near, then use the stronger
remedies

remedies, the weaker having made a way for them. Tender natures (as maids) must have but gentle remedies; as Aloes one dram and a half, Agarick and Rhubarb of each one dram; Myrrh, Gum *Ammoniack* dissolved in Vinegar, Gentian Root, Asarum, of each half a dram; Cinnamon, Mastich, Spikenard, of each one scruple; five grains of Saffron, make a mass of the fine powder, with sirrup of Mugwort, the Dose is one dram.

To urge the terms in strong Country people, take pills *Aurea* and *Aggregativa*, of each two drams; pill *Foetid* and *Hiera*, of each four scruples, at the *Apothecaries*, *Diagrid* one scruple, *Trochischi Alhandal* half a scruple, with a hot pestle mix them well in a Mortar; adding sirrup of Damask Roses, one dram, oil of Anniseed olympical half a scruple; dissolve Gum *Dragant* in Cinnamon water and make your pills, and let the woman take two scruples every morning, before the time of their terms, at least three or four drops.

Ointments and Plaisters are good also, and pessaries made of Aromatical things, and sweet smells, and Fumes; as take *Benzoin*, *Storax Calamita*, *Bdellium*, *Myrrh*, what you please; mingle them, and strew some on a pan of Coles; the woman so placed, that she may receive the Fume by a Tunnel, broad at the lower

lower end, to keep the smoke in: but left these Fumes cause the head-ach, keep the Fumes down with clothes about the woman, that they come not to her head. But do none of these things to women with child, for that will be Murder: give your remedy a little before the Full Moon, or between the New and the full, for then blood increaseth: but never in the Wane of the Moon, for it doth no good: Sometimes, but seldome the courses stop with Fulness; such must, saith *Riolanus*, be let blood in the arm, but with great care.

CAHP. X.

Of the overflowing of the Courses, or immoderate flux thereof.

THis distemper is contrary to the former, and Women are often subject to it; and it brings many diseases, great weakness, loss of appetite, ill digestion, dropsies, consumptions, pains in the back and stomach: Their ordinary continuance should be two or three daies, or four or five daies in large People;

but

Book V. *The Midwives Book.* 297

but if they stay longer it is not good; or if they come oftener than once a month, I mean the Moons Month, passing through the twelve *Signs*, that is twenty seven daies and odd minutes.

The causes may be falls, or blows, or strains, or hard labour, over-heating the body, which makes the blood thin; or from weakness of the retentive faculty, and too much strength of the expulsive faculty; or from crude raw blood and weakness, or too much moisture: and this is the cause that some women have their terms by drops, and it lasts long, and there is pain, and the secrets are alwaies wet; if this be not remedied it may cause Ulcers and inflammations: if the blood be superfluous open the arm, not the ancle vein; if it be Cacochymical correct it; if too thin and sharp, correct and amend it, by coolers and thickeners; and strengthen the wombs retentive faculty by astringents, and convenient driers.

Many think that the overflowing of the Terms and Issues in women are the same diseases; but that is not so (as *Galen* shews) for by superfluous Flux of the courses only blood is voided, but in too great a measure: But womens continual Issues send forth not only blood, at certain periods, but various hu-

humours, that cause the disease.

The Terms exceed when they flow in too great abundance in a short time or continue longer than is needful ; the one resembles violent rain, the other flow rain, but lasts long. If too much blood be the cause of this superfluity, the blood will be whitish and pale ; if choller, the terms will be yellow : if melancholly, they will be dark coloured, black or blew: it weakeneth all the body, and the Liver and Bowels ; dip a clout in the blood, and dry it in the shade, and then the colour of the blood will shew the humour that offendeth, and accordingly prepare your remedies. Sometimes it causeth swounding, paleness, the whites or the dropsie : If fulness be the cause, abate blood, opening the Liver vein of the right arm; repel, cool, bind, bleed little, but often use cuppings to the back and breast against the Liver, below the paps, to draw the blood back; but scarifie not under the breasts : upon the Salvatella, bind and rub the arms and shoulders. Waters of *Plantane*, *Purslain*, *Shepherds Purse*, *Sorrel*, sirrup of *Pomegranates* or dried *Roses*, will cool and thicken the blood; and so will *Bole* or *Sealed Earth*, sirrup of *Poppeys*, *Philonium*, *Laudanum* are good. If it proceed from choller, purge with sirrup of Roses, of Rhubarb, or with Senna, or Manna na: if watry blood be the cause, the Reins and Liver are out of temper, sweat with China, and strengthen those parts.

Do not force veins, but use astringents; take the juice of ass dung, sirrup of Myrtles, of each half an ounce, with an ounce of *Plantane* water, let the woman drink it and not know what she takes, lest it offend her; or give every day a dram of the powder of Mulberry tree roots. When you use cold astringents temper them so, that you stop not the Veins; use no *Pessaries*, except the Veins of the neck of the womb be open. Cold and binding fomentations are better than baths, for baths make the humours to flow more: wash the legs and hips in cold water. If choller persist, Rhubarb powder in conserve of Roses is very good. The principal causes of this overflowing are but four; viz.

1. Some of the Vessels broken, or much dilated.
2. Violent *Purgation*.
3. Corroding humours.
4. Hard travel in Childbed, or the *Midwives* unkind handling.

First, if the Vessels be broken, the blood gusheth forth in heaps; if flowing of humors they

they come with much pain, though the quantity be small.

Secondly, All *Physicians* almost wish to stop the Courses first that are too many, before you strengthen the woman ; But I think it more reasonable to strengthen nature first, and nature will help her self with less means; but strengthen the womb, and annoint the reins and back with oils of roses, Myrtles, Quinces; do this every night. lay a piece of white bays then next your reins, upon the bare skin, and keep it there constantly; inject the juice of Plantane into the Matrix, it seldome fails: You may drink of the decoctions of Sage, Bistort, Tormentil, Knotgrass, Sannicle, Ladies-mantle, Golden Rod, Loosestrife, Meadow Sweet, Archangel, Solomons Seal, Purslane, Shepherds Purse, red Beets, Bark, and Cups of Oak and Acorns: But I commend this medicine; take of Comfry leaves or roots, of either a handful, and of Clowns all-heal the same, bruise them and boil them well in Ale, drink a good draught when you please, and it will help you, though the mouths of the Vessels be open. Too much blood is lost in the overflowing of the courses when the faculty is hurt by it, otherwise the quantity cannot be defined. The immediate causes are the opening of the Vessels; but the

mediate

mediate cause is the blood offending in quantity or quality: Vessels are opened three or four wayes by *Anastomosis*, when the mouthes lye open, by reason of a moist distemper, or use of Aloes or hot and moist bathes; or from *Diapdesis*, when the blood sweats through the Coats, this is not often; or from *Diaresis*, when the sharpness of the blood eates the Vessels in sunder; if a Vein be broken, Coral, Bole, Myrtles, Comfrey, are good to bind; or a Poultis with astringent powders, and the White of an Egg.

Thirdly, If a vessel be Corroded, a dram of the roots of Dropwort in a new Egg will glutinate: Sleep long, use little Exercise, nor Venery; but eat little: if it come from Plethory, use thin Nutriment, beware of hot things, alwayes purge the humour that offends; vomits are good to stay, and turn the course of the humours: Take Conserve of Roses two ounces, of water Lillies one ounce, prepared Pearls and burnt Harts-horn, of each half an ounce, Bole Armoniac, and *Terra Lemnia*, of each half a scruple, make an Electuary with sirrup of Plantane, this is cooling, thickning and binding: or, in case of great necessity take a Bolus made with old conserve of Roses, half an ounce, *Philonium*, or *Requies Nicolai* two scruples, or but a scruple

ple of each; let them drink Red Wine, or quench steel in their drink, or boil Plantane Seeds, Leaves and Roots in their drink.

CHAP. XI.

Of the whites, or Womens Disease, from corruption of humors.

WHen the body grows Cacochymical, womens Courses stop, or run very slowly, and sometimes they abound; sometimes all humours run thither to a general vent, and the whole body is purged by it: but the womb is not affected, it is a filthy disorderly Evacuation, either before or after Terms, or when they are wholly stopt, the colour of the matter is blew, or green, or reddish, few maids have this Disease, women with child may: it is not the running of the Reins, for that is in less quantity, whiter and thicker; nor from nightly Pollutions, which come onely in sleep: The cause is some excrementitious humor, sometimes like watry blood; a cold and moist womb breeds this Disease: or, when ill humors are gathered in the whole body, or Liver, Spleen or stomach, they are sometimes thus voided; nature, that useth to send forth good blood by the Veins, casts forth these ill humours by them; they are of divers colours, and stink: If it be from a Phlegmatick humor, the Ligaments of womb grow loose, and the womb falls out in time; they make thick veins, and they are discoloured in their Faces, short breathed: if the humor be not bred in the womb, it comes from a Cacochymy of the whole body; if it comes from the whole, it is more in quantity; if onely from the womb it is but little: Many have had this Disease long, and found no great hurt, but if it be not timely looked to, it will do mischief; causing Consumptions, Faintings, and Convulsions, when the matter is sent to the nerves and brain: You must not stop it suddenly, for so it will find a way to the nobler parts. Bleeding is naught in this case: general Evacuations, are good; and after particulars, according to the part diseased: The whites, and over-flowing of the Terms, I say, are a disease; and although it resemble the Gonorrhæa, it is not the same; it is also like the matter that flows from an Ulcer of the womb, but it is not that neither.

The running of the Reins in Men & women

is not the same disease with this; the running of the Reins is peculiar to unchast women: but b this flux of whites may proceed from too much cold, or too much heat, and hath many differences, as will appear by the colour of the matter sent forth; the colour shews the peccant humor; it is necessary for the cure to search whether it be a Gonorrhæa or involuntary flux of seed; which both women and Men are subject to, and the remedies are the same, as the causes are in both. Women commonly call the whites the running of the Reins; but the running of the Reins comes most commonly by unlawful Venery, or excess in that Act: but the proper cause of the whites is too much superfluity of Excrement; but where those Excrements are bred, is doubted: Some say these corrupt humours are daily bred in the principal parts; others say they come onely from the womb, and seed Vessels; others say from the Reins onely, and the womb is unaffected: But *Galen* plainly shews that the whole body is affected, that dischargeth it self by the womb, and therefore weak and flegmatick women are most subject to have the whites.

To cure it, first observe a strict Diet; cleanse the whole body by purging, letting blood, Sweating, and Diureticks; in very moist

moist bodies, prepare the humours three or four dayes before purging; or take *Cassia* new drawn one ounce, powder of Rhubarb one dram, with sirrup of water Lillies or Violets, take it in the morning, dissolve it if you please in Posset drink, and about two hours after take some broth: You may take every day a dram of *Trochisci de Carabe* in Plantane water; or give every second or third day a dram of the filings of Ivory in Plantane water, a very laudable remedy. To sweat also is very laudable in this case; take Barley water three ounces, strong wine two ounces, drink it warm, and lie and sweat. Conserve of Roses and *Marmalade* are excellent for this disease: drink the decoction of Comfrey Roots, with Sugar to sweeten it, take three or four ounces at a draught. Whites of eggs well beaten with red Rose water, and made with Cotton, or Linnen into a Pessary, and put into the *Matrix*, with a string tied to it to pull it out again, is commended.

Diureticks are not good till the body be well purged, and then they will help to drive the ill humour forth by Urine: Lest the womb be hurt with ill humours, inject a decoction of Barley, Honey of Roses, and Whey with sirrup of dried Roses. Take red Saunders two drams and a half, yellow Saunders one dram

X and

and a halfe, red Roses three drams, fine Bole a quarter of an ounce, burnt Ivory one dram, Camphire half a dram, white wax one ounce, oil of Roses three ounces, make an ointment: This is not only good to anoint the secrets, but also to cool the inflammation of the kidneys, stomach, liver and other parts.

If the Whites flow from abundance of superfluous humours, you may evacuate much through the skin, by often rubbing of the body; but first rub easily, and by degrees rub harder.

Of these fluxes there are three sorts, White, Red and Yellow; and there are three kinds of Archangel, or dead nettles to cure them.

First, The White Flowers helps the Whites.

Secondly, The Red are to cure the Reds.

Thirdly, And the Yellow flux is cured by the Yellow.

Half a dram of Myrrh taken every morning is commended, or a scruple of the Pills of Amber at night, often taken; they will not work till the day following.

Many strange things are oftentimes voided by the Womb, as Stones and Gravel: And *Peter Diversas* relates, that a *Nun* voided a rugged Stone as large as a Ducks Egg, and
it

it gave her some ease ; but there followed a foule flux of the Womb that killed her.

Garcias Lopius saw a Woman that voided many Ascarides, or small Worms, by the Womb.

When stinking humors are cast forth this way it is not properly the Running of the reins, for both sexes have sometimes the running of the reins; and most commonly it comes from a foul course, whereas the whites come from a corruption of humours: if it run white, and little, and thick, it is a true flux of seed; if it last, and be not cured, it brings a wasting of body and barrenness: if this flux grow from fulness of Seed, the buds of willow stept in wine will cure it : if it proceed from a weak retention, give half a scruple of Castor, and use astringents to the reins and belly; or a bath of willow leaves, Myrtles, Quinces, each two handfuls ; red Roses, Rosemary each a handful, Cypress Nuts three ounces; let her sit up to the Navel, apply bags of the same to the Loins and Privities, and anoint the said parts with oil of Mastich and Myrtles.

CHAP.

CHAP. XII.

Of the Swelling and Puffing up of the Body, especially the Belly and the Feet of Women after Delivery.

THe Swellings of these parts in Childbed women come either from a depraved diet, used whilest they were with child, or else drinking immoderately after delivery; or it may be they abound with more blood than the child could retain, or her purgations discharge; wherefore it grows crude, being superfluous, and makes the parts swell so much that a man would think she were with child again: but it commonly ceaseth if the woman be once largely purged, either by the womb or the belly. Hysterical, or Mother fomentations are sufficient oftentimes to cure it; or take a Sheeps-skin of a Sheep new killed, and wet it with sharp Wine, and lay it on.

If in travel they keep ill diet, the humours turn to Wind, and they fall down to the legs, and make them swell: take heed of drink, and when the purgations are over, use things that expel wind: take wormwood, Betony, Southernwood, Origanum, Cammomile
Flowers

Flowers, Calamint, Annis-seed, Rue, Carroway seeds, boil them, and make a fomentation for the feet.

If too much drinking be the cause, let her abstain from that; Medicaments that heat and resolve, and are good for Dropsies, are very good in this distemper: the infusion of Rhubarb is much commended, especially if the humour proceed from ill habit and course of life. *Hippocrates* prescribes a Goats or Sheeps Liver made into powder and taken with wine of the infusion of Elecampane; also Treacle taken with Fumitory and Fennel waters: and to abate the swelling of the Feet, make a decoction of Rose stalks and Cammomile Flowers, excellent to bath them in: and for her belly swelled, lay on a Plaister of Bay berries, or of Melilot; or take Bay berries and Juniper berries, of each one handful, Goats Dung four ounces, Cammomile Flowers powdered half a handful, Cummin seed two drams, pour spirit of wine upon them as you bruise them in a Mortar, make a Plaister with a little oil of Spike added, and lay it over the womans belly.

For the swellings of the Bellies of maids, if it come not by a masculine blow, take Dittany root, and Cubebs, bruise them, and Cummin seeds, and Cow Dung, and lay it to their bellies

bellies as hot as can be endured. Women after Delivery, are also subject to have their Wombs inflamed, when the birth is very great, and their labour hard, and the mouth of their Womb narrow, so that great violence stretcheth it wider than they can suffer; and sometimes there is great loss of blood, and the womb is torn by putting forth of the child; it must be cured by such things as ease pains, as Baths and Fomentations, and such softening things as are proper for the belly: This following Anodyne is very effectual; take Flowers of Mallows, Marshmallows, Vervain, and Rue of each a handful, Self heal, Agrimony, Cammomile Flowers, Melilot tops, red Roses, of each a handful; cut them very small, sew them up in fine linnen bags, boil them in Goats milk, or equal parts of Plantane water and Wine, press them well between two Trenchers, and make application of one after the other hot to the place affected; but first anoint the part with Poplar ointments, or with oil of Roses: after this cleanse all the secret parts with a spunge dipt in water of Oaken Leaves, Self Heal, and of Plantane made luke warm, and injections put up with a Syring, are effectual also; of Mel Passium, and Plantane water mingled, and cast in warm; or take Galls, Lentils, Flowers of Pomegranates, Seeds of Kneeholm, Saunders and Roses, of each a like quantity; boil all in water, and strain it, and with a Syring inject the decoction, and it will cleanse the Womb. When the Mother is cleansed it will be proper to make the flesh incarnate, if it be corroded; as take Centaury six ounces, Orris, Comfrey Roots, Agrimony, of each three handfuls, Gum Tragant, Sarcocolla, Dragons Blood, Frankincence, Hypocistis, Mummy, of each a dram, boil all in a sufficient quantity of water to the consumption of half; then put to it Iron refuse prepared one ounce and a quarter, boil it a while longer, and bath the part with it.

If the womb be too hard, and she feel pain between the Navel and the Matrix, then take Ducks grease, Deers, or Ox marrow, Neats Foot oil, Yolks of eggs, Bdellium, of each a like proportion; two drams of Saffron, dissolve all in wine, and mix oil of Lillies with them, and dip a tent of Linnen or Cotten in this, and thrust it up into the place; use this often, for this will ease it and take away the pain.

And if the womb be foul with Ulcers, or the like, take half an ounce of Oxymel of Squils, sirrup of Vinegar and Bizantine of each three quarters of an ounce, Agrimony and

Lovage Waters of each one ounce, water of Cichory two ounces, let her drink this every morning early, and sleep upon it; and fast four hour after it; the Urine will in a weeks time, or somewhat longer, become clean, and well cleansed, and the party cured.

Womens bellies use to be mightily stretched in Child-bearing, in so much that they will be plaighted, and full of wrinkles ever after, that were plain and smooth before, growing lank when they are delivered; but if it be but four months past it may be helped by laying a linnen cloth over the belly dipt in oils of sweet Almonds, Lillies, Jessamine; and if the belly be already wrinkled, then take Goats and Sheeps Suet, and oil of sweet Almonds, of each one ounce, *Sperma Ceti* two drams, and with a little wax make an ointment: when the Flux is past you may lay on the Cataplasie of *Ætius*, or anoint with oils of Mastich and of Roses.

CHAP.

CHAP. XIII.

Of Cold, Moist, Hot, Dry, and of all the several Distempers of the Womb.

THe wombs of Women should be alwaies kept temperate, that they exceed not in any preternatural quality; if they do, the mans Seed will be like corn sowed upon sand, and will prove unfruitful, if the womb be too hot, or cold, or moist, or dry.

Those that have hot wombs have but few courses, and those are either yellow, or black, or burnt, and fiery, that come disorderly; and such persons will fall into Hypochondriacal Melancholly, and rage of the womb; if this be from their birth, it will be hard to cure: yet it may, by good Diet, and proper means be much mended by Medicaments, that cool and asswage Choler; but take heed you do not cool too fast, and stop the courses: you may safely use conserve of Succory, Violets, Water Lillies, Borage, of each one Ounce, Conserve of Roses half an ounce, *Diamargariton Frigidum*, and *Diatrion Santalon*, of each half a dram, with sirrup of Lemmons or Oranges, or juice of Citrons; take a Nutmeg in quantity at once, twice or thrice in a day: and anoint the back and loins with

Poplar Unguent, or oyl of water Lillies, Roses, *Venus* Navel wort. Let her wear thin cloaths and use the cold Air; let her avoid hot and salt meats, Wine, and strong drink; eat Lettice, and Endive, and cooling herbs, that she may sleep well.

The contrary to this is a cold womb; and these are not fruitful, they are too cold to nourish the seed of Man: it is from the birth in some, but in others by accident; from cold Air, cold Diet and Medicaments, or from too much idleness: the signs are quite contrary to the former, for the other are extreme desirous of Venery; and, these abhor it, and take no pleasure in it: they have few or no hairs about their Secrets; and their seed is watry and Slimy, their wombs are windy, and they are subject to Gonorrhæas, and the Whites. The Cure is long, and hard to be done; but, they must use such things as warm the womb, with drinking good wine, and sometimes Cordial Waters, and good warm nourishing Meats, and of easie digestion; with Annifeed, Fennel feed, and Time: And Fumigations are good, of Myrrh, Frankincence, Mastick, Bay berries, of each a dram; *Libdanum* two drams, Storax and Cloves of each a dram, Gum *Arabick* and wine, make Troches; put one or two upon a Pan of coles, and

and let her receive the Fume at the Matrix.

   Then take Labdanum two ounces, Frankincence, Mastick, Liquid Storax, of each half an ounce; oyl of Cloves and of Nutmegs of each half a scruple, oyl of Lillies and Rue of each one ounce, Wax sufficient, make a Plaister, and lay it over the Region of the womb. But if the womb be moist (and this is commonly joyned with a cold distemper) it drowns the seed, like as if a Man should sow Corn in a quagmire. The causes are almost the same as of cold; for it is Idleness that is the cause in most women that are troubled with it, and such women have abundance of Courses; but they are thin and waterish, and the whites also; their Secrets are alwayes wet: they cannot retain the mans seed, but it slips out again. This must be cured as the cold distemper, by a heating and drying Diet, and Medicaments, Baths, Injections, Fomentations, wherein Brimstone is mingled; but take heed of Astringents, for they will make the Disease worse, by stopping the ill humours in.

   The fourth is a dry Distemper of the womb, this is natural to some, but to most it comes when they are old, and past childing, when the womb grows hard; if it be from any other drying causes, such women will be barren before they be old: It may proceed from diseases, as Feavers, Inflammations, Obstructions, when the blood goes not to the Matrix to moisten it; so that if they void any blood, it comes from the Veins in the neck of the womb, and not from the bottom; they have but few courses, little seed, they are of a lean, dry Constitution; their lower Lip is of a blackish red, and commonly chapt: This Distemper, if it be long, is seldom cured; moistning things must do it, as Borage, Buglofs, Almonds, Dates, Figs, Raisins: Moistning and nourishing Diet is good, and to forbear salt and dry meats; avoid anger, sadness, fasting, and use to sleep long, and labour but little: rub the parts with oyl of sweet Almonds, Lillies, Linseed, sweet Butter, Jesamine, Hens or Ducks Grease.

Besides these four, there are compound distempers, as cold and moist wombs, and hot and dry; but I presume I need not in particular speak of them, because I have given sufficient remedies in the several qualitis already, which will be easie to apply: I confess a compound distemper is harder to be cured than a simple; therefore I shall add one or two remedies more.

First, If then the Womb be cold and moist, cure this with surrup of Mugwort, Bettony, Mints,

Mints, or Hyssop; then purge the cold humor with Agarick, Mechoachan, Turbith and Sena: Sudorificks of *Guaicum, Sarsa*, and China are very good.

Secondly, If the womb be subject to a hot and dry distemper, you must put away choler from the Liver, and from the whole body: those things that will do it are Manna, and Tamarinds, Sirrup of Roses, Rhubarb, Senna, Cassia, and the like, which are very safe, gentle, and effectual Remedies.

BOOK.

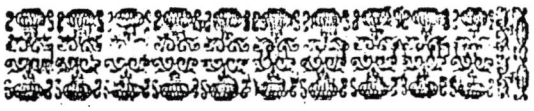

BOOK VI.

CHAP. I.

Of the Strangling of the womb, and the effects of it, with the Causes and Cure.

THe womb, by its consent with other parts of the Body, as well as by its own nature, is subject to multitudes of diseases; and it is not to be uttered almost what Miseries women in general, by meanes thereof, be they Maids, Wives, or widowes, are affected with: But amongst all diseases, those that are called Hysterical Passions, or strangling of the womb, are held to be the most grievous: Swounding and Falling Sickness are from hence, by the consent the womb hath with the heart and brain; and sometimes this comes to pass by stopping of the Terms, which load the heart, the brain and womb

Womb with evil humors; and sometimes it ariseth from the stopping in of the seed of Generation, as is seen in Antient Maids and widowes; for by reason hereof, ill vapors and wind rise up from the womb to the Midriff, and so stops their breath: it is most commonly the widowes disease, who were wont to use Copulation, and are now constrained to live without it; when the seed is thus retained it corrupts, and sends up filthy vapours to the brain, whereby the Animal Spirits are clouded, and many ill consequents proceed from it, as Falling Sicknesses, Megrims, Dulness, Giddiness, Drowsiness, Shortness of breath, Head-ache, beating of the Heart, Frenzy and Madness, and indeed what not. The same woman may be tormented with several of these at the same time, when the seed and the Courses are mingled with ill humours, being once corrupted. The Menstrual blood and seed are noble parts; but the best things once corrupted, become the worst, and degenerate into a venemous nature, and are little better than Poyson.

When the Vessels of the womb lye near the Vessels of other parts of the body, or there is near affinity of one part with the womb; then, by consent, are many grievous Diseases produced.

The

The womb is of a membranous nature, and for that reason it consents exceedingly with the nerves and membranes, and so the parts that are near are soon offended by it; and it conveys its ill qualities to the whole body, by Nerves, Veins and Arteries; the Brain hath it by the membranes of the marrow of the Back, and by Nerves; the arteries they carry it to the Heart, and the veins to the Liver, and these are large in the womb; and by them all the noxious blood, and poisonous vapours return.

The Veins of the Mesentery give it a consent with the stomach; and so do the arteries carry all to the Spleen, which is the cause that some women in age grow hypochondriacal by heat of their blood, because their courses did not flow sufficient when they were young. It will be hard to distinguish these two diseases in women, or to cure the one, and not cure the other.

The Breasts they consent with the womb by Nerves and Veins, that go from it to them: so then it is clear that it holds a correspondence with the heart, the Midriff, the Brain and Head, and all the instruments of motion and sense; likewise with the Stomach, Liver, Spleen, Bladder, Belly, Mesentery, Hips, Back, Straight Gut, Legs and arms, and some

cause

cause of strange symptomes in them all. For *Galen* saith well, the strangling of the Mother, or Hysterical Passion, is but one by name but the symptomes are scarce to be numbered. It alters womens complexions, & they grow sandy, or pale and yellow, or swarthy, and now and then their eyes and faces shew red, and very sanguine.

When this strange affection falls upon them, they will gnash their teeth, and become speechless, for their breath is stopt: and it hath been often observed that they have been supposed to be dead; neither breath, nor Pulse, nor Life, to be found for that time: and sometimes their breath is stopt so close and it holds so long, that they have died of it.

The causes of this disease are very many; for a sudden fear, a bad news related, hath cast divers women into these fits; for by this Melancholly gets the mastery of them: it were but reason therefore for men to forbear relating any sad accident to them, but with great proviso.

When the womb is strangled, no one disease can determine it; for that seldome comes alone: sometimes only the breath is stopt, sometimes the speech and animal actions of the brain fail, and the whole body is chill,

Y and

and almost dead by ill vapors that choke it rising from the womb.

The Malignant Vapors then sent from thence by the Nerves, Veins and arteries, are the immediate causes of all the hurt that is done; and these vapors are much like the wind, very powerful, and almost unperceived; they are so subtil and thin, that they pass in a moment of time through the whole body: it will choke the Patient when they flie to the Throat, as people are that eat White Hellebore, or venomous mushromes. Ofttimes you shall see the woman to loth and vomit, and draw her breath short, and her heart akes; if the vapour strike the heart first, it will cease from moving, and she falls into a swound: but if it flie to the brain, she is void of all sense and motion.

There is nothing worse than corrupt seed to offend the Body, Women with Child are not free from this disease when corrupt humours rise from an unclean womb.

The chief seat of this ill humour lieth in the Trumpet of the womb, and in her stones; for the substance of it is loose and hollow, and the Stones lie in bladders full of water; and women that have strangling of the womb, have this water of a yellow colour, and grosser than it should be.

Many *Physicians* have miſtook the ſtones and the Trumpet for the womb it ſelf, when putrified rotten ſeed makes them ſwell, and windy humours cauſe them to riſe as far as the Navel; but I ſpoke of this before, when I ſhewed the reaſon how the womb is thought to aſcend higher than nature hath placed it: It hath ſometimes a long time to breed in, and ſometimes it comes ſuddenly, according as the corruption of the humours is, which ſometimes alſo lie ſtill; and ſo ſoon as they are but moved they evacuate, and ſend a poiſonous fume into other parts of the body: And nothing will ſooner ſtir theſe vapours and humours in women (who are ſubject to this diſeaſe) than anger, or fear, or ſuch like paſſions; or ſweet ſcents, and ſmells applied to their noſes, which is an argument that the womb is delighted with ſweet ſcents, but cannot away with ſtinking things; for let Musk or Civet be held to ſuch womens noſes, they are preſently ſick till they be taken away.

What Diſtemper this ſtrangling of the womb is, *Phyſicians* agree not; ſome ſay it is a cold diſtemper: but coldneſs is not the chief ſymptome, though cold be great; others ſay it is a convulſion, or Syncope, or breathing ſtopt: but it cannot be ſet forth by any one ſymptome; for though the venomous vapor be small that breeds it, it goes many waies, and spreads through all the body. But the true causes of this Disease are the poisonous vapours that rise from the womb: it is not an apparent quality that this vapour works by, but a secret quality; as the *Torpedo* or *Scorpion* small creatures prevail with to do great mischief, as they are enemies to the natural heat and vital spirits: and when the heart suffers, there can be no good animal spirits bred, because the vital are corrupted; but blood and seed, whilest they are in their own proper vessels, hurt not, unless they are mingled with ill humors.

Fernelius saith, that the womb and seed, the place and matter of life, are the breeding of the most deadly poisons.

Hippocrates, in these fits, bids give them wine to refresh their weakness: *Avicenna* bids give them no wine, but water, and forbids eating flesh, because they ingender more seed and blood: but when she is in the fit, wine is best; for a little wine will not presently get to the womb.

Sometimes both maids and widdows, from such like causes, are troubled with the rage of the womb, that they will grow even mad with carnal desire, and entice men to lie with them; they are hot, but not feaverish, and

they

they are inclined to madness.

Modest women will die of consumptions, when they have this rage of the womb, rather than declare their desire, but some women are shameless.

The cause is great store of sharp hot seed, that is not natural, but the next degree to it, that bites, and swells, and provokes nature to expulsion: the brain suffers by consent; the womb in the Nymphe is most affected, which swells with heat, but the Clitoris, and not the Nymphe is the seat of lust: hot blood and humours in the womb breed this, and they are increased by hot spiced meats and drinks, idleness and bawdy acts and objects; at first it may be cured, but the end of it is frenzy and madness if it be neglected.

Maids must marry that cannot live chast, or draw blood to abate the heat and sharpness of it; let them purge these humours gently, and use cooling and moistening meats and drinks, and all with moderation. Lettice, Violets, and water-Lillies, and Purslain are good coolers, and take away the windiness of the parts: the seed, leaves and flowers of *Agnus Castus* strewed in their beds, or Camphire smelt unto are very good in such cases.

Let them use this Electuary; take conserve of water Lillies, Violets, tops of *Agnus Cast-*

us, of each one ounce; of red Roses half an ounce; of red Coral, and emralds in powder, of each half a dram; of Coleworts, and Lettice candid, of each one ounce, with firrup of Violets and water-Lillies, make an Electuary: lay a plate of lead to their backs.

Nuns, and such as cannot marry, may use things, that by a hidden quality diminish seed, but they cause barrenness: let them eat no eggs, nor much nourishing meats, and sleep little.

Camphire, that is so much commended against this preternatural desire, is hot and sharp, and bitter, it will burn and flame, and being of thin parts penetrates deep; but it hath cold operations, for it will cure burns and hot swellings, and head-ach that comes of heat, by a likeness and affinity it hath to draw hot vapours to it; so Linseed oil is good against burnings.

Scaliger affirms that Camphire increaseth Venery; it may do so if it be used seldome, but often used, it is certain that it will destroy it.

There is moreover (from ill tempered seed, and melancholly blood, in the vessels near the Heart, which contaminates the Vital and Animal Spirits) a melancholy distemper, that especially Maids and Widows are often

troubled

troubled with, and they grow exceeding pensive and sad: for melancholy black blood abounding in the Vessels of the Matrix, runs sometimes back by the great arteries to the heart, and infects all the spirits: when this blood lieth still, they are well; but if it be stirred, or urged, then presently they fall into this distemper, they know not why: and the arteries of the spleen and back beat strongly, and melancholly vapours fly up. They are sorely troubled, and weary of all things; they can take no rest, their pain lieth most on their left side, and sometimes on the left breast: in time they will grow mad, and their former great silence turns to prating exceedingly, crying out that they see fearful spirits, and dead men; when it is gone so far, it is hard to cure: it is vain then to try to make them merry, they despair and wish to die; and when they find an opportunity, they will kill, or drown, or hang themselves: At first when the blood is hot and fiery, open a vein in the arm, if they have their courses; if not, in the foot or ancle to bring the courses down. Cooling, moistening cordials, and such things as revive the spirits, and conquer melancholy, wil do much; driers are naught, for melancholly is dry. *Confectio Alkermes* is commended for those that can away with it; but *Confectio de Hyacintho*

Hyacintho is better: use a moistening diet. To breed mirth, give her waters of Balm and Borage, of each three ounces; sirrup of the juices of Borage and Buglosse of each one ounce and a half; take this at twice, and use it often.

To purge melancholly, take six drams of Senna, Agarick one dram and a half; Borage and violet flowers of each a small handful, two drams of Citron peels; infuse all six hours in good Rhenish wine, strain them, and put to them sirrup of Violets one ounce.

CHAP. II.

Of the Falling sickness.

WHen Women, by reason of the ill affections of the womb, fall into Epilepsies, and Falling sickness, it is worse than any other cause, as the symptomes prove: for the poisonous vapor is not only in the Nerves as when it is from the brain, but also in the membranes, veins, and arteries.

The same foul vapour that causeth strangling of the womb, produceth this; for it causeth divers diseases, according to the parts it takes

takes hold on: but when it lights forcibly on the Nerves, then it causeth the Falling-sickness.

Sometimes there is a convulsion of the whole body, and sometimes but of some parts; as of the head, or tongue, hands, or legs, eyes, or ears; some cannot hear, others cannot see, all lose the sense of feeling: some cry out, but know not wherefore. They that fall, if the vapour be not too strong, when they rise, they go to their work again, as if they had no harm: but here is not only convulsions, as in those that have the Falling-sickness from other parts, but stopping the breath, as in the strangling of the womb; but these seldome some at the mouth, as those do, for the brain is entire, or not much offended; nor is their hearing taken away quite by the vapour fastening upon the roots of the Nerves of the ears.

Rue and Castor that cure fits of the Mother, are good here; the cure is almost the same, only you must add some things that respect the nerves and the Brain: Use these Pills twice in a week, before supper one hour, and take a scruple, or half a dram; Take Senna and Peony root, of each half an ounce, Mugwort, Rue, Betony, Yarrow, half a handful of each; boil them, & then clarifie the decoction;

put

put to it Aloes one ounce and a half, of juice of the herb Mercury one ounce let it stand and settle, pour off the clear liquor, then add two drams of Rhubarb, sprinkled with water of Cinnamon, Agarick half an ounce, Mastick and Epileptick powder, of each half a dram, make the pills with sirrup of Mugwort.

To mend the distemper of the head and Womb, take conserve of Rosemary flowers, and of the Tile tree, of Balm and Lillies of the valley, of the root Scorzonera Candied, of each one ounce, *Diamoscbu dulce* one dram with two drams of the roots of Peony, and seeds of *Agnus Castus*, and sirrup of Stœchas, make an Electuary to take at your pleasure.

Nor are these all the ill consequences of the wombs distempers, but sometimes violent head-ach springs from it, which is the greatest pain of all the rest; and sometimes it is all over the head, or but upon one side, or in the eyes, the ill vapours rising by the veins and arteries of the Womb to the membranes and films of the brain; when the vessels are full of a thin sharp blood, that is carried from the womb to the membranes, it stretcheth and rends them, and corrodes and bites so, that the pain is intollerable: the cure is to purge away

away the peccant humour that lieth in the Womb; for this is not as other head-ach is, that comes from other causes: the pain runs also to the Loins and the Membranes there, by some capillary veins from the womb. The pain of the head by affection with the womb, is in all the head commonly, but is chiefly in the hinder part of the head, because the womb being Nervous consents with the membranes of the brain, by the membrane of the Marrow of the back: & hence it is that women are more subject to the head-ach than men are, because of the womb that holds such affinity with the Nerves of the head.

The violent beating of the heart and Arteries both in the Sides and Back, is by consent from the womb, when evil humors therein contained, pass by the Arteries, and Poysonous vapours arise to those parts; Cordials are good, as Cinnamon Water, and *Aqua Monefardi*, or *Mathiolas* his water: the Disease seems small, but it is not safe, because the cause of it is very ill.

In this Disease the Artery that beats in the Back beats strongly, because it is part of the great Artery; but the Arteries that beat in the Hypochondrion beat not so strongly, for they are smaller branches from the Spleen and Mesentery, but the cause is the same. The

Arteries

Arteries are inflamed by the ill vapours and humours sent from the womb, and the heart is exceedingly heated by them: but this hot humor sometimes beats by reason of the great Artery quite over the whole body, but it lasts not long, for there is little corruption of the humors. Some say the blood in the Veins is too hot, and over-heats the Artery; but if this heat of the Artery affect the Brain, the Patient will be mad; if it go over the whole body she falls into a Consumption: lay your hand on the left side, and you shall feel the Arteries beat much. So then, this Disease hath several considerations, and must be cured partly as hypochondriacal Melancholy, partly as in the cure for stopping of the Courses, and partly as Melancholy, arising from the womb.

Physitians can hardly tell which way to proceed oftentimes in these Distempers, because it is hard to say what Disease the woman is sick of, when the Spleen and left Hypochondry are afflicted from the womb.

The womb hath two Arteries, the one from the Hypogastrick Artery, and another from the preparing Arteries; that which comes from the Hypogastrick runs almost through the whole Abdomen: when the foul corrupt blood in the womb runs backward

Book VI. *The Midwives Book.* 333
ward to the Hypogastrick Artery, it passeth to the Cæliac Artery, and so to the Spleen, and the parts near it: and it is Natures present way to thrust ill humors to the ignoble parts. When the courses are stopt, these ill humors are thought to be onely in the Veins, but the veins and Arteries mouthes are so joyned, that they pass from the Veins to the Arteries, and that is the reason that elderly women, whose courses were stopt when they were young, are troubled oftentimes with the Spleen, & hypochondriack Melancholy; These cannot endure to smell to sweet Scents: they are short breathed, Costive, and Belch often; they have pain in the left side, and are very sad, when the thin part of the blood is inflamed they grow very hot, and red in the Face, but that lasts not long; the disease it will produce (if not cured) is chiefly a Schirrhus of the Spleen; open a Vein, if the blood be hot, and the Courses stopt, use Leeches to the hæmorroids; and Purge often, but very gently, with *Quercetan's* Pill of *Tartar*, or *Fernelius* his *Cum Ammoniaco*, and Birth-wort; or prepared Steel to open the Courses, and to cure Melancholy that ariseth from the womb.

When the liver is hurt by the gross blood running back to the holow vein from the womb, as it often doth if the courses be stopt, & blood

abound

abound; it breeds raw flegmatick blood, and causeth the Green-sickness: for there are many more great veins in the womb than in any other part of the body, and they are often obstructed: and sometimes, by this stopping, not onely sundry Diseases, but Hair will grow over the whole body; for hairs grow from the Excrementitious part of the blood, and if that Excrement be sent over the body, it will produce hair: So *Hippocrates* tells us of a woman with a great beard; and it is not long since there was a woman to be seen here in *England* which had not onely a long beard, but her whole Body covered with hair.

It is also by reason of the womb, or by consent from it, that many women have no stomach, others have a very large Appetite; and sometimes a desire to eat strange things, not fit for Food: they Vomit, and have the Hiccough, & many such ill symptomes: as the vapors are, so are the Diseases; if Cold, then they breed cold diseases; if hot, such diseases as proceed of heat: For these filthy vapors, when the way is large, easily ascend from the Arteries of the womb, and get into the Hypogastrick, and Cæliac Arteries: hot vapors cause Thirst, cold vapors destroy concoction, and are the cause of many cruel diseases by their Malignity. When the stomach is hurt

by

by the womb, it is easily perceived, for the signes of it go away sometimes, and come again, onely when the Fumes fly to the stomach: There is no cure for this, but by first curing the womb; for this disease is worse than if the stomach were originally the cause of the distemper: Cure the womb, and if there be no other cause, the stomach is cured; first give a vomit to cleanse the stomach, and use often to take pills of Aloes and Mastick, for these fortifie the stomach.

If one womb in a woman be the cause of so many strong and violent diseases, she may be thought a happy woman of our sex that was born without a womb: *Columbus* reports that he saw such a woman, and that her secrets were as the secrets of other women; and part of the neck out.

It will be needless to tell you what some have written, that it hath been often seen, that worms, and Hair, and Fat, and Stones, and many other strange things have been found in womens wombs; but what a miserable case is she in that was born with two wombs? Such a woman *Julius Obsequens* related that he saw,: and *Bauhinus* speaks of a maid who had a Matrix like that of a *Bitch* divided in two parts: But some perhaps may think these things fabulous; I confess they are monstrous,

and

and out of the ordinary courſe of nature; and I know no cure for them, if ſuch things ſhould happen: I forbear therefore to ſpeak any more of them, and ſhall proceed to ſome things more material to be known, and ſuch things as few women living but have frequent occaſion to be provided with remedies for.

CHAP. III.

Of Womens Breaſts and Nipples.

NAture, within ſome convenient time after the Child is conceived in the womb, begins to provide nouriſhment for it ſo ſoon as it ſhall be born. The breaſts are two in number, leſt by accident one Breaſt ſhould fail, and ſometimes women have Twins, and more children than one to give ſuck to.

Some women faith *Cardan*, have been ſeen with more than two breaſts for they have had two breaſts on each ſide, but that is very rare. The form of the breaſt is round, and ſharp at the Nipples; yet theſe differ in many women, for ſome have breaſts no bigger than men, and ſome have huge overgrown ſwoln breaſts,

by

by reason of much blood abounding, and strong heat to draw and to concoct it.

The breasts should be of a moderate size, neither too great nor too small; not too soft nor too hard; it is not necessary to have them over-big; though they can hold but little milk, thee may hold sufficient: but large breasts are in danger to be cancerated and inflamed; besides that the milk is not so good, because their wants a moderate heat. The immediate causes of great Breasts is partly natural by birth, the passages being loose and large; and sleep and idleness furthers it, and much handling of them heats and draws the blood thither: their causes are not many. It is best to prevent their growing too big at first, for it is not easily done afterward: Cooling Diet, and drying and astringent repercussive Topical means are the best. Binding things help loose breasts, and make them hard; all cold Narcotick stupefying Medicaments are forbidden, they will bind the Vessels, but they abate Natural heat, and will let no milk breed.

When children are weaned, Discussers and Driers will do well to consume the Moisture that is superfluous. Take the Meal of Beans and Orobus, of each two ounces and a half; Powder of Comfrey roots half an ounce,

Mints three drams; Wormwood, Cammomile Flowers, Roses, of each two drams; when they are boiled with two ounces of oil of Mastick, make a Cataplasme: or take red Roses, Myrtle leaves, Horstail, Mints, Plantain, a handful of each; Flowers of sowr Pomegranates two Pugils, boil all in Vinegar and red wine, and with a spunge lay it warm to the breasts, and let it dry on.

If Milk be too much in the breasts after the child is born, and the child be not able to suck it all, the breasts will very frequently inflame, or Imposthumes breed in them; they swell and grow red, and are painful, being overstretched, whence hard tumours grow: too much blood is the cause of it, or the child is too weak, and cannot draw it forth. Sometimes it goeth away without any remedies, but if you need help then hinder the breeding of more milk, and try to consume that which is bred; if the child cannot draw it forth, Glasses are made to suck it forth. The woman must eat and drink with moderation, and use a drying diet: if she nurse not the child her self, or if the child be weaned, to dry up the milk, take a good quantity of Rozin, mingle it with Cream, and being lukewarm lay it all over the breasts; or make a plaister to dry up the Milk, with Bean meal,

red

red Vinegar, and oil of Roses, lay it on warm.

If the Breasts be inflamed, keep a good reasonable cooling Diet, moistening and comfortable; it is blood and not milk that causeth inflamation: for milk, when it grows hot, makes pain; and thereby the blood that staies in the small capillar veins, being out of the vessels is inflamed and corrupt: it may also come from Falls or bruises, or strait lacing of the breasts; if there be a Feaver and a throbbing pain, and a red hard swelling, the breasts are inflamed. Inflammations may be without danger, but the breasts that are loose and full of Kernels, will soon turn to a Schirrhus, or a Cancer: If the body then be full of blood open a vein, but if the Courses be stopt open a vein in the Ancle, and after that in the arm. You may purge bad humors easily with Manna or Senna.: if the blood be over hot, eat Endive, Lettice, Water-Lillies, Plantane, Purslain, use repercussives, and moderate cooling things.

Apply a cloth dipt in oil of Roses, with Honey and Water; when the strength of the inflammation is past use Discussers as well as repercussives; as, take white-bread Crumbs, Barley-flour, of each one ounce and a half: flour of *Beans*, and Fenugreek of each half an ounce: Powder of Cammomile Flowers, and red Roses, of each tow drams, boil them, then mingle Rose Vinegar one ounce, and as much of oyle of Roses and Camomil, lay it over the breasts; then use onely Discutients, as take *Bean* Meal, Lupines, Fenugreek, Linseed, and Powder of Camomil Flowers, each an ounce, make a Cataplasme; if the Matter begin to grow hard, use things that soften and attenuate; as take a handful of Mallowes and boil them soft, Powder of Linseed, Marshmallows and Camomil Flowers each one ounce; boil all again, and with an ounce of oyl of Jessamine make a Cataplasme: If you find that it will come to suppuration, lay on a Plaister of Diachylon, if it turn to Matter, and the Impostume break; otherwise open it, with a Lancet, and let out the Matter; then cleanse it thus; Take Turpentine, and Honey of Roses, of each one ounce, Myrrh a scruple; it will be hard to cure the Ulcer unless you dry the Milk in the other breast, because much blood will run thither to breed Milk.

An Erisipelas of the breasts comes from great Anger, or some Fright, which turns to an inflammation, and is cured as the former: apply no fat things nor cold repercussives to discuss the thin blood that makes the inflammation; lay on a clout dipt in Elder-water, and give her Harts-horn, *Terra Sigillata*, and Cardnus duus, with Elder-water to make her sweat.

Some womens breasts are too small, when the blood cannot find a way to the breasts, but is repelled, and forced some other way; or when the Liver is dry, and the woman Feaverish, toils over much, or watcheth, or from some cause that wasts the body: Therefore feed well, and foment the breasts with Warm water and white-wine, wherein softning things have been boiled, then anoint them with oyl of sweet Almonds, and rub the Breasts often to attract the blood.

Sometimes hard cold swellings will breed in womens breasts, and Phlegmatick swellings, as we see in persons that have the Greensickness, their breasts will pill, for the part is loose and spungy; it is larger when the terms are like to flow, and when they are gone it abateth for a while: If it come from an ill habit of the body, derived from the womb, it is to be feared; otherwise it may be discust, or dissolved: dry, and hot meats and means are best. If the Courses be stopt open them, and cure the ill habit, then use Topicks to discuss, and strengthen the part; they must be temperately hot, otherwise you will cause a Schirrhus by resolving the thin parts, and leave the thick to grow harder. Make a ly of Colewort and vine Ashes, and brimstone;

or a decoction with Hyssop, Sage, Origanum, and Camomile Flowers, then anoint with oyl of Lillies, Bays, and Camomile; or take four ounces of *Barley* Meal, and half an ounce of Linseed, and of Fenugreek, Dill and Camomile Flowers as much,: one ounce of Marshmallow Roots, with oyl of Dill and Camomile, make an application. These Phlegmatick swellings must be discust at first, or they may turn into Cancers: She must eat Bread well baked, parched Almonds, dryed Raisins; let her drink a decoction of China Roots, Sassafras and Sarsa; forbear Milk-meats, unleavened Bread and Sleeping presently after meat.

Besides watry and Hydropick humours, there are Kernels growing in the breasts, which are small round spungy bodies, and sometimes swell by humors flowing thither: there grow sometimes other hard swellings caused by that they call the *Kings-evil*; it is engendred of gross Phlegm, or thick mattery blood, and grows hard under the skin; the stopping of the Courses is the ordinary cause, when the Menstrual blood runs back to the breasts, this will soon become a Cancer, if it be not prevented by softning means, and a moderate thin Diet, keeping her self warm, and using good exercise before Meats; avoid idleness,

and

and meats of hard digestion; Baths of Brimstone are good to be prescribed against windy and watry swellings.

But *Celsus* saith, That the Scrofula of the Breasts is seldome seen, for that must proceed from a thick Phlegmatick humor, mixt with a melancholy humor; it is sometimes painful, and somewhat like a Cancer, or will soon be turned to one; but stands often times at the same pass for many years: It comes from disorder, or stopping of the Terms, there being so great consent betwixt the breasts and the womb; you may feel the small kernels of the breast, but that I speak of now is one unmoveable humor, but the other are small: If it lye near the skin it is soon dissolved, but if it lye deep it will hardly be dissolved, because the substance of it is so earthy: first Purge, then bleed, after that apply softning and discussing remedies that are strong, as you must do for a Schirrhus humor; Take Orris Roots and boil them in Oxynel, and stamp them, mix them with Oyntment of Marshmallowes and Turpentine, of each three ounces, and one ounce of Mucilage of the seed of Fenugreek; If you cannot discuss it, ripen it, or cut it open, but take heed how you do it for this is troublesome and dangerous.

All these humors, if they be unskilfully handled

handled will soon turn to a Schirrhus, from melancholy in the veins flowing to the breasts, and it is thick flegm dried; there are two kinds of it, one is bred of Melancholy blood, which is gross & feculent, or thick flegm mixed with it, and this feels no pain: but the other is not so hard, for it is not yet fully come to its perfection; and it is probable that it is mingled with other humors.

A perfect Schirrhus grows from the stoppings of the Spleen, whereby the Melancholy blood is retained, and being in great quantity falls upon the Breasts, or else the courses stopt fly thither.

There is a double intention for the cure:

First, Use emollient means to soften all that is hard and knotty in the breasts, then keep a good Diet; and beware of salt Meats, and such as are smoak'd, and hard of digestion, and moreover all things of a sharp corroding faculty; use moderate Exercise and Mirth, provoke the courses if they be stopt, and let on Leeches, or bleed in the foot.

Sena and Rhubarb are good to purge the body well; and when you have purged, do so no more till you have used some Cordials, as Conserve of Bugloss, and Orange Flowers, *Confectio Alkermes, Electuarium Degemus*, and *Trisantales*. Sometimes flegm and melancholy

choly are mingled to cause this Schirrhus, but then it is but a bastard Schirrhus; if burnt humors abound most it will be a Schrrhus, if Melancholy a cancer.

Secondly, The perfect signs of a Schirrhus are, that it is very hard, and feels no pain; if it feel any it is not yet fixed: it is coloured according to the humor, white, or black, or blew; a bastard Schirrhus is hot and painful, if it go on it will be a Cancer, and the Veins will swell and look blew: if hairs once grow upon it there is no hopes of cure; and the bigger and harder it is the more incurable. Let general medicaments proceed, and cure the cause from the Matrix and from the whole body: soften, attenuate, and discuss the hardness, but take heed of hot things that will discuss the thin parts, and leave the thick behind; neither use too many moistning softning means, for that will ferment the matter, and change the Schirrhus to a Cancer, that is far worse; but either soften, and moisten, and digest together, or by turns: A Fomentation of Mallows, Marshmallows, brank Ursine, Camomile Flowers, Linseed and Fenugreek are good; anoint afterwards with oyl of sweet Almonds, Hens grease, Marrow of a Calf, oyntment of Marshmallowes, lay on the great Diachylon, or the Plaister of Frogs, take

the

the Fume of a hot ftone, fprinkling wine upon it; lay on a Plaifter of *Gum Ammoniacum* diffolved in Vinegar of Squills, a baftard Schirrhus will foon Cancerate. Bleed, & purge away the humor that breeds black blood; to hinder humors from flowing to it; anoint with oyl of Rofes, and juyce of Plantane if it be hot, beat them well in a mortar of Lead till they fhew another colour; then mix Cerufs, and Litharge of filver one ounce, with wax make an oyntment: or take one ounce of Mallow Roots, boil & bruife them, let Sheeps Suet, and Capons greefe, of each two ounces, be added to it, with wax fufficient to make an Oyntment.

But the difeafe (worfe than a Schirrhus) is a Cancer of the breafts: and *William Fabricius* faith, that if it be not an Ulcerated Cancer, the woman may live above forty years with it, and no pain moleft her; but if you lay on any thing to foften and ripen thefe fwellings, fhe will dye in half a year. Many orderly women have lived long with Cancers as if they ailed nothing.

Hippocrates bids not to cure an occult Cancer, if you do, the perfon will dye of the cure: becaufe the breafts are loofe and fpungy, Cancers are foon bred there. Burnt blood flowing from the womb of one who is of a hot and dry

dry Conſtitution, and the Terms ſtopping, after a Tumor, they make an Internal or External Cancer.

A Cancer that comes naturally undiſcerned, is hardly known at firſt, being no greater than a Peaſe, and daily increaſeth with roots ſpreading, and Veins about it; when the skin is eaten through it becomes a loathſome Ulcer: the Matter is black, and the lips are hard; it is ſcarce curable, becauſe it is bred of black burnt blood that is malign; and the Veſſels are looſned and relapſed by ſoftners and ripeners miſapplyed to it; ſo that the paſſage is made for the humors to paſs to and fro, and ſerve to infect the reſt.

Purge melancholy, and draw blood, but uſe no Topicks to ripen or rot the part; onely Anodynes that will take away pain; as oyl of Frogs and Snails, with Frogs aſhes made to an oyntment, with Nightſhade water. Aſhes of Crayfiſh, or of the herb Robert, or the inward Rind of an Aſh-Tree.

Aretæus ſhewes the way to cut them forth, and to burn the part if the Ulcer be deep. *Fabricius* bids burn the roots firſt, and afterwards to conſume the Reliques, and to ſtop the blood when the root is cut up.

You muſt often Purge away melancholy humors, and provoke the Courſes, or the

Cancer will return. Mithridate and Treacle, with juyces of Sorrel and Borrage, and Crayfish Broth, and Asses milk are approved good to palliate the Cure, and to keep it from going farther, and ease pain.

This water is commended; Take *Scrofularia* roots and herb Robert, of each one handful, Lambs Tongue, Nightshade, Buglos, Borage, Purslane, Bettony, Eybright, of each half a handful, one Frog, two whites of Eggs, with Quince seeds, and Fenugreeck, each one ounce, a pint of rose water, & as much of Eybright water, distil them in a Leaden still.

Cancers must not be handled like other Ulcers, for softners, Drawers and healers exasperate, and kill the woman with great dolour.

Fichsius his blessed powder against a Cancer is this; take white arsenick that shineth like Glass one ounce, pour on Aquavitæ on the powder of it, pour it off again, and put on fresh Aquavitæ every third day, for fifteen dayes together; then take roots of great Dragon gathered in *August* or *July*, slice them, and dry them in the wind, two ounces; and take three drams of clear Chimney Soot, make a powder, keep it close stopt in a glass, to use after one year, and not before.

For the cure of any other Ulcers, or Fistulaes

Book VI. *The Midwives Book.* 349

laes of the breasts, first try to dry up the milk, and when the breasts hang down bind them up, that the humours fall not down to them; cleanse them with a decoction of Rhapontick, Agrimony, and Zedoary, to heal take six quarts of strong wine, and boil in it Rhus Obsoniox, Cypress Nuts, of each four ounces, and two ounces of Green Galls, to the thickness of Honey: If the Fistula be Callous, and hard about the edges, open the Orifice with a Gentian root, and take the redness away, then cleanse and heal as ordinary Ulcers.

Sometimes stones, hair, or worms are bred in the breasts from corrupt blood, or milk, and so they may breed in the back, or Navel. Sometimes the Veins and Arteries of the breasts are so streight that they can contain no blood to make milk; it is either gross humors that stop them, as they do the Vessels of the womb, or they are made so by the wombs vessels being stopt, or from hard humors bred there.

Sometimes the Nipple hath no hold for the child to draw forth the milk by, and it was so made at first; or else it is from a wound or ulcer that leaves a scar that stops it: The breasts then must needs pine away; but if the milk cannot be suck'd forth, & the breasts are swoln, the reason is that the Paps, or veins for

the

the milk are not as they should be.

When gross humours only obstruct, that may be cured; but a Nipple naturally without a hole, or the hole stopt by a Schirrhus, or Scar, after an ulcer is cured, cannot be healed; often rubbing of the breasts will open the veins for milk : but the Nipples for the child to suck by are oftentimes deficient or lie tied, either one or both, that women can hardly give suck; if an ulcer have eaten away the Nipple, or it was not made at her birth, it will never be otherwise; if the hole be never so small, so there be a hole, often sucking will make it larger, especially by a sucking instrument

Clefts and Chaps of the breasts are troublesome, and usual to Nurses; and in time those Chaps grow to foul Ulcers, and hinder giving of suck: You may prevent this mischief if in the two last months they go with child you lay two cups of wax made up with a little Rozin, to cover the Nipples.

To cure the Nipples take oil of Myrtles, of wax, ointment of Lead and Tutty, or take Tutty prepared one scruple, and half a dram of Allum, Camphire six grains, with ointment of Roses, and Capons grease make it up; or take Pomatum one ounce and a half, Mastick a scruple, Powder of red roses, and Gum
Traganth

Traganth of each half a scruple; before the child sucks wash the breasts with Rose water and White-wine; and that it may suck without pain, cover the sore pap with a silver Nipple covered with the pap of a Cow new killed: You may take what quantity you please of Mutton Suet, or Lambs Suet, and wash it in Rose water, when it is melted and clarified, and annoint the paps with it.

CHAP. IV.

Directions for Nurses.

But there is one consideration more for the Nurse before I leave this; and that is, that she may not want good milk in her breasts, for if she do, the child will suffer more than the Nurse, because he draws it from her to feed him: Those that are fretful, lean, or sickly, have bad Livers and Stomachs, and ill digestion, that they can have neither much, nor yet good milk, and bad diet hinders much.

Such as want milk should drink milk wherein Fennel Seed hath been soked, and feed on good nourishment, and drink good drink, Barley Water and

and Almond milk are good for hot cholerick people; let her eat Lettice, Borrage, Spuriache, and Lamb sodden, and eaten with Vervine, Calves or Goats milk nourish and breed milk in the breasts; the eating of Annifeeds, Cummin feeds, Carraway feeds or their decoction drank will help well; all things that increase feed ripen milk: when you go to bed drink two drams and a half of bruised Annifeeds in the decoction of Coleworts. Use this Plaister, take Deers suet half an ounce, Parsley herb and root the like quantity, barley meal one ounce and a half, red Storax three drams, boil the roots and herbs well, and beat them to Pap, and incorporate all with three ounces of oyl of sweet Almonds, and lay them to the breasts and nipple.

There are many things hinder milk, either little blood to breed it, or the faculty of the breasts is deficient and cannot do it, or the Organs are not right as they should be; also much watching, & fasting, & labour, & sweating, and great evacuations by stool or Urine, strong passions, or great pains, sorrows, cares, or strong Feavers, and other discussers may destroy or hinder milk in the breasts, so may also the childs great weakness who cannot draw it thither; it is easily known by any of
these

these causes; when the breasts swell not but flag, and lie wrinkled, you know there is no great store of milk in them: if the fault be in the Liver, that it breeds not good blood, you must rectify the Liver; yet she may be in good health, sufficient as to other things, but then the infant will be ruined by it; and it is for that end that nature provides milk that the child may be fed.

The usual way for rich people is to put forth their children to nurse, but that is a remedy that needs a remedy, if it might be had; because it changeth the natural disposition of the child, and oftentimes exposeth the infant to many hazards, if great care be not taken in the choice of the nurse.

There are not many Women that want milk to suckle their own children; so there are some that may well be excused, because of their weakness, that they cannot give suck to their own children: but multitudes pretend weakness when they have no cause for it, because they have not so much love for their own, as Dumb creatures have.

Nature indeed hath provided some helps where milk is wanting for the child, but those are not many; to shew women that nature commonly doth her part with most mothers, to furnish them with milk without farther means than by good wholesome meats and drinks: but there are abundance of things that will hinder milk, or destroy it. For all things that are cold, or else hot and dry, are enemies to womens milk; but none will breed it but such things, as are hot and moist, or not very dry, and of such things there are no great plenty.

Also they must be of easie digestion, and that will breed good blood, that the milk that is bred may have no strong qualities with it to offend the infant. You may lay a plaister of Mustard all over the breasts, and change it often, and lay on another; all such things as being eaten (breed milk) will do the like if you lay them on outwardly: or foment the breasts with this decoction, as Fennel, Smallage, Mints, pound them, and lay them on, with Barley meal half an ounce, the seeds of Gith one dram, and with two drams of Storax Calamita, and two ounces of the oil of Lillies to make a Poultis.

Some say that by sympathy a Cows Udder dried in an oven, first cut into pieces, and then powdered, half a pound of this powder to an ounce of Anniseed, and as much of sweet Fennel-seed, with two ounces of Cummin seed, and four ounces of Sugar, will make milk increase exceedingly; or boil a

handful

handful of Green Parsly, and a handful of Fennel, with a small handful of Barley, and half an ounce of red Pease in chicken broth, or sweeten the former decoction with fine Sugar, and so drink it: Dill, and Basil, and Rochet, and Chrystal also, but this must be warily taken, not too often not too much, are good to cause milk in the breasts: some prescribe the hoofs of a Cows forefeet dried and powdered, and a dram taken every morning in Ale; I think it should be the hoofs of the hinder feet, for they stand nearest the Udder, where milk is bred. I mislike not the experiment, but our Ladies thistle is by Signature, and (the white milky veins it hath) well known to be a very good help to women that want milk.

A woman may be of a good complexion, and yet want milk in her breasts: and there is a Royal Person now living, that I will not be so bold to name here, that when his Nurse wanted milk, the Physicians, Doctor *Mayhern* and others, were desirous to put her off from being nurse, because (they said) she had not milk sufficient to supply the child with; but his Sacred Majesty of Blessed and Glorious Memory spoke in the womans behalf: when the Physicians confess, That the milk she had was very good; What saith his Majesty, is not a pint of Cream as good as a quart of Milk?

Some women there are that are full of blood, lusty, and strong, and so well tempered to increase milk, that they can suckle a child of their own, and another for a friend; and it will not be amiss for them, when they have too great plenty to do so, if they be poor, for it will help them with food, and not hurt their own child: for if a child suck too much milk, it will soon fall into Convulsion fits, if the children be full bodied; and if milk be too much in the breasts, it will clodder and corrupt, and inflame the blood if it be not drawn forth.

When blood first comes to the breasts to make milk, though it come in great plenty we may not stop it, but afterwards labour to diminish it by a slender diet, and eating things that breed small nourishment; or else lay repercussive medicaments to the veins under the arms, and above the breasts, to drive the blood back; you may also open a vein: Calamints and Agnus Castus, Coriander seed and Hemlock are enemies to breeding of milk.

When you suspect that the blood will be inflamed by too great plenty of milk, then make a Poultiss of Houslcek, Lettice, Poppies, and
Water-

Water Lillies, this will drive it back.

They that are desirous to put forth their Children to Nurse may use this decoction; of Bays, Mallows, Fennel, Smallage, Parsley, Mints, half a handful of each, to foment the breasts, and afterwards they must anoint them with oyl Omphacine made of sowr grapes; then take Turpentine washt with Wine and Rose-water three ounces, and two or three Eggs, with one scruple of Saffron, and a sufficient quantity of wax to make a Plaister; lay this on upon the breasts fresh every day before Supper; but leave a hole in the middle of the Plaister for the Nipple to come forth.

If the milk be much, and stay long in the breasts, it does curdle, when the thinner part evaporates, and the thick stayes behind and turns into kernels and hard swellings, which being the Cheesy part of the milk will soon grow hard, and this will easily inflame and impostumate; besides the plenty, it may be salt or sharp, or exceed in many other ill qualities: when milk is too much it will cause pain in the breasts, and clefts; but to hinder it from clotting and congealing, make a pap of grated white bread, new milk, and oyl of Roses, seethe them all together, and lay it warm over the breasts; let her use to eat

Saffron, Cinnamon, and *Mints* with her *Meats*, and observe a moderate Diet with moist *Meats*, which breed but thin milk: but if the milk be clodded and inflamed, pound Chickweed and lay it warm over the breasts, or annoint them with the mucilage of Fleawort, Purslane seeds, and Fenugreek, made up with wax to an ointment.

But sometimes the woman takes cold, and falls into an Ague, then lay on a Poultis to the breasts made with Melilot, Camomile, Fennel seeds, Anniseeds, Dill seeds, Linseeds, Fenugreek, Southernwood, Basil, and Ginger, with oyl of Camomile; to hinder the curdling, take two ounces of Coriander seed, and as much of Mints, and one ounce of oyl of Dill made to a Livint, with a little wax: and to dissolve what is already curdled, take an ounce of each of these roots, Fennel, and Eringos, and half a handful of green Fennel tops, and one dram of Anniseeds, boil all to a pint, add Oxymel Simple two ounces, and as much of the sirrup of the two opening roots at the *Apothecaries*.

It is a thing to be wondered at, how Nature sometimes will find strange conveniences & passages that are not ordinary in some women; for some have voided their breasts milk by their Urine, and sometimes by the womb;

and

and it hath been a great Dispute by which of the two the milk came forth: the shortest way for the milk to return, is the way the blood came to the breasts to make the milk, not from the veins of the breasts to the hypogastrick Veins, and next to the womb, but from the breast veins to the epigastrick veins, and from them to the hypogastrick, and so to the womb; but this is seldome seen or heard of: but strange things have come forth of the breasts, and sometimes the menstrual blood unchanged runs forth this way at certain seasons.

Hippocrates Writes that when the blood comes out of the Nipples, those women are Mad: yet *Amatus Lusitanus* tells us, of his own experience, that he saw two women at whose Paps their Monthly Terms came forth and yet neither of them was Mad. But we must rightly understand *Hippocrates* meaning, for he doth mean of her fiery blood that flies up and enflames the party; whereof part goes to the breasts, and much to the the brain, causing pain and inflammations, and that is a forerunner of Madness: but it is not menstrual blood will do this, unless it be endued with some extraordinary malignant quality; for that is ordained to go to the breasts to make milk, which is the reason that Nurses have few or no Courses, because the blood goes to the breasts to make milk, as I said.

But if this accident fall out, that the blood runs forth at the breasts undigested, not changed by the faculty of the breasts into Milk, as it ought to be, then open the Saphæna vein in the Foot; and that will pull it back again; and cure this Distemper.

There is so near agreement between the breasts and the womb, that any distemper of the womb will change the very colour of the Nipples; and therefore it is not well to prejudicate, and to think they are not Maids when their Nipples change colour, when it is onely a sign that their wombs are distempered.

The Nipples are red after Copulation, red (I say) as a Strawberry, & that is their natural colour: but Nurses Nipples, when they give Suck, are blew, and they grow black when they are old.

If there be pain in the breasts from abundance of milk onely, the pain is not very great, it is onely by overstretching them; but if the milk be sowr, or sharp, or salt, or corroding, the pain is more, and will be greater if there be inflammation; but when there is an Ulcer, or a Cancer, the pains are out of measure great: you may know the cause of the pain by the great-

greatness of it; and you have sufficient directions before how to cure them.

But having made way for it, I shall now proceed to speak a few words of Nurses, and Nursing of Children.

CHAP. V.

How to Chuse a Nurse.

THis dispute about Nurses, who are fit for it, and who are not, is much handled by Physicians; and some there be that will tye every woman to Nurse her own Child, because *Sarah*, the wife to so great a Man as *Abraham*, was, nursed *Isaac*: And indeed if there be no other obstacle the Argument may carry some weight with it; for doubtless the mothers milk is commonly best agreeing with the child; and if the mother do not Nurse her own Child, it is a question whether she will ever love it so well as she doth that proves the Nurse to it as well as Mother: and without doubt the child will be much alienated in his affections by sucking of strange Milk, and that may be one great cause of Childrens proving so undutiful to their Parents.

The *Lacedemepians* chose the youngest son
after

after his Father to succeed in the Kingdom, & rejected all the rest; because the mother gave suck onely to the youngest.

Tacitus gives a reason why the *Germans* are so exceeding strong; because (saith he) they are commonly sucked by their own Mothers.

Yet *Alcibiades*, a strong and valiant Captain, was thought to have come to his great strength, by sucking the breasts of a *Spartan* woman: for they are great, vigorous, and usually very strong women.

I cannot think it alwayes necessary for the mother to give her own Child suck; she may have sore breasts, and many infirmities, that she cannot do it.

Moreover a Nurse ought to be of a good Complexion and Constitution; and if the Mother be not so, it will be good to change the milk by chosing a good wholesome nurse, that may correct the natural humors of the Child drawn from the ill complexion of the Mother.

Many children dye whilest they are sucking the breasts, or else get such Diseases (if the milk be naught) that they can hardly ever be cured, and the chief cause is the Nurses milk. If a Nurse be well complexioned her milk cannot be ill; for a Fig-Tree bears not

Thistles;

Thistles: a good Tree will bring forth good Fruit.

But few can tell, when they see a Nurse, whether her complexion be good or not: wherefore I shall give you such Rules whereby you may be able to know that; and I have gained most of it by my own experience.

Many *Physicians* have troubled themselves and others with unnecessary directions, but the chifest is to choose a nurse of a sanguine complexion, for that is most predominant in children; and therefore that is most agreeing to their age: but beware you choose not a woman that is crooked, or squint-eyed, nor with a mishapen Nose, or body, or with black ill-favoured Teeth, or with stinking breath, or with any notable depravation; for these are signs of ill manners that the child will partake of by sucking such ill qualified milk as such people yield; and the child will soon be squint-eyed by imitation, for that age is subject to represent, and take impression upon every occasion: but a sanguine complexioned woman is commonly free from all these distempers, unless by accident it fall out otherwise; and her milk will be good, and her breasts and nipples handsome, and well proportioned; she is of a mean stature, not too tall, nor too low; not fat,

fat, but well flesht; of a ruddy, merry, cheerful, delightsome countenance, and clear skin'd that her Veins appear through it; her hair is in a mean between black, and white and red, neither in the extream, but a light brown, that partakes somewhat of them all: Such a woman is sociable, not subject to melancholy, nor to be angry and fretful; nor peevish and passionate; but jovial, and will Sing and Dance, taking great delight in children; and therefore is the most fit to Nurse them: whereas all the other tempers, except sanguine, as Flegm, or Choler, or melancholy, breed milk that will agree well with no child; and their own constitutions are not agreeable to the nursing of children: though her complexion then be not exactly sanguine, for that is seldom found, let it suffice if blood be predominant above the rest. Moreover, be her temper naturally never so good, yet if she be diseased she is not for your turn; or if she be above fourty years old, or under eighteen years: she must be of ability to live well, that there be no want; and one that hath had good Education to instruct her; for if she be not well bred, she will never breed the child well: she must have prudence and care to see to it. But there is one rule from the Sex; That a female Child must suck the breasts of a Nurse that had a Girl the last child she had, and a Boy must suck her that lately had a boy. But the Nurse must not company with Man so long as she gives suck to the child, for if she conceive, the child will suffer by it: she must live in a well-tempered pure Air; she must sleep well when she is sleepy, that she may soon wake if the child cry. She must use moderate exercise, and indeed the Dancing and Rocking of the child will hardly suffer her to be idle: and therefore all such as put their children to Nurse, should do well to consider the great care and pains of the Nurse, by well rewarding them, when they have made a good choice: for, if the Nurse be not good, they had better be without them.

Nor is it onely a present Gratification from the Parents that is answerable to the Nurses pains: But children should remember, when they come to years, to be thankful to their Nurses that bred them up, and to requite their great care and pains, having them in little less esteem than their own Mothers that bore them.

The Nurse on the other side must not neglect her Duty, and doubtless some nurses are as fond of their nurse Children as if they were their own.

If the nurse use good Diet and Exercise, it will

will breed good blood, and good blood makes good milk: but let her forbear all sharp, sowr, fiery, melancholy meats; or Mustard, and Onyons, or Leeks and Garlick: and let her not drink much strong drink, for that will enflame the Child, and make it cholerick: all Cheese breeds melancholy, and Fish is Flegmatick. Gross and thick air make gross blood, and heavy bodies, and dull wits. Places that are near the Sea side, and Bogs, are very sickly and unwholsome; but a clear air, that is pure, is as needful as Meat and Drink, it makes the body sprightful, and the reason and understanding ready, good vital and animal spirits are bred by it, whereby all things to reason become more subservient; opinion, fancy, judgement, resolution, apprehension, imagination, memory, knowledge, mirth, hope, trust, joy, urbanity, and what can be said almost are produced: Meats and Drinks feed the body, but the air guides the mind in almost all its actions; and life and health, sickness and death depend most upon it.

If the nurses milk be too hot, Succory, Purslain are good herbs for her to eat; and if it be too cold, then Vervain, and Mother of time, Cinnamon, Borrage and Buglofs, and all wholesome Herbs and Meats and Drinks,

that

that a little exceed in heat mend her milk.

If the child be ill the Nurses milk is commonly the cause of it; if wind oppress the child, let the Nurse but put Fennel seed, and Anniseed into her meats or broths, and the child will be well; but of that more by and by, as I pass on to speak of the diseases and infirmities of children: but before I part with the Nurse it will be but reason to enquire when the Nurse should part with her child, and wean it from the breasts.

I know there can be no general rule for all, because some children are weak, and must stay longer before they be weaned.

Avicenna saith two years is the time children should suck: I have seen some in *England* that have kept their children sucking near four years, who would carry their stool after their Nurses to sit down on to give them suck; but a year old is sufficient to most children; yet they are loth to leave the Dug till they be driven from it.

Breast milk is very sweet, & of good digestion and therefore some that are fallen into consumptions in their riper years, are cured by sucking a wholesome womans breasts: but sucking is not proper for children so soon as they can concoct other nutriment. Milk is for Babes, but strong meat for men.

I have

I have known some women so fond of their children, that they would never wean them by their good will: But when children suck so over-long, as three or four years, I seldome hear of any of them that ever come to good; insomuch that many women have repented of their folly when it was too late. Their children by overcockering, growing so stuborn and unnatural, that they have proved a great grief to their parents.

It seems God sometimes thus punishes women for their folly; and the children thus tenderly bred, for want of stronger meat than breast milk in their child-hood, grow lame, and weak, and sick of the Rickets.

Some women will not be contented with such children as God sends them, but they will be mending the feature of their noses, and their bodies, till they make them very ill favoured, that would have grown in good shape: and some though they have Daughters, will not be contented unless they may have a son.

God sometimes hears their prayers, and sends them a Boy, it may be a Fool, that will be a boy as long as he lives.

I have shewed you that children, be they Boys or Girls, unless they be weak, should not suck the breast above a year; and if it be a nurses breasts, and not the own mother that they suck, it is the same thing for time; yet the Nurse should be chosen as near to the constitution of the mother as possibly you can, for then there will not be so great alteration in the constitution and manners of the child; a Nurse is best after her second child, if she be but between twenty and thirty years of age, her milk must not be above ten months old when you chuse her; nor under two months old, for that will be too new.

If the nurses milk prove ill, she must take a gentle purgation; but if it be to purge the child, it must be very gentle indeed, for that purging quality of the Medicament passeth to the milk, and will operate upon the Child, which cannot otherwise be purged by Physick.

It hath been much argued whether the mother or some other women be best to nurse the child; surely I should think the mother, in all respects, if she be sound and well; because it agrees better with the childs temper; for the milk of the mother is the same with that nutriment the child drew in, in the Womb. But yet it will do good sometimes to change the nurse, if the mothers milk contract any ill qualities, or be too sharp, or salt, or otherwise offensive to the child; for if the child do not take rest well, or cry and complain, doubtless the milk it feeds on is distempered: Good milk is neither too thick nor too thin; too thin is raw and breeds crudities; too thick is hardly concocted by the infant: it must be white and sweet scented; if it smell sowr, or burnt, it will corrupt in the stomach; and so it will if it taste salt, or sowr, or bitter, or have any ill tast: drop a drop of breast milk on your nail, or upon a Glass, and if it shew very white, and neither stick like glew nor run off like water, but be off a middle nature, you may conclude that it is good.

When the blood is too full of Whey it breeds thin milk, which gives little nourishment, and the children by sucking of it fall into Fluxes, and looseness of the belly; and sharp milk makes them scabby: purge away the whey of the blood if it be too hot & cholerick with Rhubarb, otherwise with Mechoachan, or sirrup of Roses: cold and moist breasts are mended by the contraries, that is by hot and dry things: If wheyish humours come from the Liver, that must be mended: hot and dry things (that profit) are bread, well baked with Aniseed, and Fennel seed; Roast-meat, Rice, sweet Almonds: but broth, and Fish and Sallets, and Summer fruits must be avoided: good exercise breeds good
blood

blood; gross diet makes thick and gross milk; and sometimes a hot and dry distemper of the breasts will burn up the thin part of the milk: purge away thick humours from the blood, & eat meats of good digestion, as Veal, Chickens, Kids flesh; and use a moistening and attenuating Diet; Fryed Onions, and all sowr spiced meats, will communicate their qualities to the milk, that you may find both by smell and tast.

Strong passions of anger, or fear will cause chollerick and melancholly milk, which makes the child lean, that it cannnot thrive: Hence come gripings, and wringing pains in the belly, Thrush in the mouth, and Falling-sickness; good wine moderately drank sometimes, will help the ill smell and taste of the milk. Let the Nurse be sure to observe a Diet that is most proper for her milk, and may not corrupt it; and also to avoid all passions and venereous actions during the time she is a nurse; and if for all this the milk prove ill, she must purge away evil qualities, according to my former prescriptions.

CAAP. VI.

Of the Child.

CHildren that look white and pale when they are born, are weak and sickly, and seldome live long, but if it be of a reddish colour all over the body, when it is first born, and this colour change by degrees to a Rose colour, there is no doubt of the child but it may do well: if it cry strongly and clear, it argues a great strength of the breast. Take notice of all the parts of it, and see all be right; and the Midwife must handle it very tenderly and wash the body with warm wine, then when it is dry roul it up with soft cloths, and lay it into the Cradle: but in the swadling of it be sure that all parts be bound up in their due place, and order gently, without any crookedness, or rugged foldings; for infants are tender twigs, and as you use them, so they will grow straight or crooked; wipe the childs eyes often, to make them clean, with a piece of soft linnen, or silk; and lay the arms right down by the sides, that they may grow right, and sometimes with your hand stroke down the belly of the child toward the neck of the bladder, to provoke it to make water; But the first work to be done, so soon as it is born, is to cut the Navel-string, and to bind that up right; I shewed you how to do it before; when the Navel-string is cut off, strew upon it a powder of Bole, Sarcocolla, Dragons blood, Cummin and Myrrh, of each the same quantity, and bind a piece of Cotton, or Wool over it, to keep it from falling off again; and if the child be weak after this, anoint the childs body over with oil of Acorns, for that will comfort and strengthen it, and keep away the cold; wash the child next with warm water; pare your nails, and pick out the filth from the childs nostrils; open the Fundament that it may encline to go to stool, and keep it neither too hot nor too cold, nor in a place that is too light; let not the beams of the Sun or Moon dart upon it as it lieth in the Cradle especially, but let the cradle stand in a darkish and shadowy place, and let the head lie a little higher than the body; for a child that is very young to look upon the light of a candle will make them pore blind, or squint-eyed: So will the light of the Sun; set not a candle behind the head of it, for the child will turn its eyes to the light. Take heed the child be not frighted, for it will soon be fearful if you let it sleep alone, so soon as it

B 3   awakes

awakes and misseth the Nurse; keep it not waking longer than it will, but use means to provoke it to sleep; by rocking it in the cradle, and singing Lullabies to it; carry it often in the arms, and dance it, to keep it from the Rickets and other diseases: let it not suck too much at once, but often suckle it as it can digest it.

After four months let loose the arms, but still roul the breast, and belly, and feet to keep out cold air for a year, till the child have gained more strength. Shift the childs clouts often, for the Piss and Dung, if they lie long in it, will fetch off the skin, and put the child to great pain: you may suffer the child to cry a little, for it is better for the brain and lungs, that are thus opened and discharged of superfluous humours; and natural heat is raised by it; it doth most good before they suck, and when the former suck is digested; but too much crying will cause rheums to fall, and oftentimes the child will be broken bellied by its overstraining: change the breasts as you give suck; sometimes let it draw one, sometimes another; and for the first month let it suck as much as it can, so the stomach be not too full. Give it some pap of barley bread steeped a while in water, and then boiled in milk; children that are lusty may be fed with

this

this betimes, but they must not suck till it be a full hour after it, and thus they should be dieted till they breed teeth. So soon as the teeth come forth, let it eat more substantial meat, that is easily chewed and of quick digestion; also give it Cows milk and broths: let not the child rest too soon upon its legs, for if the legs be weak they will grow crooked, by reason of the weight of their bodies. When the child is seven months old you may (if you please) wash the body of it twice a week with warm water till it be weaned, Let the teeth come forth most part, especially the eye-teeth, before the child be weaned, for those teeth cause great pains when they are breeding, and Feavers, and grievous aking of their Gums proceed from them: the stronger the child is, the sooner he is ready to be weaned; some at twelve months old, and some not till fifteen or eighteen months old; you may stay two years if you please, but use the child to other Food by degrees, till it be acquainted with it. Let the child drink but little wine, that it do not over-heat the blood: the best time to wean the child is either the Spring or the Fall of the Leaf, the *Moon* increasing.

For seven years give the child nourishing meats and an indifferent plentiful diet to make it grow; cocker them not over much, nor provoke them to passions: I cannot tell which may do most hurt. Too much play, as children are prone to, will over-heat the blood; and want of play and idleness will make them dull: Some Parents are too fond of their children, and leave them to their own wills: some are too froward, and dishearten their children; the mean is best for them both, and so they shall be sure to find it.

 I have as briefly as I could, touched upon all occasions for women and their children; and some things may seem to be needless to to tell those that knew them before: but by their leave, they that know some things may be ignorant of other things: what one knew before, it may be another knew not: and what she knew not, another might know.

 There are many things here that most women desire to know: the reason is the same why all meats are eaten, and all *Maids* may be married; for if we all were taken with the same thing, there could be no living in the world.

CHAP.

CHAP. VII.

Of the Diseases that Infants and children are often troubled with.

I. Sometimes the child, so soon almost as it is but new born, will fall into strange throws and convulsions.

Hippocrates divides childrens diseases according to their several ages; Children (new born) are subject to inflammation of the navel after it is cut, to moistness of the Eares, to Coughs and Vomitings, and Ulcers in the mouth; to Feares and watchings. When the Teeth begin to breed, there are Feavers, Convulsions, and Fluxes of the Belly, chiefly when the Eye-Teeth breed: When they grow older the Tonsils are enflamed, the Turnbones of the neck are laxated inwardly, they have short breath, and are troubled with the stone in the bladder, round wormes, and Ascarides, Strangury, Kings-evil, and standing Yards; as they grow, still new diseases come on: as the Measels, Small-pox; some are Tongue-tyed until the Ligament be cut that is too short, and hinders their Speech. Use no strong Vomitings, or purgings, or Glisters to children, nor bleed them; but give them gentle means, such are Suppositories, and mild Glisters, with a little Sugar and Milk: give stronger Physick to the Nurse, if need require, to purge the child: strong medicaments given to the nurse may endanger the child that sucks the breasts; but weak purges are sufficient to do it good. You may give the child a Glister thus; take Mallows, and violet leaves, of each one handful, flowers of violets and camomile of each a small handful, boil them, and take four or five ounces of the decoction, and with four or six drams of sirrup of roses, and half an ounce of oyl of Violets, make it ready to give luke-warm, or something more hot, as it may well endure.

II. If a Child be troubled with flegme, lay it not on the back, for you may soon choak it; but turn it to lie on one side or the other. Keep the belly loose; thrust up a suppository of Castle sope, rubbed over with fresh butter, to make it more smooth & gentle to pass into the body; a spoonful of sirrup of Violets afterwards will force down the flegme: you may, if the child be temperate in heat, mingle half the quantity of sweet Almond oyl, with half so much sirrup of Violets; but rub

the

the belly down with sweet butter, as often as it is undressed.

III. If the childs Codds be swoln, observe whether wind or water be the cause of it; the water will sweat out if you chafe the part with fresh butter: if it be wind swing the child well and dance it, and put the decoction of Anniseeds in their drink: but there may be many causes of the swelling of the Codds; if wind be the cause, the Codds will shew thin as a horn, and be as stiff as a Drums head: too much crying may cause an inflammation, or bursting. If the swelling arise from heat, cooling herbs will cure it; but for wind, boil a handful of bay leaves, of Dill, Camomile, and Fennel, of each a handful, Rue half a handful boil all in a quart of Beer wort to a pint: strain it out hard, and with the liquor boil as much Bean meal as will make a poultis, putting to it two or three spoonfuls of oyl of Camomile, apply it hot to the Codds.

IV. If the childs Fundament slip forth, as it will oftentimes in many children, when they are bound, and strain to go to stool, or have taken cold, or the Muscles are relaxed by moisture, when there is a looseness of the Belly, and a Tenesmus or Needing, then the Muscle

Muscle that bindes up the hole will come forth; if it come from straining it is easily cured at first; but too much moisture causing it, will be hard to overcome, especially when the belly is loose, for then the Medicaments are driven off.

For the cure then; if it be swoln, and will not be put in, bath it first with a decoction of Mallows, and Marshmallows; or annoint it with oyl of Lillies; then try to put it up, having cast some astringents upon it; or take Galls, Acorn cups, Myrtle berries, dryed red Roses, burnt Harts-horn, burnt Allum, and flowers of sowr Pomegranates, of each a like quantity; make a strong decoction in water, and whilest it is warm bath the Gut with it, and put it into its place: and, to make it flag up, spread a little melted wax, Frankincense and Mastick together, upon a Linnen Clout, and lay it to the Fundament, so bind it on, and take it off onely when the child goes to stool: sprinkle the Gut with this following powder: Of red roses and sowr Pomegranate flowers, of each half a dram; Frankincense and mastick of each one dram.

V. If the Infant be too loose bellyed, and cannot contain its Excrements; this proceeds either from breeding of Teeth, and
that

that is usually with a feaver, or from concoction depraved, and the nourishment corrupted, or from much waking, or great pain, or Feaverish humors stirring in the body: or when they drink or suck too much, being over-hot : taking cold may also bring a Looseness; if the Excrements be yellow, and green, and stink, some sharp humor is the cause of it : When children breed teeth it is good to have the belly somewhat loose; but if it exceed it must be stopt, for the child will consume. If the Excrements be black, and the child feaverish, it is an ill sign. But a Sucking child needs not be cured so much as the Nurse; mend her milk, or get another Nurse; and let her avoid green fruit, and Meats of hard digestion. When the child is past sucking, then purge, things that leave a binding quality behind will do it; such are sirrup or honey of red Roses: You may give a Glister of two or three ounces of the decoction of Milium and Myrobolans, with an ounce or two of sirrup of dried red Roses. If it proceed from a hot cause, cleanse first, then give sirrup of dried roses, Quinces, Myrtles, Currants, Coral, Mastick, Harts-horn, or powder of Myrtles, with a little Dragons blood, and annoint the belly with oyl of roses, of Mastick, of Myrtles. In a cold cause the Excre-

ments

ments will be white; then give sirrup of miſlick and Quinces, with mint water; and take half a scruple of Frankincenſe, and of Nutmeg as much, temper it with the juyce of a Quince, and give it the child: Lay a plaiſter to the childs belly, made with the ſeeds of red Roſes, Cummin, Anniſeed, and Smallage, Barley meal, and Juyce of Plantane, with a little Vinegar, boil all together: When the ſtools are red, or yellow, a ſpoonful or two of red Roſe ſirrup, or of Pomegranates, with Mint water, may do much good; or beat some Sorrel-ſeeds to powder, and give it to eat with the yolk of a roaſted Egg; or bruiſe the ſeed, and boil it in fountain water, and let the child drink of it twice a day.

If the child be coſtive and cannot go to ſtool, this comes oftentimes from a cold and dry diſtemper of the Guts, from the birth, or form ſlimy flegme that ſticks to the Guts, and wraps up the Dung: this laſt comes from the milk, when the Nurſe drinks little, or eates hard meats, or aſtringent diet; or elſe it may come from a hot diſtemper of the Kidneys and Liver, that drieth the excrements; or want of choler to provoke expulſion.

A dry diſtemper of the Guts is not eaſily helped: when there wants choler the body looks yellow, and the dung is white, becauſe the choller is gone ſome other way. When the

the child is bound, the Head will ache, and there is pain in the belly: wherefore it is more healthful if the belly be loose, so it be moderate.

A hot distemper is remedied by bathing it often in a bath of boiled Lettice and Succory, to mosten and cool it: In a hot cause use coolers, in a moist drying things; let the nurse abstain from binding meats in dry causes, as from Quinces, Medlars, Pease, Beans; and annoint the stomach and belly of the child with fresh butter, oyl of Lillies, hens grease; if the child be grown give it the decoction of red Coleworts, with a little Honey and salt: Flegme is cured with sirrup of Roses, or with Honey; and to cool, sirrup of Violets is effectual, or emulsions of the four cold seeds: When choler will not come from the Gall to the guts, to move the expulsive faculty, let it drink a decoction of Grass roots, Maidenhair, Fennel, and Sparagus; if it will not yet void the Excrements, make a suppository of Honey boiled hard, let it be as big as a date stone, or a little bigger, and as long as your little finger; or you may make it of the stalks, or roots of Beets, or flower de Luce, dip them in oyl, and thrust it up into the Fundament; lay a piece of wool dipt in oyl to the childes navel, and give it the quantity of a Pease of good honey: When the child sucks give the Nurse a gentle purge to loosen the belly,

belly, if foluble meats will not do it; you may fafely lay a plaifter over the childes belly, made of Mallowes and Marfhmallowes, of each one handful, Holyhocks two ounces, ten Figs, Fenugreek and Linfeed of each one ounce, boil all in water and then ftamp them in a mortar, make it up with butter and hensgreafe, of each two ounces, Saffron one fcruple; fpread it on a Linnen Cloath; or apply to the navel a walnut fhell full of hens-greafe and Oxe Gall, and anoint the belly with foftning things, as with oyl of fweet Almonds and of Linfeed; bran, with the juyce of Dwarf Elder will make a loofning Poultis for the belly.

VI. The child may be troubled with worms that breed in their Guts, fome like mites of Cheefe, and fome like earth worms; and fome children have been obferved to have them in their Mothers bellies, for they have voided them fo foon almoft as they were born: but the chief caufe is by mingling milk with other meats, when the conftitution is hot and moift; or from Summer Fruits, and fweet Meats that worms love. Thefe worms are broad and fmall, or round and long: you may know when they have worms, when their Mouthes water much, and their breath ftinks;

stinks when they gnash their teeth, and start in their sleep, and cry, when they have a dry cough; loath their meat, are very thirsty, when they vomit and hicket, when their bellies swell, and they are much bound, or very loose, when they make thick white water with pain: when their belly is empty, and the worms want meat, their face is covered with a cold sweat, and their cheeks flush with red colour, and suddenly become pale; by this you may know what worms they are, for these signs shew round worms commonly rather than flat: sometimes children have no great hurt by it when they have worms, till the worms grow too strong, and then dangerous symptomes follow. Long round worms are worst, for they will eat quite through the belly; and when there is a Feaver the danger is greater. Those that do least hurt are white; but the fewer and smaller the worms are, the less is the danger.

It is best to eat meats of good juice, with Oranges and Pomegranates, forbearing all slimy sweet fat meats, Fish, and milk, and Summer fruits; and to take some powder of hartshorn, and drink thin wine mingled with Grass and Sorrel waters; these will keep worms that they breed not, which is better than

than to let them breed; and drive them out afterwards.

Keep the childs belly loose with Glisters, when you know they have worms; or give them the decoction of Sebestens before meat; Scordium and Wormwood are good, but children will not be perswaded to take bitter medicaments; wherefore you may give them Grass water, with juice of Lemmons, or one or two drops of Spirit of Vitriol.

These things following will kill Worms, and cast them forth; eight grains of *Mercurius Dulcis* steept all night in Couch-grass water, strain it finely, and give nothing but the water. Wormseed, Harts-horn, or Coralline are good; lay Peach-leaves bruised to the Navel, or a little Ox Gall; Saint Johns wort, and Wormwood; Knot-grass water drank with milk; Ox Gall and Cummin-seed laid to the Navel are good against great worms; mingle with your juice of Wormwood, and Ox Gall of each two ounces, of Coloquintida one ounce, made into a Cataplasme with Wheat meal, lay it over the Belly and Navel. If there be a Feaver withal use such cooling remedies as are here prescribed against a Feaver; you must use several medicaments, for the worms will quickly grow familiar with any medicament, and will not stir for it: the best time to administer

minister your remedies is about the new, or full of the Moon, for then they will sooner move than in the quarters; let the child be fasting, and go to stool first if he can, and give the medicament to destroy the Worms when they are hungry, , and the time the child (that is of age) is wont to eat his breakfast, for the worms will look for it.

VII. Sometimes children have Convulsion Fits, and the Falling-sickness; it is natural to some from their birth, but others have it by accident; the nurses ill milk may breed it, let her cleanse her body, and not use too much moist and cooling diet; nor let the child suck too much at one time, to over-charge the stomach. The Male-Peony root hanged about the childs neck, and a small quantity of the powder of the same given to the child (in any convenient way) with milk, or pap, or broth, or drink is much commended, and so is the seed: it is good for the child to smell to Rue, and Assafætida, and sometimes rub the Nostrils with a drop of oil of Castor, or of Costus; it may proceed from ill milk in the childs stomach, or by consent from other parts, or from worms in the Guts, or from ill vapours that ascend where bad humours abound: These prick the Films of the brain, and cause the childs distemper; it may be originally

nally bred in the brain, or arise from some sudden fright, or from breeding of teeth; this last will be gone when the pain of the teeth is over.

Many young children die of this disease it may come with the Small Pox or Measles, and when they come forth it will be cured, if nature be strong; the Nurses good diet is a great furtherer to the cure: in the fit you may give Peony or Lavender Water, and rub the Nape of the neck with a drop of oil of Amber, and touch the Nose with it; an Elks hoof, or an Emrald are useful to hang about the neck, and may be given inwardly.

If it proceed from corrupt milk in the stomach, dip a feather in oil of Almonds, and thrust it down the Throat to cause vomit.

The *Florentines* with a hot Iron burn the child in the nape of the neck to dry the brain; and *Celsus* maintains it to be the very last remedy.

But *Paulus Æquinita* saith, It would be sure to kill him with waking pain; he would scarce be able to sleep after it.

To prevent this mischief, so soon as the child is born give him this following powder; male-Peony roots, one scruple, gathered in the Moons decreasing, magistery of Coral half a scruple, with Leaf God.

VIII.

VIII. Convulsion Fits come when the brain labours to cast off what offends it; many die of it, for the cause lieth in the nerves and marrow of the back; wherefore wash the body and back with a decoction of Marshmallows, Lilly roots, Peony and Cammomile flowers: The Sun-flower boiled in water is good to wash the Infant with, and annoint the back with mans grease, or Goose grease, or with oils of Foxes, or of worms, or of Lillies, or of Mastick, or Turpentine: This disease comes either of indigestion, or of weakness of the attractive faculty, especially in such children as are fat and moist; the back may be anointed with oils of Rue, or of Flower de Luce; or bath the Limbs with a decoction of Primroses, or of Cowslips, or Cammomile flowers; if you find great heat then mingle oil of Violets, and oil of sweet Almonds, and anoint with that.

IX. Sometimes the childs navel swells, and sticks out, that should lie in; the reason may be because the navel-string was not well tied, and too much of it was left behind which sticks forth, sometimes it may come from the childs crying, or coughing, and that looseneth the Peritonæum, it is without inflammmation: but sometimes the navel hath an Ulcer, and the Guts fall into it. It falls out often so soon as the string is cut, wherefore take Spike and seeth it in oil of sweet Almonds, mingle a little Turpentine with it, dip in a piece of Wool, and bind it on the part: but if crying, or coughing, or bruise, or fall, be the cause of it, then use bitter Lupines mingled with the powder of an old Linnen cloth burnt to ashes, mingle all with red wine, dip in Cotton and apply it to the Navel: if the navel be inflamed the Navel feels hard, else it will feel soft, and is neither hot nor red, but will last longer than when it is enflamed: if the Peritonæum be loose only, and not broken, it will be no bigger when he cryeth, nor doth the Navel come forth much; but it will increase if it be broken, if he either cry or stir much, but it will not be seen when he lieth on his back: ill cutting of the Navel string is not so much dangerous, as it is troublesome to the child; it may be cured at first, though it be too long, or hath an Ulcer; but in time, if it be neglected, the guts will fall into it, and cause inflammation, and an Illack passion, which will kill the child: wind puffs up the Navel when the Peritonæum is loose; then take the powder of Cummin-seed, Bay berries and Lupines, with red wine; or a bag of Spike and Cummin-seeds boiled in red wine

for

for a Cataplasme, and roul it on.

If the Peritonæum be broken, let the gut be first put in, then lay on astringent Powders of Cypress-nuts, Mirrh, Frankincense, Sarcocolla, Mastick, Allum, and Isinglass, of each a like quantity, and make a Poultiss of it with Whites of eggs: give the child inwardly such remedies as are good against Ruptures. When the Navel is inflamed, it looks red, and is hard, hot and pants much; this shews it was not well tied, for the pain draws the blood to it: If it turns to an Imposthume and break, the guts will come out, and kill the child. To ease the pain take two ounces of Mallows boiled and stampt, Barley meal half an ounce, with two drams of Lupines and Fenugreek, make a Cataplasme of them with oil of Roses; drive back the blood with an application, made of one dram of Frankincense, with Fleabane seed, and Acacia of each half a dram, incorporated with the white of an egg: Keep it if possible, from imposthumation: but if it cannot be kept, then take half an ounce of Turpentine, two ounces of oil of Roses, and with the Yolk of an Egg lay it on.

X. If the child be burst, as young children often are, it may be easily cured at first, the Peritonæum

Peritonæum is either loose or broken, and the small guts fall into the Cods; when the child coughs much, or cries, or by some violent fall, or straining to go to stool; elder people are not so easily cured of this. Sometimes it is only a rupture which falls out of the belly into the Cods, and the Peritonæum is well.

If a Gut be fallen, it is but of one side the right or left Groin, and you may see it and feel it, and the hole too through which the Gut fell; but the watry rupture is all over, even alike; this will vanish of it self so soon as the water is consumed. Keep the child loose, and from crying and violent motion; lay it upon the back, and thrust up the gut gently, the head lying low, and the heels up; then take *Emplastrum ad Herniam*, or an ointment made of Comfrey roots, with a thick bolster steeped in Smiths water, and lay it on: keep the child quiet, and see the Bolster come not off; never unbind it, so in time the hole will grow narrow, and the gut larger, and will stay in its place.

You may lay on a Plaister made of *Gum Elemi* steept in vinegar, till there be a cream on the top, with that and oil of eggs make it up; or take Frankincense one dram, Aloes, Acacia, Cypress nuts of each two drams, with a dram of Myrrh and Isinglass make a Plaister.

The watry rupture is cured with oil of Elder, of Bays and of Rue; or else make a Cataplasme of Bean flower, Fenugreek, Linseed, Cummin seed, Cammomile flowers, and the oils aforesaid.

XI. Sometimes children are weak, that they are long before they can go; wherefore it is good to strengthen their legs and thighs, that they may be able to go betimes; and that may be done thus, take the juice of Marjoram, of Sage, and of Danewort an equal quantity of each; fill a glass viol with these juices, and with Past lute it round; and when you set in houshold bread in the oven, then set in your glass, when you draw it forth break the glass, and save the ointment you shall find in it; melt this with some Neats-foot oil, and rub the Childs Legs and Thighs with it, on the hinder parts.

XII. Children have many diseases, that chiefly happen about the head outwardly, as many ulcerous risings and pushes, which come chiefly from the Nurses ill milk; wherefore purge the nurse, and give the child some sirrup of Borrage, or of Fumitory; bath the Scabs with softening decoctions, then dry them with *Album Camphoratum*.

If these milky Scabs called Achores and Favi be not well cured, they turn to a Scald, or scabby stinking Ulcer, called Tinea a moth, because like a moth it will fret as they eat Garments.

The milk scab comes at the first sucking, and after that the Achores, which are scabs that are not white, and are only upon the head; but the white scabs run over all the face and the body: Those Ulcers in the head especially still run with matter; they are of several colours, as white, red, yellow, black; but they all come from excrementitious, watery, salt, thick, and thin humours, that itch, and make them to scratch; they were gathered in the womb, and bad milk increaseth them, in time they cure themselves, if the cause be not too bad, but if the matter be too fierce, it will pierce the Scull; when it runs it doth children good, if it stink it may cause the Falling sickness.

Carduus and Scabius water, and good cordials will drive them out; coolers and binders are naught, for they strike them in.

The nurse must keep a good diet, and prepare her self with Buglofs, Borrage, Fumitory, Succory, Hops, Polypody, and Dock roots; then purge with Senna, Epithymum and Rhubarb; forbear salt, spiced, and sharp meats

meats: Conserve of Succory roots and Citrons candied of each half an ounce; of Borrage, Bugloss, Violets, Fumitory, and Succory, of each one ounce; Harts-horn, Diarrhodon, Diamargariton frigid, of each a scruple, make an Electuary with sirrup of Gilliflowers; let the nurse take daily two drams.

Purge the child with Manna; wash the Head with a decoction of Mallowes, Barley, Wormwood, Celandine, Marshmallow roots boiled in barley water, and boys piss; make an ointment to use after it with oyl of bitter Almonds, oyl of Roses, and some Litharge: or wash the head with Soap, if you fear it may turn to a Scald head, or eat into the skull; and then with the former decoction: or take Ceruss, Litharge of each two drams; of Agarick and Pomegranate flowers of each one dram, oyl of Roses and Vinegar make an oyntment.

If it come to be a Scald head, it is a dry Ulcer in the head onely, called Tinea; but Achores are moist Ulcers in the head and body sometimes.

A Scald head is infectious, it proceeds from a salt sharp melancholick humor, from the Mothers blood, or from corrupt Milk: These Scabs are like bran sometimes, or Scurf, with Scales; sometimes slimy; and when the

Scab

Scab comes off you shall see red quick knobs of flesh, like the in-side of a fig, some of them are malignant; they run but little, but that which comes forth stinks much. An old, black or ash-coloured scab is hard to cure; the other is not so when it is new, and yellow matter comes from it; The hair will scarce ever come again when it is cured, the skin is so exceeding hard; rub the skin and if it will not seem red, there is no hopes of hair. The salt humours make the skin thick and dry, wherefore it will be good to moisten with laying on a Beet, or a Colewort leaf spread with Hogs grease, and remove the scab with such things as cleanse and are somewhat sharp.

When the child comes to age, and is able to bear it, purge with Senna, Rhubarb, and Agarick, then take Brimstone two drams, Mustard half a dram, Briony roots, and Staves-acre, of each one dram, Vinegar one ounce, Turpentine and Bears grease of each half an ounce; this ointment will make the scab fall: or if you beat Hogs-grease, and Water-cresses together, and lay it on the scab, it will fall off in four and twenty hours: when the scab is fallen use a pitcht Cap to pull out the hair by the roots; then use softeners to correct the dry distemper.

Apply things that will consume the excrements

ments that lie deep in the skin; as take one ounce of each of these following roots, of Docks, Lillies, and Marshmallows; of Mallows, Fumitory, Sage, of each two handfuls, and boil all in vinegar, and Ly, and wash the head daily with it. Then make a Cerot of Tar and Wax; or take salt-Peter one ounce, Oxymel one ounce and a half; or mingle with Hogs grease live Brimstone one ounce, with Hellebore, and Staves-acre, of each two drams; but beware of poisons, such as are Arsenick, or Pigment, or Mercury, for they are dangerous to corrode the part that lieth so near the brain.

XIII. Sometimes childrens heads swell with water, and are very big; the water is either without the skul, or within the skul; for this water lieth either between the skin, and the *pericranium*, or between the bone and the *pericranium*; or between the bone and the membranes, called the *Dura* and *Pia Mater*. Sometimes abundance of vapours get between the bones and skin of the head, & make the head so great, that they kill the child; if it be water the child will be giddy, and have Epileptick fits, nor can it rest. If it be only, wind between the skin and the *pericranium* a decoction of Sage, Betony, Calamint,

lamint, and Origanum, of each one handful, of Anniseeds and Fennel seeds of each two drams, with a handful of Cammomile flowers, and of Melilot and red roses the like quantity boiled in water with some wine will cure it. The watry humour is hardly cured. A humour from water within the brain is smaller and harder than when it is out of the skull, but it is more hard to cure, and almost incurable. A humour of wind is seldome without water that breeds it; apply discussers that make the humours thin, to the head, the nose, and the ears; as Cammomile, Rue, and Origanum. Take thirty snails in their shells, of Mugwort, and Marjoram of each one handful, stamp them, then put to them Saffron half a dram, and a scruple of Camphire, and make a poultiss with oil of Cammomile: Also take Nutmegs, Cubebs, Cloves of each one scruple; Frankincense Bark, Calamus, of each half a dram; Marjoram water three ounces, snuff up this water often, and drop hot oils into the ears. If the water be not dissipated in twenty daies, you must open the skull, and let out the water by degrees; and beware that the child take no cold: If such means as are outwardly applied will not help it, the last remedy is by the Chirurgion.

XIV

XIV. Sometimes children are much vexed with the Hiccough, or Hickets, or Huchets as they call it, it comes commonly from too much repletion, and fulness; wherefore dip a feather in oil, and put it down the childs Throat and make it vomit: It may come from a cold stomach; then anoint the stomach with oil of Cammomile, of Wormwood, of Mastick and Quinces, and dissolve a scruple of the Troches of Diarrhodon in the Nurses Milk, and give it the child.

If this disease come from too much Milk, the belly swells, and the child vomits: if the Nurses Milk be bad, it comes from thence: and the Excrements will smell of stinking Milk.

This is no dangerous disease unless the cause be violent, for then it will flie to the Nerves, and cause a Convulsion, Falling sickness and death.

Give the child sirrups of Mints and Betony, to strengthen the stomach, and anoint it with oil of Mints, of Mastick, and of Dill.

There is a disease like the Hickets in children, from grief, or anger, when the spirits flie from the Heart to the Midriff, and stop the breath, but it is soon over.

XV. Chil-

XV. Children are sometimes subject to vomiting from too much, or from ill milk, or from flegm that falls from the head to the stomach; a moist loose stomach is the immediate cause; if they vomit *milk* they are better for it: if the *milk* be naught, the matter that comes forth will shew that, for it is yellow, green, or filthy coloured, and it stinks.

Worms may make them vomit, but that will be known by the signs: children that vomit often are best in health, and thrive best, because their stomach is kept clean of ill humours; but to vomit too much will make them waste away: cleanse the stomach with honey of Roses, and strengthen it with sirrup of Quinces, and of Mints.

When the humour is too sharp and hot, give the sirrup of Pomegranates, or of Coral, or of Currants: Coral hath a hidden vertue, and some hang it about their necks.

Anoint the stomach with oils of Mastick, Mints, Quinces, Wormwood, of each half an ounce; oil of Nutmegs (by expression) half a dram; oil of Mints chymically extracted three drops; or dip bread in hot Wine, and lay it to the mouth of the stomach.

XVI. If

XVI. If the child be griped, and pained in the belly, you shall know it by the great unquietness, and crying, and turning it self from side to side; it is oft with a scowring, and from bad milk, that breeds sharp windy humours; it gets to the guts and gnaws them; and sometimes it is from worms: if it be wind it will cease when they break wind; but ill humors cause a constant pain. Tough flegm binds the belly, and the Dung is slimy: sharp humours cause a green and yellow flux; if this pain last long, it casts them into convulsions, and falling-sicknesses, and is dangerous: Foment the belly with a decoction of Lavender, Fennel, and Cummin seed; or take oil of Olives, and Dill seed, and dip a piece of Wool in it, and lay it over the belly warm.

Give the child some oil of sweet Almonds, with Sugar-Candy, and a scruple of Annifeeds; and purge it with Honey of Roses, which is good also when the body is swoln with wind, or too much milk not digested: and use a decoction of Cardiaca, Cammomile flowers, and Cummin seed; or boil the top of dwarf-Elder, and of Elder in white wine, and bath the parts that are swoln with it.

If the griping pain comes from the sharp milk

milk; firrup of Succory with Rhubarb, or firrup, or Honey of Roses; or a Glister of the decoction of bran, and Pellitory of the wall, with firrup of Roses is very good, using an outward Ointment of oil of Dill, and Cammomile.

XVII. Sometimes children will sneeze mightily, it may come from an imposthume in the head; then cooling oils and ointments are commended; but if any other cause produce it, put the powder of Bazil into the nostrils.: If heat cause it the childs eyes will sink in; then bruise Purslain leaves, and with oil of Roses, Barley meal, and the yolk of an egg mingled, make an Application to the Head.

XVIII. When the child is Feaverish and hot, the nurse must eat cooling and moistening things; and anoint all the parts of the child with oil of Roses, and Unguent Populeon; and lay to the breasts clarified juice of Wormwood, Plantane, Mallows, Seagreen, made to a Cataplasme of Barley meal.

XIX. It falls oftentimes out that children are squint-eyed, and that comes when they lie in their Cradle, and the Candle, or light

stands

stands behind them, or on one side: It may come from the Falling-sickness, or by birth, but that is seldome and not curable: if ill custom have bred it, put your candle on the other side, or a Picture, till the childs eyes come to look right; but you may prevent all if you set the candle before the child, and not on either side, for the child will stare after the light; you may when you find the childs eyes distorted, hang cloths of all colours on the other side, to make the child to turn the eyes the contrary way, to gaze on them till it be cured.

XX. Sometimes children have sore eyes with great pain, with Ulcers, and Worms, and inflammations; for childrens brains are very moist, and there are many excrements which nature casts forth at other places, because the natural Emunctories will not carry them all out; much of this goes to their ears, which will be very sore, that they will cry, and not suffer them to be touched; it is dangerous, for it will not let them sleep, the heat and pain is so great; it causeth the Falling-sickness, and fouls the spongy bones, and breeds Worms, and sometimes makes children deaf so long as they live; you cannot use strong remedies to children; drop a little hemp seed oyl with

Wine

Wine into their ears; to allay the pain, use warm milk about their ears, or oil of Violets, or the decoction of Poppey tops: to dry up the moisture use honey of Roses, or water of honey to drop in their ears.

XXI. The usual painful disease of all children is the breeding of their teeth; it is very dangerous to some: about the seventh month, first come forth the fore teeth, then the ey-teeth; lastly the grinders: first the Gums itch, then they prick like needles, by reason of the sharp bones, which causeth watchings, and inflammations of the Gums, Feavers, Convulsions, Scourings; especially when they breed their eye-teeth. The beginning of the seventh month is the time that discovers it, and the childs putting his finger into his mouth, and holding the nipple faster than they were wont; when the tooth is coming forth, the Gum is whiter than in other parts: the watching breeds cholerick humours, and inflames the body, and brings a Feaver.

If the teeth be long before they can come forth, children commonly will die of Feavers, and Convulsion fits: they that scowr have seldome any Convulsion.

When the gums are thick, the teeth can scarce get forth; wherefore soften the Gum with

with rubbing it with Honey and Fresh Butter; or let the child chew a candle of Virgins Wax: Let the Nurse keep a moderate Diet, inclining to cold, as Barley Broths, Water-Gruel, Lettice, Endive, Rear-eggs: take heed of salt spiced meats, and wine; but anoint the childs Gum with a Mucilage of Quinces, made with Mallows water, or with the brains of an Hare.

XXII. If the Gums be ulcerated, let the Nurse rub the childs gums, and Wheals, and Pushes with her finger, and anoint them with Hens grease, Hares brains, oil of Cammomile, and Mel Rosarum, or sirrup of violets, with Plantane water; and if the inflammation be great, boil Pomegranate flowers, Roses, and Sanders of each two drams, Allum half a dram, in water, strain out three ounces, and dissolve in it the sirrup of Mulberries half an ounce. If the Pushes and Wheals be white, take Pomegranate flowers, Amber, Cypress nuts of each two drams, Roses, and Myrtle flowers of each half a handful, boil them in water, add to the decoction one ounce and a half of honey of Roses. Sometimes there riseth between the Gums, and the great teeth a little fleshy substance, to consume that wash it with a deccoction of the roots of Plantain, Bugloss, Agrimony of each a handful, Barley a small handful, and red Roses a handful; four Dates, Flowers of Pomegranates two drams, Liquorish one dram and a half.

XXIII. Children are very much molested with destillations, Coughs, and Catarrhs: if the humour be sharp and hot that falls from the brain, the child will look red in the face; if it be a cold humour much matter will run forth at the nose and mouth; then keep the child resonably warm, and give it Sugar-candy, with oil of sweet Almonds: wash the childs feet with Ale boiled with Betony, Marjoram, Rosemary, then anoint the soles of the feet with Goose grease: rub the breast with fresh butter, and oil of sweet Almonds, and lay on warm linnen cloths; for slimy humours give it a spoonful of sirrup of Maiden-hair, or of Liquorish and Hyssop mingled; Take also Gum Traganth, Arabick, Quince seeds, juice of Liquorish, and Sugar Pelets, mingle them, and in new milk let the child take of it every day. Where the cause is cold that makes the Cough; beat a little Myrrh to powder and give it the child, with oil of sweet Almonds, and a little honey: when it comes from heat, make a decoction of Raisins in water, and with white poppey seed, and Gum Dragant

each

each two drams; seeds of Gourds four drams, beat all together, and give the child a four penny weight in the foresaid decoction.

XXIV. If the breath be short let it take an Electuary of Honey and Linseed, and anoint the ears and parts about them with Olive oil.

XXV. If the childs nose be stopt, put a little Ointment of Roses, and good Pomatum into the Nostrils to soften the hard matter.

Wash the inflamed, or Gummy eyes, that will not open, with breast milk, or Plantain and Rose Water: Childrens moist brains breed moist humours that run to their ears; make them clean with a rag, and drop in Honey of Roses mingled with oil of bitter Almonds.

XXVI. If the child new born be in great pain, then rub it with Pellitory of the Wall and fresh Butter, or with Spinach and Hogsgrease, and lay it to the Navel, take care it be not too hot; or make a cake of oils of eggs and of Nuts for the Navel; give it a Glister if it need with Milk, Sugar, and the yolk of an Egg.

XXVII. Chil-

XXVII. Children are subject to all sorts of Feavers, but chiefly to Feavers from corrupt milk, and Feavers with breeding of teeth.

They have epidemical Feavers sometimes that cast forth the Meazles, or small Pox; the mothers menstrual blood is the original cause, but the corrupt air stirs it up; for as the air is pure, or impure, so these diseases are more raging, or less: It is oftentimes infectious, and the humours so corrupt, that worms breed under the scabs, and corrode the bones and inward parts, as hath been proved by opening some that died. If it be a Feaverish time, that it spreads much, give good Antidotes, and change the air; but all children almost will have them first or last: Before there is a Feaver you may fortifie nature, and give a gentle purge; but for my part I approve not of purging, or bleeding in these distempers, unless it be long before: So soon as you see the feaver, drive them out by Cordials, and prefer the eyes and throat, and prevent deformity.

The first signs of this disease (for they are both from one cause) are pains of the head, redness in the eyes, a dry Cough with a feaver, then little pimples break forth all the body over; but chiefly they aim at the throat and face.

The

The small Pox is dangerous to all, but most to those that are of an ill habit of body; and if they come forth in heaps and not orderly; or if they look blew, black, or ill coloured, they are exceeding dangerous. If the child suck, the nurse must use a moderate diet; she may eat Hen broth, with herbs of Succory, Borrage, Buglos, and Endive boiled in it: Let her drink this drink following to make them come easily and quickly forth; take peeled Lentils half an ounce, fat figs two ounces, Gum Lac two drams, Gum Traganth and Fennel seed of each two drams and a half; boil this in fountain water, strain it, and sweeten two pints of it with Sugar, and sirrup of Maiden-hair, let her drink half a pint fasting. If the child be weaned give it a Julep of cordial waters two ounces and a half, sirrup of Lemmons one ounce, use this often; and four or five hours after, give it some Unicorns horn and Oriental Bezoar in powder.

To preserve the eyes anoint the Eye-lids with Plantane and Rose water, and a little Saffron: To preserve the nose take Rose water, and Betony of each one ounce, Vinegar half an ounce, and as much powder of peels of Citrons, add to it Saffron six grains, let the child smell to it often; dip some cotton in it, and stop the ears to keep the Small Pox from

from thence. You may preserve the mouth, the tongue, and the throat with a handful of barley, and leaves of Plantain, Sorrel, Agrimony, and of Vervain, of each a handful, all boiled in water to six ounces, dissolve in it sirrup of Pomegranates, and of Roses of each half an ounce, Saffron half a scruple, make a Gargarisme: sirrup of Juniper, of Violets, and of water-Lillies preserve the Lungs.

When the Pox are fully out, then to make them die quickly rub the face with fresh hogs-greafe, old Lard melted, and strained, and mingled with water, or with oil of sweet Almonds.

When the Pox are dead, and begin to fall away, to keep them from Pock-holes anoint the face with a feather dipt in an Ointment made of Chalk and Cream, use this two or three daies, it will smooth the skin handsomely, and take away the spots.

XXVIII. Children are exceedingly prone to breed Lice more than men of age, though all people are troubled with them: They breed from the Excrements of the head and body; it is not only filth that breeds Lice, but a certain matter fit for them; for fleas will not breed of the same that lice are bred of. Children and women that are hot and moist have many excrements to breed such things withall. Some meats breed Lice, as figs by their gross juice, which naturally tends to the skin, and variety of meat. Lice breed most in Childrens heads, and stick fast to the skin, and roots of the hair; some have died of Lice: and Lice will leave some when they are dying. To prevent Lice comb and keep childrens heads clean, let them eat no figs, but meats of good juice, and purge them with hot drying, thin medicaments: Use no Mercury, nor Arsenick to childrens heads, but use this Lotion, take parts alike, of round Birthwort, Lupines, Pine and Cypress leaves, boil them in water, then anoint the head with powder of Staves-acre three drams, of Lupines half an ounce, of Agarick two drams, quick brimstone one dram and half, Ox Gall half an ounce, all made up with oil of Wormwood.

XXIX. If the child fright in the sleep, give it good breast milk, but not too much; let it not sleep presently, but carry it about till the milk descend to the bottom of the stomack: give it sometimes the oil of sweet Almonds, or honey of Roses two spoonfuls. To cleanse the stomack strengthen it with magistery of Coral, or Confection of Jacinths with milk

milk; anoint the stomach with oil of Wormwood, Nard, Mints, Mastick, Nutmegs; if it be from worms, you have the remedies before: It is for the most part ill vapours that ascend by the Weasand and veins to the head, when children cannot concoct what they have in their stomachs.

XXX. Sometimes children cannot sleep, it is by reason of corrupt milk that disturbs the animal spirits; hence arise Catarrhs, Convulsions, Feavers, driness; let better milk be given it; the Nurse must eat Lettice, sweet Almonds, Poppey seeds, but sleeping medicaments are not good for infants. Wash the feet with a decoction of Dill tops, Cammomile flowers,, Sage, Osiers, Vine leaves, Poppy-heads; to the Temples use oil of Dill, or oil of Roses, with oil of Nutmegs, with Poppey seeds, Breast milk, Rose, or Nightshade water, with Saffron. If the Childs brain be very dry, moisten the covering of the Cradle.

XXXI. Bad and sharp milk hurts the childs stomach, for it cannot endure it, for it breeds bad humours: all these diseases spring from it, the Thrush, Bladders in the Gums, and inflammation of the Tonsils.

Bladders in the Gums are cured with powder of Lentils husked, and strewed upon them; or with a Liviment of the flour of Milian, and oil of Roses.

The inflammation of the Tonsils (I suppose) it is, that disease in children called the Mumps, that commonly comes between eleven and thirteen years old; the parts being then so hard, that the humour cannot breath forth: alwaies keep the belly loose, and anoint outwardly with oil of sweet Almonds, or Cammomile, or St. *John*'s wort inwardly; first repel, secondly mix resolvers with repellers, and lastly only resolvers, but not too hot; in age Gargarismes are best. Infants may take Diamoron, Honey of Roses, sirrup of Myrtles and Pomegranates.

XXXII. Sometimes childrens string of the tongue is so short that they cannot suck, a skilful Chirurgeon must help it: or use this Liviment; boil clarified honey till you can powder it, then dry yolks of eggs in a Glass in an Oven, powder them, take a dram weight, Mastick and Frankincense, of each one scruple, burnt Allum six grains, make it up with honey of roses. The Frog is, when the veins under the tongue swell with gross black blood; and if the flegm sweat forth, and stick in the

passages

passages, the swelling is like Mushromes, and make them stammer; take Cuttlebone, Sal-gem, Pepper of each one dram, burnt Spunge three drams, make a powder; or of Honey of Besome; rub it under the tongue, and lay a plaister of Goose dung, and Honey boiled in Wine till the Wine be consumed, under the Chin.

XXXIII. Some children grow lean, and pine away, and the cause is not known; if it be from Witchcraft, good prayers to God are the best remedy: yet some hang Amber, and Coral about the childs neck, as a Soveraign Amulet. But leanness may proceed from a dry distemper of the whole body, then it is best to bath it in a decoction of Mallows, Marshmallows, Branc-Ursine, Sheeps heads, and anoint with oil of sweet Almonds; if it be hot and dry add Roses, Violets, Lettice, Poppey-heads, and afterwards anoint with oils of Violets, and Roses. The child may be lean from want of milk, or bad milk from the nurse, remedy that, or change the nurse; for little, or bad milk will breed no good blood, and the children cannot thrive by it: sometimes worms in the body draw away the nourishment, sometimes very small worms breed without the body, all over, and in the Musculous

lous parts, and stick in the skin, and will not come quite forth; but after you rub the child in a Bath they will put forth their heads like black hairs, and run in again when they feel the cold air; they breed of slimy humours, shut up in the Capillary veins, which turn to worms for want of transpiration;if you rub the child with Yarhound on the back,and especially with Honey and Bread, you shall see their black heads; when you see the heads come forth,run over them with a Rasor,do it often.

XXXIV. Children used to be galled with lying in piss'd clouts, and the scarf skin comes from the true skin; the skin looks red, change the clouts often, and keep the child clean by washing it, then anoint the sore with Diapompholix, or cast on this powder finely sprinkled, of burnt Allum, Frankincense, Litharge of Silver, and seeds and leaves of Roses.

XXXV. Some children cannot hold their water, but piss the bed when they sleep, the bladder-closing muscle being weak; so when piss pricks it, it comes forth. The stone in the bladder may hurt the Muscle; the cause of weakness is a cold moist humour, from superfluity, or from tough and gross meats; in

Age

Age it will be hard to be cured; but in infants it easily may. The nurse must use a hot drying diet, with Sage, Hyssop, Marjoram; the child must drink little, anoint the region of the bladder outwardly with oil of Costus, or Flower de luce, and other like driers; use Sulphur and Allum Baths, with oaken leaves: And give it this powder, take burnt Hogs-bladders, Stones of a Hare roasted, and Cocks throats roasted, of each half a dram, and two scruples of Acorns, Mace and Nip of each a scruple, give half a dram with Oaken leave Water.

XXXVI. Childrens Urine is sometimes stopt, either by gross matter, or the stone; you may try with the Catheter; you must purge the humours with honey of Roses, Cassia, Turpentine, with a decoction of red Peaso, also Grass-water, and Restharrow, and Dropwort water are good; take Hares blood one ounce, Saxifrage roots six drams, calcine them, the Dose is a scruple, of half a dram, with White-Wine, and Saxifrage Water. The Stone in the bladder is as common with children as the Stone of the Kidneys with men and women, crude gross meats and unclean milk breed it; there is also a weakness in the Liver and stomach when they do not well part gross blood from the pure, but much earthy juice remains in the child; sometimes it is natural from the Parents; they piss by drops, and what comes forth is like clear water, or whey, or milk, and sometimes blood comes forth; it grows daily, and at last they must be cut if they be not cured in time. Let then the belly be alwaies kept loose, and the nurse eat no slimy gross meats; anoint the bladder with oil of Lillies, and of Scorpions, and lay on a Cataplasme of Pellitory of the Wall boild in oil of Lillies, or give two drops of Spirit of Vitriol, with half a dram of Cypress Turpentine. Take Magistery, or Crabs eyes, white Amber prepared, Goats blood of each a scruple; give it frequently, with water of Parsley.

XXXVII. There is one disease more I shall end with, and that is called Siriasis, an inflammation of the membranes of the brain; it is from phlegmatick blood putrified, and grows hot and cholerick; hot weather, windy milk, and nurses ill diet may cause it: The forehead grows hot & hollow, the face is red, they are dry & Feaverish, want an appetite. The fore part of the head is hollow, where the sagittal and Coronal Sutures meet, for there the bones are membranous, and harden in time; it is

dangerous

dangerous and some say deadly. When this bone or membrane falls there is a pit and the brain falls down, they commonly die in three daies. Give a glister of sirrup of Roses, or Violets, lay on coolers of the juice of Lettice, Gourd, Melons, or split a Pompion in two pieces, and lay it on, but cool not the brain too much, anoint it with oil of Roses, let the Nurses diet be cooling, or change her for a better. Take oil of Roses half an ounce, Populeon one ounce, the white of an egg, and an emulsion of the cold seeds drawn with Rose water two drams; after the inflammation is abated, and the flux stopt, lay on oil of Cammomile one ounce and a half, of Dill hal half an ounce, with the yolk of an egg.

Thus by the blessing of Almighty God, I have with great pains and endeavour run through all the parts of the *Midwives* Duty; and what is required both for the *Mother*, the *Nurse*, and the *Infant*; desiring that it may be as useful for the end I have written it, to profit others, as I have found it beneficial to Me in my long *Practice* of *Midwifery*. To God alone be all Praise and Glory, *Amen.*

FINIS

Books Printed for, or Sold by Simon Miller, at the Star, at the West-end of S. Pauls.

Quarto.

PHysical Experiments, being a plain description of the causes, signs and cures of most diseases incident to the body of man; with a discourse of Witch-craft: by *William Drage* Practitioner of Physick, at *Hitchin* in *Hartfordshire*.

Bishop *White* upon the Sabbath.

The Artificial Changeling.

The Life of *Tamerlane* the Great.

The Pragmatical Jesuit, a play; by *Richard Carpenter*.

The Life and Death of the Valiant and Renowned Sir *Francis Drake*, His Voyages and Discoveries in the *West-Indies*, and about the World; with his Noble and Heroick Acts. By *Samuel Clark* late Minister of *Bennet Finck London*.

Large Octavo.

Master *Shepherd* on the Sabbath.

The Rights of the Crown of *England* as it is Established

Established b͟y Law; by *E. Bagshaw* of the *Inner Temple.*

An Enchiridion of Fortification, or a handful of knowledge, in Martial affairs, demonstrating both by Rule and Figure, (as well Mathematically by exact Calculations, as Practically,) to fortifie any body, either Regular, or Irregular. How to run approaches, to pierce through a Counter-scarf, to make a Gallery over a Mote, to spring a Myne, &c. With many other notable matters belonging to War, useful and necessary for all Officers, to enrich their knowledge and Practice.

The Life and Adventures of *Buscon*, the witty *Spaniard*.

Epicurus's Morals.

Small Octavo.

Daphnis and *Chloe*, a Romance.

Merry Drollery, complete; or a Collection of Jovial Poems, Merry Songs, Witty Drolleries, intermixed with Pleasant Catches, Collected, By *W.N. C.B. R.S. J.G.* Lovers of Wit.

The Midwives Book, or the whole art of Midwifry discoverd, directing child-bearing women how to behave themselves in their Conception, Bearing, Breeding, and Nursing of Children, in six Books.

Butler

Butler of War.

Tractatus de Venenis; or a Treatise of poisons. Their sundry sorts, names, natures, and virtues, with their symptoms, signs diagnostick and prognostick, and antidotes. Wherein are divers necessary questions discussed; The truth by the most Learned, confirmed; by many instances, examples, and stories Illustrated; And both Philosophically and Medicinally handled; By *William Ramsey.*

The Urinal of Physick. By *Robert Record* Doctor of Physick. Whereunto is added an ingenious treatise concerning Physicians, Apothecaries, and Chirurgeons, set forth by a Doctor in Queen *Elizabeths* daies; with a Translation of *Papius Abalsissa* concerning Apothecaries Confecting their Medicines; worthy perusing and following.

Large *Twelves*.

The Moral Practice of the Jesuites Demonstrated by many Remarkable Histories of their Actions in all parts of the World, Collected either from Books of the Greatest Authority, or most certain and unquestionable Records and Memorials by the Doctors of the *Sorbonne.*

Artimedorus of Dreams.

Oxford Jeasts Refin'd, now in the Press.

The third part of the Bible and New Testament.

A Complete Practice of Physick, Wherein is plainly pescribed, the Nature, Causes, differences, and signs, of all diseases in the body of man. With the choicest cures for the same; By *John Smith*, Doctor in Physick.

The Duty of every one that will be saved, being Rules, Precepts, Promises and Examples, directing all persons of what degree soever, how to govern their passions and to live vertuously and soberly in the world.

The Spiritual Chymist; or six Decads of Divine Meditations on several Subjects; with a short accouut of the Authors Life; By *William Spurstow*, D. D. Sometime Minister of the Gospel at *Hackney* near *London*.

Small Twelves.

The Understanding Christians Duty:
A Help to prayer.

A new method of preserving and restoring health, by the vertue of Coral and Steel.

Davids sling.

P-219594

219594
RECORD OF EXHIBITION

Date	Opening
9/21/87 - 3/20/83	
8/28/97 - 2/2/98	tp

Elizabeth Cellier's *To Dr.—* (*Wing* C1663) is reproduced, by permission, from the copy at the Folger Library. The text block of the original measures 112.5 × 157.5 mm.

To Dr. ——— An Answer to his Queries, concerning the COLLEDG *of* MIDWIVES.

TO answer your Query, Doctor, *Whether ever there were a Colledg of Midwives in any part of the World?* According to my Promise made the 12th Instant, I will now prove, there was some Hundreds, if not Thousands of Years before you can prove one of Physicians; As appears both by Sacred and Prophane Histories. I will begin with the first; and desire you to read the first Chapter of *Exodus*.

Vers. 15. *And the King of Egypt spake to the Hebrew Midwives, of which the Name of the one was* Shiprah, *and the other* Puah.

Vers. 16. *And he said unto them, When ye do the Office of a Midwife to the Hebrew Women, and see them upon the Stooles; if it be a Son, you shall kill him: but if it be a Daughter, then she shall live.*

Vers. 17. *But the Midwives feared God, and did not as the King of Egypt commanded them, but saved the Men Children alive.*

Vers. 20. *Wherefore God dealt well with the Midwives: and the People multiplied, and waxed very mighty.*

Vers. 21. *And it came to pass, because the Midwives feared God, that he made them Houses.*

I believe no Rational Person will think that these two Women could in their own Persons act as Midwives to all the Women of that *mighty People*, who about 100 Years after, went up out of *Egypt* 600000 Fighting Men, besides Women and Children, and a great mixt Multitude, but rather that they were the Governesses and Teachers of other Midwives, which could not be a few; and as I am informed by a Learned *Rabbi*, now in Town, their Names signify the same.

And the Apostle faith, *That God built them Houses, and blessed them.*

Now if it were, as some think, that these were not *Israelites* but *Egyptians*, appointed Governesses over such as should assist the Hebrew Women, who by Conversation among them *learned the knowledg of the only true God, and fearing him, did not impose those bloody Orders of destroying the Males.*

Then it was plain that the Government of that Art was regular, under Superiours, as the *Magi* and Priesthood of that Nation was, and must have some certain place for consulting in, from whence they might issue their Directions. Which, by your leave, Doctor, without Absurdity in the Language of these Times, might well be called *a Colledg*.

But for the Piety of the Ruling Midwives God built them Houses: that is, they were Incorporated into the Body of the Jews, and reckoned *Honourable Families among them*: As *Rahab* and others for their singular Service to that Nation afterwards were. *Which Families of the Faithful Midwives,* some Hebrews say, *continue in Honour among them at* Thessalonica *to this Day.*

And such a favour from God of *building Houses for them,* we do not read the Physicians ever received; nor was Physick then a regular Study, nor brought under Government in that Learned Nation of *Egypt*, in *Herodotus* his time, which put together, proves the Antiquity of the Midwives Government so much antienter than that of the Doctors.

For your further Satisfaction be pleased to read *Origen* his 11*th* Homily upon *Exodus*, which will inform you, that *Shiprah* and *Puah* were not only the *Governesses of the Midwives,* but also Women of Great Learning, and excellently
skill'd

skill'd in Physick, which was then practised by Women to Women.

And you cannot deny at our last Conference, but that *Hippocrates* swears by *Apollo* and *Escalapius*, and by *Hygea* and *Panacea* the *Gods and Goddesses of Physick*: And pray, Doctor, who were the Gods and Goddesses of Antiquity, but Men and Women, who first found out and taught Arts and Mysteries so beneficial to Mankind, as made them think they could not but be guided by a Divine Spirit to the knowledg of things so useful and so far above the Vulgar Capacities This? *Hippocrates* is so ingenuous as to confess, and doth not part the *Gods* and *Goddesses*, but had them in equal Veneration, as appears by his Oath, to which I refer you, because I perceive you have forgot it; For he swears *he will not cut those that have the Stone, but will leave it to the skilful in that Practice.* But you, tho you understand nothing of it, pretend to teach us an Art much more difficult *(And which ought to be kept as a Secret amongst Women as much as is possible.)*

'Tis true among the *subtile Athenians*, some Physicians being gotten into the Government, and Miscarriages happening to some Noble Women about that time, they obtain'd a Law, that for the future no Woman should study or practise any part of Physick on pain of Death. This Law continued some time, during which many Women perished, both in Child bearing, and by private Diseases; their Modesty not permitting them to admit of Men either to Deliver or Cure them.

Till God stirred up the Spirit of *Agnodicea*, a Noble Maid, to pity the miserable condition of her own Sex, and hazard her Life to help them, which to enable her self to do, she cut off her Hair, Apparelled her self like a Man, and became the Scholar of *Hyrophilus* the most Famous Physician of that Time; and having learn'd the Art, she found out a Woman that had long languish'd under private Diseases, and made proffer of her Service to cure her, which the sick Person refused, thinking her to be a Man; but when *Agnodice* had discovered that she was a Maid, the Woman committed her self into her Hands, who cured her perfectly: And after her many others with the like Skill and Industry. So that in a short time she became the Successful and Beloved Physician of the whole Sex, none but she being called to assist them.

This so incensed the Physicians that they conspired her Ruin, saying she shaved off her Beard to abuse the Women, who feigned themselves Sick to enjoy her Company; *and there being Witnesses to be found then* (as of late Years, that would swear any thing for Money) she was upon their Testimony, condemned to Death for *committing Adultery* with *Agisilea* one of the *Areopagites* Wives; it being easy to make Old Men, who had beautiful Wives, believe any thing of so young and handsome a Doctor.

This forced *Agnodice* to discover her Sex to save her Life; and then the enraged Physicians accused her of transgressing the Law, which forbid Women to Study or Practise Physick. And for this Crime she was like to be condemned to Death; which coming to the Ears of the Noble Women, they ran before the *Areopagites*, which were the Chief Magistrates, and the House being encompassed by most Women of the City, the Ladies entred before the Judges, and told them they would no longer account them for Husbands or Friends, but for cruel Enemies, that condemned her to Death, who restored them to their Healths; protesting they would all die with her if she were put to Death.

This caused the Magistrates to disanul that Law, and make another, which gave Gentlewomen leave to Study and Practise all parts of Physick *to their own Sex, giving* large Stipends *to those that did it well and carefully, and imposing severe Penalties upon the unskilful and negligent*: And there were many Noble Women who studied that Practise, and taught it publickly in their Schools as long as *Athens* flourished in Learning.

But

But *Phænareta* the Mother of wise *Socrates*, who was a Woman of great *Learning* and *Skill*, *deserves a particular remembrance, both for her own, and her Son's sake*; who, as it is believed by many, was a Martyr, being put to Death for professing there was but *one God*, which Wisdom himself saith he learned of his Mother. Thus, Doctor, it appears, even that Learned Idolatrous City had in it a *Midwife that knew and feared the true God*: Tho, as the Apostle saith, *there was an Altar therein dedicated to the unknown God, &c.*

This *Ambrose Perre*, Counsellour and Chyrurgion to the King of *France*, and his Ingenuous Disciple *Gulielmus*, prove fully: and that is as far as my small Learning and weak Capacity goes. But you, Doctor, may prove it more at large when you please, by the *Hebrew*, *Greek*, *Latin* and *Arabick* Books, which treat on these Subjects; in which times the three parts of Physick, *Midwifery*, *Chirurgery*, and *the making up and administring of Medicines*, were all one, tho the last, which was then the servile part, hath now usurp'd upon the other two; but we pretend only to the First, as being the *most Antient, Honourable and Useful Part*: Wherein we desire you not to concern your selves, until we desire your Company, which we will certainly do as often as we have occasion for your Advice in any thing we do not understand, or which doth not appertain to our Practice.

But to come into our own Country, it is not hard to prove by antient British Books and Writings, that before the *Romans* came hither here were Colledges of Women practising Physick, dedicated to some of the Female Deities; but whether so antient as the *Bards* I cannot tell, tho some old British Songs written in praise of the *Goddess* 𝔆𝔢𝔞𝔴𝔱𝔥, seem to prove it: but they were in the time of the *Druides*, as appears both by Brittish and French Books, and the Name of *Wise Women*, by which *Midwives* are still called in *France*, and most of the Western Parts, as they are by that of *Wise Mother* in the

Low-

Low-Countries, Germany, and most of the Northern Parts of the World.

And here in London *were Colledges of Women about the Temple of* Diana, *who was Goddess of Midwives here, as well as at* Ephesus. From whence the Grecians say, she was absent at Q *Olympia*'s Labour, who was that Night deliver'd of *Alexander* the *Great*; where she was so fully employed, that she could not defend her Stately Temple, which was burned down by *Heroftrateus* the Shoemaker, to perpetuate his Name.

Nor did the Bishops pretend to License Midwives till Bp. *Bonner*'s time, who drew up the Form of the first License, which continued in full force till 1642, and then the Physicians and Chirurgions contending about it, it was adjudged a Chyrurgical Operation, and the Midwives were Licensed at *Chirurgions-Hall, but not till they had passed three Examinations, before six skilful Midwives, and as many Chirurgions expert in the Art of Midwifery.* Thus it continued until the Act of Uniformity passed, which sent the Midwives back to *Doctors Commons*, where they pay their Money, *(take an Oath which is impossible for them to keep)* and return home as skilful as they went thither.

I make no Reflections on those learned Gentlemen the Licensers, but refer the curious for their further satisfaction, to the Yearly Bills of Mortality, from 42 to 62: Collections of which they may find at *Clerks-Hall:* Which if they please to compare with these of late Years, they will find there did not then happen the eight part of the Casualties, either to Women or Children, as do now.

I hope, Doctor, these Considerations will deter any of you from pretending to teach us Midwifery, especially such as confess *they never delivered Women in their Lives,* and being asked *What they would do in such a Case?* reply *they have not yet studied it,* but will when occasion serves; *This is something to the purpose I must confess, Doctor:* But I doubt it will not satisfy the
Women

Women of this Age, who are so sensible and impatient of their Pain, that few of them will be prevailed with to bear it, in Complement to the Doctor, *while he fetches his Book, studies the Case, and teaches the Midwife to perform her work,* which she hopes may be done before he comes.

I protest, Doctor, I have not Power enough with the Women to hope to prevail with them to be patient in this case, and I think if the Learnedst of you all should propose it *whilst the Pains are on*, he would come off with the same Applause which *Phormio* had, who having never seen a Battel in his Life, read a Military Lecture to *Hannibal* the *Great*.

But let this pass, Doctor, as I do the Discourses you have often made to me on this Subject, and I will tell you something worthy of your most serious Consideration: Which is,

That in *September* last, our Gracious Soveraign was pleased to promise to unite the Midwives into a Corporation, by His Royal Charter, and also to found a *Cradle-Hospital*, to breed up exposed Children, to prevent the *many Murders, and the Executions which attend them*; which pious Design will never want a suitable Return from God, who no doubt will fully reward his Care for preserving so many *Innocents* as would otherwise be lost.

And I doubt not but one way will be by giving him a Prince by his Royal Consort, who like another *Moses* may become a Mighty Captain for the Nation; and lead to Battel the Soldiers with the Hospital will preserve for him.

And now, Doctor, let me put you in mind, that tho you have often Laughed at me, and some Doctors have accounted me a Mad Woman these last four Years, for saying Her Majesty was full of Children, and that the *Bath* would assist her Breeding: 'Tis now proved so true, that I have cause to hope my self may live to praise God, not only for a *Prince of Wales, and a Duke of York*, but for many other Royal Babes by Her; and if the over Officious will but be pleased to let them live, *I hope in a few Years to see them Muster their little Soldiers:* Which Joyful Sight, I believe, is the hearty Desire of all Loyal Subjects, of what Persuasion soever, as it is the daily and fervent Prayer of,

From my House in Arundel-street, *near St.* Clement's *Church in the* Strand. Jan. 16. 168¾.

Your Servant,

ELIZABETH CELLEOR.

Where the Word of a King is, there is Power: and who shall say unto him, What doest thou? Eccles. 8. vers. 4.

FINIS.

Let this be Printed,

SUNDERLAND. P.

F158219
C1663

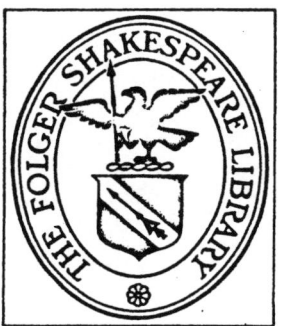

'A Scheme for the Foundation of a Royal Hospital' is reproduced, by permission, from the Clark Library's copy of *A Fourth Collection of Scarce and Valuable Tracts* (London, 1751), Volume 2, pages 243–249. The text block of the original measures 125 × 200 mm.

much Right in the first, and himself so much Right in the last, be so poorly mis-interpreted, by the unnatural Surmises of his ungrateful People. But let us blush and mend, and by giving up these Laws, do Equity in Return of Clemency and Mercy.

A Scheme for the Foundation of a Royal Hospital, and Raising a Revenue of Five or Six-thousand Pounds a Year, by, and for the Maintainance of a Corporation of skilful Midwifes, and such Foundlings, or exposed Children, as shall be admitted therein. As it was proposed and addressed to his Majesty King *James* II. By Mrs. *Elizabeth Cellier*, in the Month of *June*, 1687. Now first published from her own *MS.* found among the said King's Papers.

To the King's most excellent Majesty, the humble Proposal of Elizabeth Cellier,

Sheweth,

THAT, within the Space of twenty Years last past, above Six-thousand Women have died in Child-bed, more than Thirteen-thousand Children have been born abortive, and above Five-thousand *chrysome* Infants have been buried, within the weekly Bills of Mortality; above two Thirds of which, amounting to Sixteen-thousand Souls, have in all Probability perished, for Want of due Skill and Care, in those Women who practise the Art of Midwifry.

Besides the great Number which are overlaid, and wilfully murdered, by their wicked and cruel Mothers, for want of fit Ways to conceal their Shame, and provide for their Children, as also the many Executions on the Offenders.

To remedy which, it is humbly proposed, that your Majesty will be graciously pleased, by your Royal Authority, to unite the whole Number of skilful Midwifes, now practising within the Limits of the weekly Bills of Mortality, into a Corporation, under the Government of a certain Number of the most able and matron-like Women among them, subject to the Visitation of such Person or Persons, as your Majesty shall appoint; and such Rules for their good Government, Instruction, Direction, and Administration, as are hereunto annexed, or may, upon more mature Consideration, be thought fit to be annexed.

That such Number, so to be admitted, shall not exceed a Thousand at one Time; that every Woman, so to be admitted as a skilful Midwife, may be obliged to pay, for her Admittance, the Sum of five Pounds, and the like Sum annually, by quarterly Payments, for, and towards the pious and charitable Uses hereafter mentioned.

That all Women so admitted into the Thousand, shall be capable of being chosen Matrons, or Assistants, to the Government.

That such Midwifes as are found capable of the Employment, and cannot be admitted into the first Thousand, shall be of the second Thousand, paying for their Admittance, the Sum of fifty Shillings, and fifty Shillings a Year by quarterly Payments, towards the pious and charitable Uses hereafter mentioned, and out of these the first Thousand are to be supplied, as they die out.

That, out of the first Sum arising from the Admittance-money, one good, large, and convenient House, or Hospital, may be erected for the Receiving and Taking in of exposed Children, to be subject to the Care, Conduct, and Management of one Governess, one female Secretary, and twelve Matron-Assistants, subject to the Visitation of such Persons, as to your Majesty's Wisdom shall be thought necessary.

That such Hospital be for ever deemed, of your Majesty's Royal Foundation, and from Time to Time, subject to the Rules and Directions of your Majesty, your Heirs and Successors.

That the annual Five or Six-thousand Pounds, which may arise from the Thousand licenced Midwifes, and second Thousand, may be employed towards the Maintenance of such exposed Children as may from Time to Time be brought into the Hospital, and for the Governess, her Secretary, and the twelve Assistant Matrons, and for the necessary Nurses, and their Assistants, and others, fit to be employed for the Nourishment and Education of such exposed Children in proper Learning, Arts, and Mysteries according to their several Capacities.

That for the better Maintenance and Encouragement of so necessary and royal a Foundation of Charity, it is humbly proposed that by your Majesty's royal Authority, one fifth Part of the voluntary Charity, collected or bestowed in any of the Parishes within the Limits of the weekly Bills of Mortality, may be annexed for ever to the same, other than such Money taxed for the Maintenance of the Parish Poor, or collected on Briefs by the royal Authority for any particular charitable Use.

That likewise, by your Majesty's royal Authority, the said Hospital may have Leave, to set up in every Church, Chapel, or publick Place of Divine Service of any Religion whatsoever within the Limits aforesaid one Chest or Box, to receive the Charity of all well-minded People, who may put Money into the same, to be employed for the Uses aforesaid.

That such Hospital may be allowed, to receive the Donation, of any Lands, Legacies, or other Gifts, that pious and well-minded People may bestow upon them.

That such Hospital may be allowed to establish twelve lesser convenient Houses, in twelve of the greatest Parishes, each to be governed by one of the twelve Matrons, Assistants to the Corporation of Midwifes, which Houses may be for the Taking in, Delivery, and Month's Maintenance, at a Price certain of any Woman, that any of the Parishes, within the Limits aforesaid, shall by the Overseers of the Poor place in them, such Women being to be

subject,

subject, with the Children born of them, to the future Care of that Parish, whose Overseers place them there to be delivered, notwithstanding such House shall not happen to stand in the proper Parish.

All and every of the twelve Houses to be Members of, and Dependents on the Royal Hospital, and subject to the Government of the same, and all such Children as shall be exposed into them, whose Parents and Places of Abode cannot be found, are to be conveyed thence to the great Hospital, there to be bred up and educated, as though they had been exposed into it.

That for the better Maintenance, and encouraging the Government of the said Hospital, in the educating such exposed Children, in proper Learning, Arts and Sciences, according to their several Capacities, it is humbly proposed, that by your Majesty's royal Authority, all the Children so exposed, shall be deemed Members of, and Apprentices to the said Society, till they attain the full Age of twenty one Years, to be reckoned from their first Admittance into the same, unless by Consent of the Government thereof, they should happen to be married, or otherwise licensed to depart, under the public Seal of the same.

That likewise by your Majesty's Royal Authority, the Children exposed and educated, as aforesaid, may be privileged to take to themselves Sirnames, from the several Arts, or Mysteries, they shall be excellent in, or from the remarkable Days they were exposed on, or from their Complexions, Shapes, &c. and be made capable, by such Names, of any Honour or Employment, without being liable to Reproach, for their innocent Misfortune.

That by your Majesty's Royal Charter, the Children so educated may be free Members of every City and Corporation, within your Majesty's Kingdom of *England*, and Dominion of *Wales*.

That for the better providing sure Ways and Means, for the Instructing all present and future Midwifes, who shall be admitted into the said Corporation, fit Care ought to be taken to induce that Person, who shall be found most able in the Arts, and most fit for that Employment, to instruct them in the most perfect Rules of Skill by reading Lectures, and discoursing to them.

That on the Lecture Days, or other Times appointed for that Purpose, such Midwife, in whose Practice any extraordinary Occurrents shall happen, shall report the same to the Governess, and such of her Assistants, as shall then happen to be present, and they to be free in his, or their Instructions.

And it is humbly proposed, in the first Years before the Charge of the said Hospital can be great, that out of the annual Duties arising from the licensed Midwifes, the Sum of   may be paid to the Proposer to enable her to provide for her Children, that nothing may divert her from employing all her Industry for the Good of those poor exposed Children.

And that all Admittance-money which shall be paid after the first Thousands are settled, shall be divided between the Governess and the Man Midwife or Director of the House for the Time being, by even and equal Proportions.

That

That upon the Admitting any Woman to be Deputy to any Midwife, the Sum of thirty Shillings shall be paid, and the like Sum annually, by quarterly Payments, twenty Shillings whereof shall be as a Fee to the Governess, and ten Shillings to her Secretary, besides their necessary Lodging and other Conveniencies in the said Hospital.

That after this first Settlement, no married Woman be admitted to be either Governess, Secretary, or any of the twelve principal Assistants to the Government; and that no married Person, of either Sex, shall be suffered to inhabit within the said Hospital, to avoid such Inconveniencies as may arise, as the Children grow to Maturity; and that, as soon as any of them be found fit and capable of such Employment, the Governess, Secretary, under Governesses, Governors, Treasurer, Register, and all other Offices of the House shall be chosen, as they become capable thereof, and have entered themselves to continue Members of the said Society, during their natural Lives; and if any of these Persons do marry afterwards, then to clear their Accounts and depart the House, by being expelled the Society.

RULES *for governing the Hospital of found Children.*

THAT the Governess be appointed by his Majesty, as likewise her Secretary, and twelve Assistants, who are to name twenty-four to be of the Government.

That, upon the Death of the Governess, her Place be supplied by her Secretary, or such Person as shall be chosen by the twelve principal Assistants, or the major Part of them, and the Approbation of his Majesty; that the Secretary be chosen by the Governess, and approved of by his Majesty, his Heirs and Successors.

That, upon the Vacancy of one of the twelve principal Assistants, by Death or otherwise, one of the Four-and-twenty shall succeed, by Election of the Governess, Secretary, and the other Eleven; as also, the Number of Four-and-twenty shall be supplied, by Election of the Governess, female Secretary, and twelve principal Assistants, or the major Part of them; and, in all Cases, the Governess to have three, and the Secretary, two Voices.

That all Rules for governing the Children, under five Years of Age, shall be made by the Governess, her Secretary, and their Assistants; that the Government of the Whole, under such Rules, be in the Governess.

That all female Children shall continue under the sole Government and Direction of the Governess, untill they attain the full Age of twenty-one Years, or are married by her Consent.

That all male Children, at the Age of five Years, shall be separated from the Female, and put under Government of the several Masters, to be appointed to instruct them in learning Arts and Trades, according to their several Capacities, and the Rules of the House.

That the principal Chaplain be Governor of the male Children above five Years of Age, according to such Rules, as shall be made from Time to Time, for well ordering the said Hospital.

That all Parish-found Children, under the Age of three Years, shall be admitted into the said Hospital, as soon as it is built, for two Shillings *per* Week, or the Sum of fifteen Pounds, to be paid at the Election of the Overseers, or Vestry of the Parish, that send them, to continue there twenty-one Years.

That there shall be appointed proper Mistresses, to instruct all the Children, under five Years of Age, in Reading and Arts, according to their Capacities, who are to have Salaries and Subsistence from the House, by such Rules as shall be made from Time to Time, as Occasion happens; which Mistresses are all to be subject to the Governess.

That like Mistresses be appointed, for instructing the female Children in Plain-work, Lace-making, Point-embroidery, and all other female Arts, according to their several Capacities, and under the like Government.

That Masters, in several Mysteries, Arts, and Handicrafts, be appointed, to teach the male Children, as Painters, Engravers, Carvers, Watchmakers, Smiths, and Carpenters, of all Sorts; Salemakers, Taylors, Shoemakers, and many other Trades, according to their Geniusses, Strengths, and several Capacities.

That an able Register be appointed, to set down, and keep, a due Account of the Day of the Entrance of every Child into the Hospital, with the proper Marks of its Body, Colour of its Cloaths, and other Things about it, with its Hospital Name, and where it was found, with its own Name, if a Note be left thereof, to the End that any one may recover their lost Child, if they please; that the Register take Care to cause all Children to be instructed in fair Writing and Accounts, according to their several Capacities.

That all Names are to be given by the Governess, and that every Child, upon its being brought into the Hospital, shall be marked with a Cross of Blue under the Brawn of the Arm, with the Day and Year of its Admittance; to the End they may be found out and recovered, if they should chance to conveigh themselves out of the Hospital before the Age of twenty-one Years, to defraud it of the Benefit of the Mystery, Art, or Trade they have learned.

That a Woman, sufficiently skilled in Writing and Accounts, be appointed Secretary to the Governess and Company of Midwifes, to be present at all Controversies about the Art of Midwifery, to register all the extraordinary Accidents happening in the Practice, which all licensed Midwifes are, from Time to Time, to report to the Society; that the female Secretary be reckoned an Assistant to the Government, next to the Governess, and capable of succeeding in her Stead, if chosen thereunto by the Governess, in her Lifetime, with the Approbation of his Majesty, his Heirs, and Successors.

That the principal Physician, or Man-midwife, examine all extraordinary Accidents, and, once a Month at least, read a publick Lecture to the whole Society of licensed Midwifes, who are all obliged to be present at it, if not employed in their Practice; and he shall deliver a Copy of such Reading, to be entered into the Book to be kept for that Purpose: A Copy of which shall be made out to any Person, demanding the same, for such reasonable Fee, as shall be appointed by the Government, and shall be free, for any licensed Midwife,

wife, at all convenient Times, to have Recourse to the said Book, and to read any Part of the same *gratis*.

That no Men shall be present at such publick Lectures, on any Pretence whatsoever, except such able Doctors and Surgeons, as shall enter themselves Students in the said Art, and pay, for such their Admittance, ten Pounds, and ten Pounds a Year; five Pounds to the House, and the other Five to be divided equally between the Governess and the chief Doctor, or Surgeon, that shall be Director of the House for the Time being.

That all Physicians and Surgeons, so admitted Students and Practitioners in the Art of Midwifery, shall be of Council with the principle Man-midwife, and be capable of succeeding him, by Election of the Governess, her Secretary, twelve Assistants, and the twenty-four lower Assistants, or the major Part of them all: Elections to be made by Balloting, the Governess three Balls and the Secretary two Balls.

That the Man-register, and Secretary of the House, be under the Command and Direction of the whole Government thereof for all Business, except the Art of Midwifery which is to be meddled with by none but the Governess, female Secretary, Man-midwife, and their Assistants.

That any Child, under the Age of one Year, whose Parents are known, or not known, shall be admitted into the House, under the Rules of being there twenty-one Years; provided there be paid into the Stock of the Hospital the Sum of thirty Pounds, at the sending in of the said Child.

That any Person or Persons, who would have a Child out of the said Society, shall have Power to examine the Register, whether the Child, by its Marks, be living or dead, and may redeem the same, being under the Age of five Years, for twenty-five Pounds, or being of that Age, or under the Age of seven Years for forty Pounds; and from Seven to Ten, for fifty Pounds; but, after the Age of ten Years, every Year it continues in the House, shall advance ten Pounds in the Price of the Redemption, till such Times they attain the Age of Fifteen; after which Time, no Increase of the Price of Redemption shall be upon any Child; any one being, at any Time to be free for a hundred Pounds, or less, if the Governess of the House, her Secretary, twelve Assistants, or the major Part of them, consent to the same; the Governess hath three, and the female Secretary two Voices, which are to be given by the Chaplain, Register, and Treasurer, if it be a male Child that is to be redeemed; but, if it be a Female, then the Power to rest in themselves.

That all the Money coming to the said Hospital, either by annual Payments, Charity, Redemption, or any other Ways whatsoever, shall be placed into one common Treasury, to be kept in one or more Iron Chests, not to be opened by the Consent of the Governess, her Secratary, the chief Chaplain, or him that shall be Governor of the male Children, the Register, and Treasurer, who shall each of them have a Key to so many several Locks, and the said Monies, other than the constant Salaries of the Officers, and daily Maintenance of the Children, shall not be applied to any extraordinary Use, but such as shall be appointed by the whole Government of the Hospital, in which

Number the Keeping of thofe Keys, for fuch Purpofes, are to be accounted Part.

The Accounts whereof, and of all Monies coming into, or going out from the fame, fhall be kept by the Regifter; and free Accefs fhall be had, at all Times, to the fame, *gratis*, by the Governors, or any of the Vifitors of the faid Hofpital; and that, once a Month, all Comings-in, and Goings-out, and all other Tranfactions on that Account, fhall be, by the Regifter, fairly entered into a Book for that Purpofe, which fhall always remain with the Governefs, and not be taken out upon any Pretence whatfoever; and that any Perfon may fearch the Regifter's Book, for the Fee of Six-pence for one Year's Search.

That Rules fhall be made, from Time to Time, by the Governors, for trying the Geniuffes of the Children, and dividing them into feveral Claffes and Employments, according to their feveral Capacities, and for entering them under proper Miftreffes and Mafters, upon certain Salaries, or, otherwife, binding them Apprentices to the Miftreffes and Mafters within the Houfe, or for Cloathing them, during their Refidence in, or at their going out of the faid Hofpital;

As likewife for all other Accidents, as Lunaticks, Idiots, and other Infirmities, Difeafes, and Sickneffes; and for feparating the Infirm from the Healthful, and the infectious Difeafes from the other Sick; and for all other Contingencies, as there fhall be Occafion.

That none fhall be detained, againft their Wills, above the Time of twenty-one Years, nor turned out at that Time, if they defire to ftay; it being in the Power of any of them, at that Age, to enter him, or herfelf, fubject to the Rules and Duties of the Houfe, for their natural Lives; nor are any of them incapacitated to get their Livings abroad, nor, being within the Houfe, at any Time to be turned out; but are to be maintained by them in neceffary Meat, Drink, Cloaths, and Lodging, during their natural Lives, or till they recover of their Diftempers, fo as to be able and willing to leave the fame.

But no Perfon, once difcharged, and out of the Care of the Houfe for fix Months, fhall be capable of demanding Enterance into the fame again, or of Maintenance from it, but by the Confent of the Governors thereof; and that fuch as return to the Houfe fhall give good Teftimony, that they have fpent their Time well, and without Scandal, or be for ever expelled the Society.

That further Rules, for the Eftablifhment and Foundation of the faid Community, or Hofpital, and for Vifiting the fame, may be appointed in the Charter for endowing the fame, and fuch Penalties impofed on fuch as practife without Licence from the Corporation, as to your Majefty's Wifdom fhall feem meet.

To which All is humbly fubmitted.

With the exception of the pages listed below, Mary Trye's *Medicatrix* (*Wing* T3174) is reproduced from the copy at the Cambridge University Library, by permission of the Syndics of Cambridge University Library. The text block of the original measures 70 × 122.5 mm.

Substituted from the copy at the National Library of Medicine in Bethesda, Maryland, are the title page, pages 3–6, 31, 41, 47, 67, 69–71, 85, 87, 93, 97, 99, 101, 113, 115–117, 119, 125, and three pages of the Advertisement appended to the end of Trye's text.

MEDICATRIX,
OR THE
Woman-Physician:
VINDICATING

Thomas O Dowde, a Chymical Physician, and Royal Licentiate; and *Chymistry*, against the Calumnies and abusive Reflections of *Henry Stubbe* a Physician at *Warwick*.

Stubbe in nomination with *Cicero*.

A Recital of some Publications Mr. *Stubbe* makes in his own Life.

His malice against ingenious Scrutinies, and the advantage thereof.

The Life of Mr. *O Dowde*: His Promotion of the *Chymical Society*: His noble Acquirements in *Medicine*: His Practice in the last great Plague, and death therein.

The Second Part.

The Authors opinion of Learning; the abuse of the same, Mr. *Stubb's* Projects and Design, only his Interest, not the benefit of the sick.

Phlebotomy he so much commends in the *Small Pox*, *Pleurisie*, *Scurvy*, *Fevers*, &c. Condemned and Rejected.

A Medicinal Challenge to Mr. *Stubbe*, proffering by experiment to confute his Avow in Phlebotomy.

And to Cure by Chymical Medicines, the *Gout*, *Stone*, *Agues*, *Dropsies*, *Falling-sickness*, *Consumptions*, *Griping of the Guts*, *Venereal Lues* or *Ilmal Francese*, &c. and those Diseases, which by his *Generous Medicaments* and *Lancet* he cannot.

A Revival of Mr. *O Dowd's* Medicines, and other *Chymical Remedies*, with an Advertisement thereof.

Written by M. Trye *the Daughter of Mr. O Dowde*.

Avec tout ton scavoir cognois toy mesme.

--- For the Life of all flesh is the blood thereof, Lev. 17.14.

LONDON, Printed by *T. R.* & *N. T.* and Sold by *Henry Broome*, at the *Gun* at the West end of St. *Pauls*, and *John Leete* at *Chancery-lane* end next *Fleet-street*, 1675.

30:16

To the Glory of Her Sex, the Honour of Her Countrey, and the moſt Accompliſh'd Lady the Lady *Fiſher*, Wife to *Sir Clement Fiſher* Knight and Baronet of *Packington-Hall* in the County of *Warwick*.

Honoured Madam,

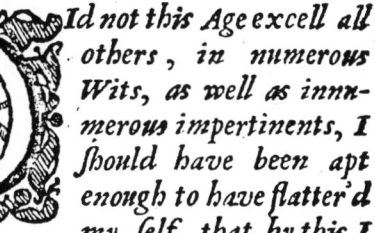*Id not this Age excell all others, in numerous Wits, as well as innumerous impertinents, I ſhould have been apt enough to have flatter'd my ſelf, that by this I* had deſigned you a *Curioſity*; but ſince it is little of Novelty to ſee a Woman in *Print*, I conceive no ſuch vain Idea's, as to Imagine, I ſhall now entertain you with any rare or more then ordinary divertiſement.

However I think it may modeſtly be ſaid, that you will find ſome things herein

The Epistle Dedicatory.

not very common, among which one is a Duty paid to the Dead, which for my part I look upon totally extinct and obliterated with the living, and that is Gratitude: another is, such a Conflict, which it may be you will pleasantly recent, and that is, That one of the Feminine Degree, in a Medicinal Contest, hath now encountered a Rhetorical and Physical Hector, an expression I confess too generous for one that deserves so little.

But that my Pen may not altogether surprise your Ladyship by these occasional and vindicatory Papers, (my misfortunes, and your distance, having interrupted that honourable acquaintance I have formerly had with you) and that you may in some measure remember; 'twill will be civil and requisite to let you know, That abiding the late great and never to be forgotten Pestilential Calamity of this City, and undergoing that mortal stroak, in which I lost Two of my dearest Friends, my Father and Mother, but surviving them my self, I received a Medicinal Talent from my Father, which by the instruction and assistance of so excellent a Tutor, as he was

to

The Epistle Dedicatory.

to me, and my constant preparation and observation of Medicines, together with my daily Experience, by reason of his very great practice; as also being Mistress of a reasonable share of that Knowledge and discretion other Women attain; I made my self capable of disposing such noble and successfull Medicines, and managing so weighty and great a Concern.

In in process to the strict Commands, and Death-bed injunction of so good a Father, which was, That his Medicines being of that value, and incomperable benefit to the World, that no Man in this Kingdom was Master of the like (notwithstanding the high malice of his Enemies and pittyfull Detractors) I should never suffer them to fall to the ground, or to dye and be buryed in oblivion, nor never to stop my Ears from the cry of the Poor, languishing for want of such Medicines; I say this Testament obliging me to the obedience of the Rechabites; I have continued his Medicines to this day, (though not in this City) to the succour of many Hundreds, more out of Charity then my private Interest, to the bright

Glory

The Epistle Dedicatory.

Glory of these Chymical, *and not to be paralel'd Medicines, and to the shame and odium of his* Galenical *opposers, as some time or other, by many laudable Instances, and miraculous examples shall be further offered,*

Yet Madam, to complete your Knowledge I must likewise add, That upon my coming to London *in* October *last, being inquisitive after the advance of Chymistry, so desirable by all sorts of People, some Papers came to my hands, subscribed by* Henry Stubbe *Physician at* VVarwick, *wherein he opposeth the* Royal Society, *and all other ingenuity, but what he commends in his own Sect; and amongst others I find many false and obusive reflections cast by him on the Urn of my deceased Father, unbecoming a Gentleman, and such an Ingagement as this Historian hath undertook, but how justly; so Charitable a Physician, and so faithful a Servant to his King and Countrey, (which without any vanity I must assert) hath deserved the affronts of this Romancer, and such —— I shall hereafter examine; perceiving also, that several*

The Epistle Dedicatory.

Gentlemen made Subjects of his scurrilous fancy, have already defended themselves: That I might at least attain to the Degree of those, mentioned to do good to such as do good to them, although I am not ignorant of my more immediate duty in this particular; I was resolved none should answer for him but my self, (not that he or his Medicines do, or ever can want Patrons or Persons to defend whatever this Campanel, *or such —— dare Honourvbly attempt) because the obligation is solely incumbent on me; being the only Child of this injur'd* Chymical Physician: *Neither do I believe it any difficult task to engage this mighty Champion, who insolently Proclaims himself, Dictater to God and Man, King and Subject, and indeed to all the World; for if I can make out his malice, and shew his ignorance, so far as is proper for me, I have my desire:* Madam, *This being the occasion of these publick Lines, at this time, that I may not prove tedious in detaining your Ladyships thoughts from more lofty Resentments, I must conclude, and beg pardon for so great a rudeness, with*

the

The Epistle Dedicatory.

the assurance, that I have embraced this opportunity only to tell you, That both this and my self are really at your Ladyships service, being the most sincere inclination of

Ever Honoured Madam,

Your Most Obedient,
and Humble Servant

Ma. Trye.

From the *Feathers* in the
Old *Pell-mell* near Saint
James's 1.Decem. 1674.

Medicatrix

MEDICATRIX,
OR THE
Woman Physician;

In Vindication of
Mr. *O Dowde* & *Chymistry* against
the Calumnies of Mr. *Stubbe.*

An Introductory Discourse.

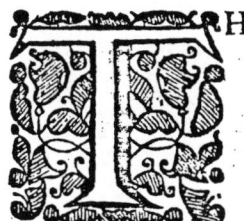Hat virtuous actions in unblameable Lives; That Noble Enterprises, and the most beneficial Arts, in as serene and candid Promoters, have been in all Ages the objects of malice and detraction, I doubt not, but is too sensibly understood by all degrees of People, without any exception of the most vulgar Capacity: And what severe,

and frequent Persecution have in all distinctions of time attended, not only just and laudable designs, but even Charity, Christian Duty, and Goodness it self, I am by some experience, and much observation, sufficiently inform'd.

But as to any Portion of this kind, that happens Relatively to concern me, I confess, I have good Divinity, and reason to content me; since, I do firmly believe, that there was once the Son of God upon Earth, that patiently endured his Temporary course, under the greatest Passion and bitter Malediction imaginable; and that not only in the general deportment of his Life, but even in this particular fact of healing, The Saviour of the World was condemned and assaulted with the Language of Devils.

And since, I must take liberty to tell Mr. *Stubbe*, That I am satisfied there is Ability enough in my Sex, both to discourse his envy, and equal the Arguments of his Pen in those things that are proper for a Woman to engage:
And

And what is more, that knowledge, and skill in Chymistry, so far as to obtain those Medicines, that neither the *Medicus* at *Warwick*, nor all his Authors he pretends he hath perused, if not conjured together, could ever paralel or procure: Neither is this so great a Mystery, nor shall I seem immodest if it be considered, that Mr. *Stubbe* abominates experiment, and all such ——

But to avoid Prolixity, which is a crime we Women are commonly guilty of; And that I may not put this Historical Gentleman, (as well as the Reader) to a second relation, how my Feminine Hand comes to be directed against him; let my Epistle to the most Honoured Lady *Fisher*, eminently known, and Eterniz'd by the particular Name of Madam *Jane Lane*, inform him; and if he requires more ample satisfaction, 'tis this; My defence is in the behalf of the injured, and what aggravates, in the cause of a deceased Father, villified by the Malice and Ignorance of Mr. *Stubbe*, and one that merits better from all Men, then what he that calls himself *Campi-*

nell, and such Phanatick Brains allow
and more then such soring Clouds, an
Tempestuous Scriblers will ever attai
too; In sum, his rude, idle Paper
blotted with Folly, and uncivilly re
flecting on this deceased Physician I hav
mentioned, together, with some othe
bold and intollerable errors, imposed o
the World by Mr. *Stubbe*, provokes
And therefore I proceed thus to Defen
and Challenge.

SECT. I.

Stubbe in nomination with *Cicer*

Although I dare not pretend to
so much a Linguist, or capable
such great Studies, Readings, and ve
bal Acquirements, as the *Medicus
Warwick* owns; whose business it
to be famous in those Accomplishmen
and who hath need enough of the
to maintain and carry on the most pr
digious and impossible Aims he dri

it; (though I do not see that all his noise of Languages and Schollarship he so much boasts of, hath furnisht him with that perfection Learning ought to produce, or what is commonly expected from it.) Yet I hope I may retain so much confidence in Mr. *Stubb's* ingenuity; That if I presume to use sometimes, only an Author English'd, as *Plutarch*, &c. or it may be *Esop*, or the like; this Age being pretty kind to us Females in such assistance; and give him likewise a reasonable measure of sense, which I believe is as much, and more, then he expects from a Woman; he will be so kind as to excuse me for the vacancy of those Masculine Capacities he himself glories in: And the rather, because he well understands, that such fine things, as are prettily term'd Philosophical in him, will scarce be thought rational in me.

This being an Age so subject to Division and Subtlety, and so full of contention, between Interest and Truth, Ignorance and Ingenuity, Purity and Impurity; and last of all Loyalty and Re-

6 *Medicatrix*, or the *Woman Physician*.

Rebellion; I made a particular consideration of this Eloquent Opiniator, and finding him depend very much on his Oratory, and perswading himself to be absolutely and uncontrollably Doctrinal, that I might the better be informed what such aims proposed, and Conceits effected by other publick Hero's, almost of this nature: I consulted with my self what Lives I had read; presently remembred *Plutarch*, and in him, the Life of *Cicero*; one that had as good an Opinion of himself, as he that calls himself the *Little Bell* of *Warwick* or the late *Physician* at *Jamaica*; I fell to the perusing the History of that generally admir'd Man of Eloquence, wherein I collect, he far surpast Mr. *Stubbe* in Wit and attain'd that Honour I fear he will never reach; and that is, by the Oration and Applause of his good friend *Cat*, the People decreed him to be call'd *Father of the Country*, it being a name never given to any before him; though it seem this unsuitable and sublime degree, did him no kindness afterwards, as the History tells: And in some other thing he was very commendable, as he gave himself to all kind of knowledge whatsoever, and there was no Art, nor any of the *Liberal Sciences* that he disdained; And 'tis said likewise, he freely extolled all *Authors* that were before him, so that in these kinds of ingenuity he much transcended his Disciple *Stubbe*, who directly opposes him in a contrary course, by not only reviling and withstanding the only Eligible and Available art in the World, which is *Chymistry*; but condemning and crucifying all *Authors* whatsoever, living or dead, not of his own lazy Tribe: And sometimes he did a little good to his Country, and such like, although it was in tendency to his own private design; and that I doubt is more then ever *Campanell* will do upon any design at all: But in many qualifications else, I think *Cicero* and the *Medicus* may very well matcht, and so its possible, the Reader will conclude, when the observations I have made, are clearly and truly weighed.

For

For I obferve, this *Roman* was very high and ambitious, recenting many good and meritorious thoughts of himfelf; His intereft was dear to him, for he would undertake any caufe to be doing; He was a *Poet*, an *Oratour*, a *Lyar*, *Mercenary*, a *Soldier*, a *Polititian*, a *Philofopher*, *Spightful* and *Malitious*, and indeed any thing; till at laft he knew not what to be, and fo fell miferably to nothing. This being fome of that account given by *Plutarch* of him, I muft leave the intelligible and knowing to judge, wherein he paralels fome of his Difciples amongft us; but to pleafure my Reader, I will recite fome eminent marks of this fam'd Oratour, mention'd by his Hiftorian, and for brevity fake but a few.

That this popular Man of *Rome* was Ambitious, and harbour'd many high fancies of himfelf, thinking much better then he did really, or the People of that City in feveral actions believe he deferv'd, evidently appears by this recital: For being concern'd to plead a caufe for fome young Gentlemen of
Rome

Rome that were accused for faults committed in the Wars against their Honour and Martial Discipline (and sent back to *Sicily*) he defended them so, that they were pardoned: *Thereupon,* (saith the History) *thinking well of himself, when his time was expired, he went to* Rome ; *and by the way, this jest hapned unto him. As he passed through the Country of* Campania *(otherwise called the* Land of Labour) *he met by chance one of the chiefest* Romaines *of all his Friends : So falling in talk with him, he asked him, what they said of him at* Rome, *and what they thought of his doings : imagining that all* Rome *had been full of the Glory of his name and deeds. His Friend asked him again, and where hast thou been* Cicero *all this while, that we have not seen thee at* Rome ? *This kill'd his heart streight, when he saw that the report of his name and doings, entring into the City of* Rome *as into an infinite Sea, was so suddenly vanished away again, without any other fame or speech.*

But after that, when he looked into himself, and saw that in reason he took
an

an *infinite labour in hand to attain Glory, wherein he saw no certain end whereby to attain unto it: it cut off a great part of the ambition he had in his head. And yet the great pleasure he took to hear his own praise, and to be overmuch given to desire of honour and estimation: Those two things continued with him even to his dying day, and did ever and anon make him swerve from Justice.*

So that the Reader may see how small occasion, and mean matter, tempted *Cicero* to swell in conceit, and to believe such publick praises were due, and attributed to him, which in reality were not; And I am apt to fancy, our *Tinckling Champion at Warwick* will be somewhat hereby resembled, when I consider the several Bravado's his Papers record; As when he rejoyces to think what a brave commendable attempt he hath put himself in abusing the *Royal Society*, Ingenuity, and all ingenious and good Men; pretending what universal encouragement and Bay's he is like to receive, not only from his Patrons and Stipendaries, but many Gentlemen of
Quality

Quality, when from the reception of a single Letter, he presently tells the World; *That he is pleased (forsooth) to understand, that so many serious and real Patriots of this Kingdom do approve, not only of his undertaking the Royal Society, but of his performances therein:* And what doth all this great boast in Plurality, that clap him on the Back and spit in his Mouth, amount to, surely but a ⸺ paucity, for I cannot find them to be above two or three, as Sir ⸺ This; and Mr. ⸺ That; whose names he mentions not, yet it may be in his writings, he may tell you of one or two more; But I shall not trouble my self to seek a Needle in a Bottle of Hay, without it were of more consequence, to peruse a long chain of confus'd Languages, and falsities which I acknowledge is beyond my *Genius* to comprehend, neither do I desire it: It is enough for me to understand, what I have undertook, and if in any reasonable degree I acquit that, I have sufficient ground to be satisfied; That Mr. *Stubbe* is as true in one thing as another;

ther; as uncertain and double as the Oracle of *Apollo*: And that he that glories of being *Physician at Jamaica*, signified as little there as he doth here, so that I hope the next voyage he makes will be to more purpose.

And in another extasie our *Medicus* is very merry, and says in a Letter to his Friend concerning the *Virtuoso's*, Thus, —— *I know a Gentleman, who in the Wars of* Ireland, *at one blow cut off a Mans head,* (I hope it was not Mr. *Stubbe*) *and the headless Trunck, clapp'd Spurs to the Horse sides, and rid about Ten Yards after;* Truly I very much doubt the *Champion of Warwick,* whatever he thinks, hath given no such fatal blow: But he proceeds, and salutes his Friend in this manner, —— *Let these Loosers talk a little, and then retire and work* —— *and endeavour to regain their Credit, which I think is irrecoverably lost, if others by my example will pursue their failings.* 'Tis well said Mr. *Stubbe,* what sentiments I have made by the way, in the behalf of the Royal Society, are but the thoughts of a Woman, so that I leave the Learned

Learned to defend themselves: And shall only repeat what is to my purpose, and that is, I think Mr. *Stubbe* wants no Opinion of himself, which will more especially appear when I have remarked one rapture more of his, and indeed that is so profound, that I shall spare him in reciting any more of that kind now: It is to be found in his rare Jewel reviv'd, called *Campanella*; where, in his Epistle to the Reader, amougst other abuses of better Men then himself, scolding against the *Virtuoso's*; And it being objected, that his Writings against one of them, contained little of matter; To this Mr. *Stubbe* humbly answers, *That they contain enough to have made Twenty* Virtuoso's *famous, and would have acquired them a memorial of ingenious and noble experimentators: they contain enough to shew the ignorance of that person* —— *They contain enough, since they contain more then they all knew.* —— O prodigious! Now whether Mr. *Stubbe* be not as conceited in this particular as ever *Cicero* was, I must leave to those that are proper to judge   Be-

Besides, if I thought I might not too much intrude on Mr. *Stubbe*; I would be his best Friend, and tell him without any flattery; if he demanded the same question of me, that his Master *Cicero* ask'd of his chief *Roman* Friend, I would thus answer, Where hath Mr. *Stubbe* lived all this while? at *Jamaica*; or where are his famous works extant, and victorious Books exposed to Sale? for I am inform'd, the Author himself, with most Book-sellers in this City, is not known; and the Books themselves scarce with any to be had; so that I am satisfied, the Generality of this Kingdom never heard his name, much less saw him; In sum, I perceive the *Physician at Warshick* is not that man of Fame he takes himself to be: but if notwithstanding this, he is resolv'd to conclude his own Acts Superlative, I must like a kind Friend tell him again; they must then be heretofore acquired by his *Neutrality* at best, not by his Loyalty, or late Conquest of the *Chymists*, or *Royal Society*.

Medicaurix, or the *Woman Phisitian*. 15.

And whether I have not now, some propable reason to imagine, that *Mr. Stubbe* is likewise deceived, in his desired Popularity, as much as ever, his Romane Master was; I shall assign to the same Judgment I have already chosen: But I have been much longer on this Paralel then I intended, and therefore least I weary my Readers, as the *Medicus* hath done his; I must omit many of those places I designed to accomodate the Reader withall, and refer him to the General account of *Cicero's* life, described by *Plutarch*, and only mention these following.

That this Roman Wit was not exempted, from Mercenary actions, (as well as pride,) taking any cause in hand to defend for advantage; Appears in the business of *Verres*, and in the cause of *Milo*, who murder'd *Clodius*; As likewise, in the case of *Munatius*, and of *Marcus Crassus*; the passages of these two last being short, and pertinent enough; I will relate, as 'tis exprest in his life: *when on a time,* Cicero *had pleaded* Munatius*'s Cause before the Judges, who shortly after*

after accused Sabinus *a friend of his*: he was so angry with him, that he told him, what Munatius, *hast thou forgotten that thou wert discharged the last day of thine Accusation, not for thine Innocency, but for a mist I cast before the Judg's eyes, that made them they could not discern the default?*

Another time also, having openly praised M. Crassus *in the Pulpit, with good audience of the people*: shortly after he spake to the contrary, all the evil he could of him, in the same place. Why, how now said Crassus: *didst thou not thy self highly praise me in this place the last day? I cannot deny it,* said Cicero: *but indeed I took an ill matter in hand, to shew mine Eloquence.*

Now, whether our *Campanel at Warwick*, be herein exemplified, or any wayes concern'd in such projects as these; it belongs to the ingenious *Chymists*, and *Virtuosi* to decide, being most able, experimentally to discern things of this nature as well as others: But I must confess, in that slender judgment I have his papers, and general abuses designed

signed therein; renders him to me as much a Juggler as an Opiniator.

 Cicero was at one time a Poet too, but, it seems that was but of the age of a *mushroom*, and of no longer date, then *Mr. Stubbs* his works, as subject to fate, as his *Viper-catcher*, and more mortal than himself; in sum, extinct as soon as written.

 Plutarch in the life of *Antonius*, reproves this great Poet for lying, in maliciously accusing *Antonius*, affirming him to be the Author of the civil Wars in *ROME*, which indeed, (saith the Historian) *was a stark lie*; *for* Cæsar *was not* —

 I shall Treat *Mr. Stubbe* more civilly, than charge him in such Language, though I have read in his papers, much worse, used to some of his Opponents; But whether, he gives me not cause enough, to charge him with the fact, particularly relating to him I defend; may be observed hereafter: What mis-representations, and sugjestions concerns (I think) many others, let the learned ingage,

C   Several

Several other acts of *Cicero*, much for my purpose may be seen in his Life at large, which to be concise, I omit: But I perceive, his *Eloquence* deceived him in his Popular projects, and Political designes, So that he was forc'd at last to pray his friends not to call him *Orator*, but *Philosopher*; saying that was his chief *Profession*.

I shall now conclude his Life, in shewing the Reader, he was for any partie that was in fashion; He could take *Pompey* by one hand, and *Cæsar* by the other; and what excellent Principles he was endued withall, as well as our *Campanell*, you will see by what follows; Upon the War, and division growing between *Pompey* and *Cæsar*; He thus sayes, ——— what way should I take? *Pompey* hath the juster, and honester cause of War, but *Cæsar* can better Execute, and provide for himself, and his friends with better safety——— In result he kept in with *Pompey*, till he was call'd Treacherous, and esteem'd despicable: Then he marched off to *Cæsar*, and ingratiated himself with him; after he dyed by the

Sword

sword, at the Commands of *Anthonius*, for his malice against him.

Thus, our English *Cicero* may, &c. I have nam'd him, with as Famous a man as himself, which is a civility beyond his merit; And although many of this *Romans* actions are ill Presidents, and some differ from the station and decree of a common Subject, and so not respect our *Medicus*; Yet if by the general observation, of this mans life, it be considered, how unjust attempts & naughty promotions for interests sake, render a Man unprosperous, and obnoxious to Justice, and an ill resentment; and by such conclusions, my friend at *Warwick*, repents, and amends, he will not only excel *Cicero* in Chronicle, but I shall likewise hope to be as Doctrinal then, as Mr. *Stubbe* believes himself is now.

And I have given the Reader, this Historical account, not only that he may see I have read in History, as well as our *Campanell*, but that I may mind him of the vast difference, between wit and wisdom, truth annd errour, justice and interest; and in sum, that it is more reasonable

sonable to expect, a just cause, to be permament and durable, though obscur'd and oppress'd, than a deceitful and unjust; though the date be old, and the name good: What else the History contains, Scholars understand, 'tis not for me to Assume.

SECT II.

An Express of the Information Mr. Stubbe *gives of his own Life, in several Particulars.*

Although M. *Stubbe* layes hold on the Hoins of the Altar, and makes the Act of indempnity to answer the second Covenant in Divinity; and that he seems to confess, beg pardon, and amend, which if truly performed, he were the more excusable: Yet since I see his confession and pretence to be no other than subtlety & hypocrisie; when 'tis obvious he still persists in his old method, to abuse His Majesties servants, and sufferers; I must take liberty to re-mention a few

Medicatrix, or the *Woman Physician*. 21

particulars of what account this *Campanell* gives of himself.

Mr. *Stubbe* fearing the *Virtuoso's*, or some of his adversaries would write a History of his Life, and what principles he is accomplish'd with, (he being as it appears by his own Relation, none of the best Subjects that ever the KING had) to prevent this design, he saith, he wrote it himself,(and 'tis scarce likely he mention'd any of the worser part)out of which, these few following I have taken.

He sayes: he was *a poor Boy at* Westminster-School, *under his Master D. Busby*: That he was after *a servant to Sir H. V. by which I believe he means Sir Henry V. he taking a liking to him*; For good reason no doubt.

Sir *H. V.* prefer'd him to be *a Kings Scholar*; but by his leave, I doubt in those times such words and Titles were not in fashion with Sr. *H. V*'s servants; but now M. *S.* uses as becomes him the language of a convert.

His *Master B. was charitable, and gave him books, clothes & schooling*, which I think was more than he deserved,

C 3   without

without he made better use of them.

He saith he was *at School at* Westminster, *but 17 years of age, and a little Stature, when the* KING *was beheaded;* Or rather (if he please)Murdered, and I am very glad to hear it was so; otherwise I should have thought——.

There being Quarrels between the Presbyterians and Sir H. V's *Friends, he sided with his Patron Sir* H. V. *His Retribution to his Generous Patron was, to promise him if ever he were able to serve him effectually,* and this he says *he did;* who questions it, and wrote *those so invidious Queries to terrifie the Presbyterians,* but protests *they contain no Tenents of his*—So 'tis like he took that Task in hand as *Cicero* did his, to shew his Eloquence.

Many other things of this nature he writes of himself, mentioning sometimes, a good deed, or two, he did among the rest; But I must desire the curous Reader, if he requires further satisfaction, to view his papers.

And lastly he tels us, he hath been his Majesties Phisitian in the Island of *Jamaica*, but that he did little service

there

there, he owneth, being sick; This I am apt enough to believe, so that if he were His Majesties Phisitian, he was far enough off Him, and I think he was rightly plac'd, and 'tis no great matter if he were sent there again, the place I am told being most fit for him.

But notwithstanding all this, Mr. *Stubbe* shall see I will do him right, and pay him more Candour then he expects, for I shall not accuse and arraign him again, since the mercy of our good King hath been so great as to pardon him: But however, this I must say, It is much ingratitude, and no good return of such an Offender, to repay his Prince by persecuting and abusing his charitable and suffering Servants, raking them out of their Graves with falsities and envy; I think they endured pretty well in their Lives, so that Good Men say 'tis pity to disturb their Ashes, except on more just occasion: Certainly this is a fiery zeal, exceeding that of *Saul*, who persecuted unto death, but there left; This, I do say in my Opinion, sounds louder of malicious principles, and ill nature, then the *Little Bell at Warwick* ever did of Ignorance, Interest, Policy, Philosophy, Phlebotomy, or what you please.

This I cannot omit the *Medicus* in, and that the World may see what great prejudice he hath really cause for, against the person I am obliged to take notice of, I shall descend to note; and inform the Reader of several occurrences in the Life of my Father.

SECT. III.

An account of the Life of Mr. O Dowde, and some of his Loyal Sufferings therein. Of his promotion of the Chymical Society.

TO revive and mention the actions of a Charitable and good Subject, is very complacent with any sober *Genius*; but by such memorial to review the many Troubles, Dangers, Imprisonments, and continual Adversity of so near a Friend; to me, is exceeding tedious

tedious and unwelcom; and a task so unsuitable to my inclination, that nothing made me more ready to decline this Tract, then the necessity I saw to recall some past passions of the deceased, in order to a vindication against such an Invective; This seemed grievous to me, so far, as sometime to disswade me; But my thoughts of Duty in general, being more prevalent then my effeminate thoughts of nature in particular, I resolved at last to enter upon the prosecution; and to avoid a prolix account of many tedious circumstances, and considerable actions, some extraordinary, and not proper for a publick relation, This Gentlemans Life being a *Series* of Trouble and Sufferings, I shall now only give the Reader this short express of him.

He descended from a Generous Family, and Heir to no less Fortune in the Kingdom of *Ireland*, but his Fathers Death leaving him in Minority, and subject to the injury and misfortune, the Second Marriage of his Mother contracted, and after the Distraction and Trou-

Troubles in that Nation compleated, he was by this means deprived of the greatest part of his Right and Inheritance, a damage not inconsiderable.

He became after a Servant to his late Sacred *Majesty*, and now Glorious St. *King Charles* the I. his Royal Master being not long after Murdered, he was then obnoxious to the lot of the banished, oppressed and persecuted, at that time the signal of Loyalty and Obedience.

Upon this Rebellion and Confusion, he going over beyond Sea, was afterwards imploy'd in the management of some affairs of his *Royal Master* His Majesty that now is: Those being at an end there, he came back privately into *England*, where he was not a little Serviceable to the Great ones of his *Royal* Masters party, *&c.* by which occasion he was never an hour safe, or free from imprisonment, losses, and dangers of Life; and to avoid these, he needed no command to remove him from one place to another; for that he was forc't to do, no place, though never so secret, was

was of longer security then a few weeks, it may be a few days, more often, much less.

He was imprison'd sometimes six Months, sometimes Two and Twenty, other times bound to a certain limit, and daily and hourly attendance of the most notorious Committees, and that for a year and more together.

To add to these kinds of persecutions, and to obtain their Bloody ends, my Mother was likewise imprison'd, and kept a close Prisoner for many Months.

This being too little, my Father was afterwards again secur'd, and examined by *Oliver* himself, and his ——— and at that time condemned upon this condition, That he should either make such discoveries as they proposed, or dye; to which I have heard his answer was, *Discoveries he should make none, Death he feared not, for he had not liv'd so ill that he was afraid to dye:* That course not prevailing, both then and several other times he wanted no offers of gain and promotion to oblige him, but that
signi-

signifying as little as the rest; In conclusion at that time, they banished him out of *England*; but sometimes returning secretly and disguised, he was again taken and imprison'd at *Nottingham*; but it pleased God before that came to any thing, the Old Usurper departed his cruel Life.

Yet the Trade went on, and after his release there, upon the accidents of that Usurpers Death he came to *London*, Then the Alternate *Successors* of the deceased *Persecutor*, upon the following mutations and transactions of the Nation, endeavouring to support as much an impossibility, as the Physician at *Warwick* in another case now promotes; He was again imprison'd by ― & *Bradshaw*, and this Imprisonment, I remember, was long and chargeable, and continued till the Weather grew fair, and the cause no longer disputeable; then he was discharged, and after returned over Sea ― And these passages so far (being too much for me) I have thought reasonable to mention; as for others in this nature, I do not think proper, nor shall I declare or expose. So

So that from the death of his firft Royal Mafter, to the Reftoration of his Second, was a continued fortune of Loyalty and Obedience, but a paffion of no fmall danger, and no lefs impoverifhing trouble; And notwithftanding all this, and more, I am contented, and do both think and fay what his own Judgement was in his Life time, That thefe things were no more then his Duty, and the Duty of every honeft and Faithful Subject.

But fince the *Campanell* urges me to things of this degree, and I am fatisfied out of his old principles, he fets himfelf to abufe thofe Men 'twere more prudence for him to forbear, I muft not omit to tell him, That he may hereby, and by what follows be affured; That *O Dowde* was no Servant nor Difciple of Sir *H. V.* no Servant to —— faid not, wrote not, did not any other then what he juftified with his Life: in few words, he was no companion for *Stubbe,* and fuch—— his principles were more Honeft, more Loyal, more Honourable, and more Ingenious: And although I cannot

not boaſt, as Mr. *Stubbe* doth, that he was ſent His Majeſties Phyſician to *Jamaica*; nor it may be of his great ſtipend reward, or brave allowance, as 'tis ſaid he hath from ſome of his Phyſical Friends, to ſupport his arrogance, and by all that I can imagine, rather to inflame the World then any thing elſe; and to abuſe and trample on all goodneſs and ingenuity, and the promoters thereof, who to their laſt breath, ventur'd their Lives and Fortunes for their *Prince* and *Country*; Actions ſo excellent, that I perfectly deſpair of ever ſeeing the *Campanell* perform.

Yet if I am not ſo plauſibly accompliſh'd as Mr. *Stubbe*, nor cannot make the moſt of a favour, as he doth, I am obliged to ſay, that His Majeſty was very kind to my Father, and I could mention wherein he particularly deſign'd him a Royal and profitable Gift, by an Order entred in Mr. *Secretary*— his Book; but my Father falling ill at that time, a great Perſon then in Office, diſpoſed His Majeſties favour other ways & much contrary to the *Royal*Command,

(the

(the more was my misfortune) which with some such things as these I omit: And I doubt not but if he had liv'd, His Majesty would have been as Condescentive and Gracious to him, as some others.

I proceed now to some other occasions of malice the *Campanell* takes against this deceased *Chymical Physician*, which account followeth.

After the happy Restoration of his now Sacred Majesty, when good Men as well as others, began to be at liberty, and to enjoy some peace and tranquility, having passed such an Ocean of Sorrows, This Gentleman being all his Life eminently devoted to Ingenuity and Industry; and his inclination leading him from his Childhood to *Medicinal Scrutinies* and *Chymical Curiosities*, to prosecute and perfect which, loosing no opportunity under all his troubles, and through his Travels, nor omitting any charge, expence, time, or labour, to obtain what was excellent, and worth his knowledge and reception; And having by an indefatigable pursuit, and diligent Elaboration, made himself Master

ster of those great secrets and particular attainments so much sought after, and only by the *Chymical Art* to be acquired; for it was a rule with him, *That if a Man could not do as much or more in an Art, then any other Professor of that Art, 'twas not worth his trouble to imploy himself therein.* That he might now both do good to his Neighbour and himself, and endeavour to provide for his Family; and in some measure make up, and regain the Losses he had sustained by so long an interruption of trouble, he put himself to Practice, and beginning presently to be famously successful and experimentally justifying his Medicines by plentiful examples to excell, and prevail far beyond the *Common Method* of contrary Practicers: He immediately meets with that fate which infallibly attends every thing that is good and excellent; and that you may easily believe was malice and envy; so that now, seeing him do good, and grow popular, those of the adverse *Physical Practice*, and some, That but yesterday were with him under a joint affliction

affliction and kind imbrace, to day a Frown was too good, so far do Men degenerate into unworthiness, and cloud themselves with disingenuity; but however, sthose that knew him, knew likewise he cared little for such accidents; and notwithstanding this, with the favour of His Majesty, who hath sufficiently express'd Himself, to be a lover of ingenuity and charity, as well as other commendable actions; he advantagiously improv'd the vertue and excellency of his Medicines, beyond the Cavill, malitious suggestions, and falsities of his adversaries, and effecting those cures never by them to be attayn'd.

Some years after His Majesties Returne, *Chymistry* growing generally in request, and the observation that the World made of the benefit, and profit the sick received by the *Chymical Physitians* of this City, induc'd many persons of *Honour* and *Quality*, to approve and commend this Art so much as to promote it, by desiring to settle, and Establish a *Chymical Society*: In order to which, he made it his bufinefs to further it, in what was proper for him, and in obedience to the commands of fome perfons of Honour, mentioned in his Book; he publisht that Tract, wherein he informs the World of this Defign, and of the Progrefs in tendency thereto, out of which, that I may the better difcourfe Mr. *Stubbe*, I have taken thefe following Subfcriptions.

Whereas after fufficient Experiment, it is found moft true, that Chymical Medicines well prepared, and afwell applyed, are above all others; the fafeſt, pleafanteſt, and moſt effectual means, both for confervation of Health, and cure of all difeafes whatfoever: And whereas fome of a different Practice from it, as well as thofe many falfe pretenders to Arcana's *of this nature; doe either malicioufly or ignorantly, hinder the clear and general underſtanding of the Vertue and Excellency of fuch Noble preparations, and by Confequence the Publique good. To the end therefore, that Patients may not fpend themfelves, their precious time and money in vain; and alfo that the Licentious abufes of* Impofters posters may hereafter be detected; Wee whose Names are hereunto Subscribed, do resolve and promise to our utermost Abilities, to preserve and advance the Honour and Credit of this profession of Chymical Physick: And in order thereunto humbly do propose, and as much as in us lyeth, endeavour an obteining of His Majesties gracious Favour by Letters Pattents, for the Instituting of an Incorporation of Professors of Physick, capable of such Constitutions and Discipline, as shall answer the ends herein propounded; Namely the Improvement of that most Laudable and necessary Science of Physick, only by Hermetick or Chymical Medicaments; and herein from time to time, to be Assistant to each other, and never to relinquish this our Engagement for any Temporal respects whatsoever.

Will. Goddard.   Febure.
Tho. Williams.   Will. Barkly.
Edw. Bolnest   Robert Bathurst.
Richard Barker.   Tho. Tillison.

Robert werdenKeſſler.
John Werden.Edw. Cooke.
John Floyd.Tho. Smart.
Mat. Clifford.James Jolly.
Geo. Starkey.Tho. Norton.
P. MaſſonetGeorge Thompſon.
Tho. Troutbeck.John Wilkinſon.
John Fryer.Jeremiah Aſtell.
Edw. Warner.Tho Yardly.
Will. Currer.Tho Barker.
John Troutbeck.Robert Turner.
Joſeph Dey.Will. Burman.
Mar. Nedham.Tho. O Dowde.
Ever. Maynwaning.

Medicatrix, or the *Woman Physician.* 37

Having perused the within written Proposals, subscribed by divers persons of Learning, experience and ingenuity, viz. for the Institution of a Noble Society, for the advancement of Hermetick Physick; We connot but give the Design condign Approbation, as tending to the Publick good; aud accordingly we shall, as occasion serves, give our Countenance, and best Assistance towards the effectual accomplishment thereof.

    Gilb. Cant.
Buckingham.   Albemarle.
  Ormonde   Lindsey.
Northampton.   Anglesey.
  Oxford,   St. Alban.   Elgin.
Pemb. & Mountgomery. Hump. London. Norwich. Carlisle. Mountgaret. H. Mansfield.
  Kenelm Digby.   G. Hamilton.
W. Killegrew. C. Harbord. J. Crew. R. Werden. J. Werden. H. Bishop. Tho. Collpeper. Jo. Ernle. Edw. Proger. Jo. Mennes. G. Shakerly. H. Proger. R. Whitfield. W. Merrick. T. Paulden. Rich. Brett. Goring Ball. Edw. Warcuppe. Freschevills Holles. Hen. Peck.
      D 3   But

But this undertaking, being of so confiderable and unfpeakable good and benefit to the Kingdom; the Reader may foon imagine, the Enterprize of courfe wanted not enemies enough to withftand it : But certainly if I may fpeak my thoughts (though the *Medicus* may fay a wamans thoughts fignifie little) if this Royally ingenious age be incompleat in any thing, 'tis in the defect of this one moft beneficial, defirable and Noble Settlement; and 'tis ftrange fo great a Concern fhould lye unattempted, and imperfect, by the vacancy and death of a few good and charitable men, who defired the prefervation and Glory of a Nation more than their own Intereft, or private profit : And if this be not conftituted in this Age, no man doubts but that it muft be of neceffity in after Ages; for 'tis certain now, *Senna, Rhubarb, Scammony, Coloquintida, Crude, Mercury,* nor *Tubbing* ; nay, *Stubbs* his *generous Medicaments,* nor Lancet it felf, will not recover the difeafes of thefe times ; what then muft be propofed to pofterity, I believe little lefs than the Golden

Golden essence of *Chymistry*.

And now having made a recital of these subscriptions, I think it is requisite to tell the *Medicus* at *Warwick*, that in one of his extavigancies, in an Epistle to the Reader, I find he imposeth on the World, much of confidence, little of Truth; when amidst his abuses of the *Royal Society*, he is pleased thus, civilly to express himself, *at first they* (meaning the *R. S.*) *would have incorporated the Colledge of Phisitians into their Society; but that the prudent and grave did decline: then they promoted the Anti-Colledge of* Pseudo-Chymists, *encouraging* O Dowde, *and his ignorant Adherents in opposition to the Phisitians; and this is not more Notorious to the World, than it is also that those objections with which* M. N. *and other Quack-salvers amuse the Age, were suggested unto them by the* Virtuosi, *and derived their repute from them.*

Thus I perceive, any language is suitable enough for Mr. *Stubbs* his mouth; any falshood for the subject of his pen; and in this kind, I believe his malicious supporters hath took a Gradual defender

der, becaufe he can write and affirm any thing, and hath folly enough to believe he can perfwade the world with his own pleafure: But 'tis time fuch a fcribler were checkt in his Race; therefore as to the firft, and laft paffages of this *Campanels* accufation, 'tis not my bufinefs to meddle with; but believe them as much of Gofpel truth as the other: As for the nature of the *Chymical Colledge*, called by him, the *Anti-Colledge*, by the Relation I have cited, the Reader may fatisfy himfelf of the fair Cafe, progrefs, and promotion therein; and of the wilful and cunning miftake of the Reipublick pretender Famous *Campanella*, and fee what fancies he is forc'd to create and juftifie; to patch up his Bleeding caufe: Thefe are thofe Gentlemen and Perfons of Honour, M. *Snbbe* out of the extract of his *Jamaica* Manners, impudently calls *ignorant adherents*: But let who will be the encouragers; and if the *Royal Society* had been the Promoters of this Noble Aim, (a happinefs too great for this Kingdom hitherto to enjoy) can the *Medicus*

flatte

Medicatrix, or the *Woman Physician.* 41

flatter himself, it is so mean a design as not to be own'd; But laying aside this supposition, He sees it hath been owned and subscribed by as good and honourable Adherents as any of his, and I believe will he by more; though he dares stile them ⸺ but because he hath been Sir *H. V*'s Servant, perhaps he thinks he may say any thing.

And I must further take liberty to tell the *Campanell*, that his Friend *O Dowde* was not to be incouraged, or put upon any attempt by the *Royal Society*, or else, (though *Stubbe* was by his Master *V.*) he was not satisfied in his own Conscience, was just, eminently advantagious, and proper for the Good of the Nation: No, since *Campanell* will have it, I will tell him Mr. *O Dowde's* reasons for his particular engagement in this business; 'twas not because he opposed the method and foundation of true Learning, as this Sophister would idly impose, and foolishly insinuate; But because Learning was made a Cloak to vail Ignorance, and cover Laziness, Learning was not suffered to answer its true,

true ends, which all defire; Men boasted of Letters, but underftood not Medicines; Words were the perfection of their Studies, not falutary Deeds the refult of their Practice: 'Twas becaufe he faw the prefent Age languifh with infupportable and grievous Difeafes; and Pofterity like to be much more; out of all hopes incurable, and not to be remedied by Vulgar Quacks: He faw neither the *generous Medicaments of H. Stubbe at Warwick*, nor yet his Lancet, fignifying any thing to the remedy and prevention of thefe great improving Calamities: He faw the Common Art of Phyfick impotent and weak, and not able to anfwer its own defign, nor the promife of the Artift: He faw poor Creatures kept a year, two, three fometimes, under the management of *Campanell's* ignorant adherents, and fuch — pretenders to that they never underftood, without any other benefit then torture and expence; And at laft the once clouded, but now bright and admir'd Chymical Medicines, were forc'd in a few days, or

weeks

weeks to be the restorer: He saw it was not in the power of *Stubbe*, or his Method, to attain those Medicines necessity required, and the high degree of *Chymistry* produc'd. These (and many more) if Mr. *Medicus* will have me inform the World, whether I will or no, were the just occasional Dictates of Mr. *O Dowdes* embracing this Honourable, and now only desirable promotion, and no other.

So that having plain enough discovered this publick Assertion of *Campanell*, to be one of his juggling disguises, and mis-representments, I shall not need to trouble my self more herein, then to conclude, when I see a Man dare question the Actions of his Prince, I must believe, That Man dare say any thing; nay, for ought I know, do any thing.

An account of Mr. O Dowdes Practice and Assistance in the last great Plague, and of his Death therein.

I shall now prosecute my promise, in giving a Relation of some further account of my Father, of his Practice in the late great Plague, and his Death therein; and trace Mr. *Stubbe* in some other of his malicious suggestions and subtlety; for I perceive he is well skill'd in the *Art of Legerdemaine*; And do believe he depended (by the freedom he useth) too much on the Common Proverb, *Si tostque l'Arbre est tombe chacun se rue dessus*, or else I can never imagine he would have so Romancingly abus'd himself, and his Readers; but if that be his conclusion, 'twill be more Wisdom for him to decline, for he will be much deceived in any wishes or hopes of that kind.

As to the general fame, and constant daily success of my Fathers *Chymical Medicines* to his death; satisfactorily prevailing without any comparison, far beyond

beyond the Common Practicers, and their Abilities; notwithstanding the Wiles and *Hocus* Mists of *Stubbe,* and such —— is so well known, I need not add any confirmation; and by his own *Printed Book*, and his *private Notes* and *Manuscripts* I have by me, will easily satisfie: Besides, the *Medicines* have ever since justified, and are still alive to justifie themselves; which to humour Mr. *Stubbe* shall hereafter appear: But in saying this, I am put in mind, That I have been several times inform'd, that the Book of my Father, the Title whereof was, The *Poor Mans Physician,* &c. hath been much desired, and sought after ever since his Death; And the *Book-seller* pressing for it, I thought proper by the way to give notice, That his Book will be revived (at leisure) by a Gentleman to whom all my Fathers *Chymical* and *Medicinal* Secrets and Preparations were Communicated.

But as to my Fathers Progress and Administration from the beginning of that great Affliction the *Pest,* untill his death, I shall inform the *Curious* in what
is

is necessary; but in order thereunto, and in tendency to explain and answer another on-set and vain Collection of the fallacious and insinuating *Champion at Warwick*, I must beg leave to mark one disguised Rapture of his more, which is this following.

In his Reply to Dr. *Thompson*, wherein he spends in one place of that Book, a whole side of Paper to tell the World the meaning of ——— a black stroak; The sum of which is no more, then to make known what envy he bears to ingenious Men; Amongst other odious, and contemptible, idle, foolish Stuffe, exclaiming against *Paracelsus*, *Helmont*, and a great many more hard Names, of (I presume) famous *Chymists*, crucifying them with ungentleman-like Language, (and indeed thereby principally forfeiting his own credit, and abusing himself) telling us, *That* Helmont *could not cure a Feaver*, *He was not known in the Street where he Liv'd*, because Mr. *Stubbes*, his Brother *Kraft*, could not find him by once asking for him, (the Mystery of which being a very

Medicatrix, or the *Woman Physician*. 47

very good one, as I have heard related by as great Travellers as the *Jamaita Physician*, I shall anon inform the Reader) endeavouring to make them as odious, as he hath made himself with such entertainments; which if those be the Glory of *Westminster-school*, the perfection of an *University* Man; I fear in time the *Campanell* may have more reason for his suggestions, then now he hath.

He at last, that he might say something more, particularly to gratifie his Masters, though to little purpose, says — *Mr. O Dowde did pretend to as great* Arcana *as any of the Fraternity:* (whatever he pretended, he had much more reason for his pretence, then you have for yours.) *God had been pleased to communicate unto him a Method in the Plague, to preserve Thousands from the Grave, which he promised to administer publickly and freely to all that did desire it.* This is true, and the only truth I find in his Papers in what is proper for my capacity. *Yet did he and his Wife die thereof in* 1665. This I dare not say, because I

think

think the contrary: But what then just nothing. For Mr. *Stubbe* will find this Plot will vanish without any advantage to his Masquerading Cause, or the noise he would make about Shadows and Nut-shells.

To which end, I shall give my Fathers own words, and the whole Paragraph, as 'tis wrote in his Book. Thus,

As to the Plague (which there hath been yet no mention) I hope Gods Mercy is such to us, there may never be occasion for experiment in that kind: But if our sins shall at any time draw down that Judgement upon us, I shall not doubt, by that Method which God hath been pleas'd to Communicate to me, to preserve Thousands from the Grave; and in that Confidence to administer freely and publickly to all that shall desire it, not excepting those persons or places, where other Physicians of the dull Road would be afraid to shew themselves.

These are the very expressions; And let the Malice or Maske of Mr. *Stubbe* and such —— make the most on't. *Yet* did he —— *dye thereof*, saith the Grave

Medicus, but he is loath to tell the World how many Lives he saved before his Death; and how many were preserv'd after by his Medicines, 'tis like, that enquiry was not pertinent to his purpose; *He is glad he dyed thereof.*

And now pray what is herein contained, but what any ingenious and able Physician, that was Master of the Medicines he was, might say and intend? what is herein said, but what was suitably perform'd? And what is herein propos'd, that was not in a proportionable measure verified? And when all this is said, the severest construction will bear, That he owns himself a Mortal Man, not an Immortal God; one that resolved as much as in him lay, to relieve and serve the Country, not to destroy it. But it seems 'tis the Method of *Stubbe, and such* —— when they cannot Eclipse the Fame and Merit of any Man justly, they catch hold of every small matter, whereby they may raise a Mist to blind the World, and stifle Ingenuity, Charity, and all good and laudable Actions.

And that Mr. *Stubbe* may be the better inform'd, or rather the World; That this *Chymical Physician* (who is so much a Mote in his Eye, and would have been a Beam if he had liv'd to this day,) did not decline his Charity, invalidate his Medicines, or revolt from his promise, in assisting to his utmost this City and Suburbs, in that great and lamentable Extremity, not to be exprest by the Tongue of a *Cicero*, or the Pen of a *Homer*; when the *Medicus* and his *generous Medicaments* fled; and at a time too, there was so much proof for such a vapouring *Champion*, and humerous *Lieutenant*: That was a time the *Campanell* would have been rung; Then Mr. *Stubbe* might have seen the Proverb in its exaltation, *A voiurd huy en chere, damain en biere*: Then he might have seen words and Phlebotomy were the least of value, and less of use, in curing a Disease. And then he might likewise have been satisfied, 'tis as easier matter to Prate and Scribble of the Pest, then to Cure it.

I shall mention what I saw, and was an Eye-witness too, being constantly with my Father in most of his Administrations and Visits at *Pest-houses*, and else, to the time of his death, and after continued his Medicines, and my Assistance to (near) the end of that never to be forgotten Calamity.

He was concern'd in the Recovery of many *Pest-sick* Patients, long before it broke out: The approaching Flame being a long time foreseen by him, before it arriv'd to any considerable appearance, or generally believ'd. But the Summer following, being 1665. there needed no Consultation for the knowledge of that devouring Disease, although there did for the Cure. The Signs were evident, the People without much Oratory easily convinc'd, and that by woful experiment; the *Town* then being hastily left by *Physicians*, as well as *Patients*, for they prudently consider'd, 'twas not Civil to send their Patients in the Country, and not attend them themselves.

The *Sickness* coming on a pace, my Father continued to give his hourly help to all that defired it, and omitted no place, perfon, nor opportunity whatfoever, where he might perfonally affift or fuccour, both in Town and out; nor refufed any condition nor occafion, wherein his perfon was demanded, or requefted; but rather freely offer'd and embrac'd all fuch vifits, of which *the Peſt-houſes* at *Fullam* had no fmall fhare: in Sum; he made it his fole and full bufinefs to expofe himfelf, to all the hazard and danger immaginable, fo that he might be as ferviceable, and as charitable as he could, to the true neceffity of thofe difmal creatures, every moment fmitten with that Fatal ftroke.

And as it is Eminently known, he was fufficiently crouded with throngs of people; fo 'tis well known, he did very confiderable fervice, and much good; and preferved, I will not fay Thoufands, but I muft fay many hundreds from the Grave. And by the view of that great Concourfe of people, that repair'd to him daily, during the
time

time before his death: There are those now alive, will say a greater Number than I have set down; and 'tis like there was some reason for it, because it was confidently reported, he got above a 1000 *l.* before his death; so it seems there were sick people enough, and no question but receiv'd some benefit; but I doubt there was not money enough to make up that summe.

I am obliged to say that his business was very great, and too much in that he spent and destroyed himself, by the continual care, trouble, and Administrations he was forc't to go through; and that the importunate and urgent necessity of the sick, induc'd so much true compassion, and diligent attendance from him, that the extraordinary care he had to save his Neighbours life, was the only loss of his own, I am too sensibly acquainted with, but I cannot say his Gain was so great, because I know the contrary, and I as well know his charity, and that his relief was very considerable to the poor sick; the Pest-houses, and many streets & places in & about this City were a Testimony, I am sure, and so much that for my part, since I see so ill a Return for his Life and Charity; I think he better had with-held it for his own Concerns: And such kind of grateful Notices, I fear will by degrees, make ingenious and serviceable Persons more cold in their Charity, and less Obnoxious to the loss of their lives, so that I am put to a stand, whether *Stubbe and such* —— that carry part of the Moon in their heads, will notwithstanding their Vizards and pretences, do their KING and Country more prejudice than Service; but I leave that to a better Pen.

The *Plague* mightily increasing, and devouring with variety of Methods; and my Father still carrying on his assistance, and the Relief to the sick, resolving not to leave this City where there was most necessity, although he was earnestly press'd by other places in the Country; and in particular by *Southamton*, as by the Mayors letter appears, with an allowance of threescore or fourscore pounds a Month, but he refused it. He

He was thrice infected with that doleful sweeping stroke, and still recover'd himself; aud might last of all (when infected) been as easily saved, (if it had pleased GOD to have seen it best for him) but that being at the heigth of the Plague, and those affairs prest so hard upon him, which he was willing to indulge, that he neglected, and consum'd himself till past the help of Art; And I believe it was the fate of several other Chymical Physitians, that were then in Town, under a diligent and proper publick practice and aid of the sick, who by reason of their great pressure, and charge they had upon them, (able Physitians being then scarce) and out of charity, Christian compassion, and earnest Zeal of succouring, and saving the lives of others, lost their own: Not the inability or insufficiency of their Medicines, as unquestionably appear'd by the effect of their applications to, and preservations of their numerous Patients, they weekly recovered.

His death was after this manner, The week before the sickness was at the

Higheſt pitch, which was in *Auguſt* 1665. My Father paſſing over to *Chelſie*, to viſit a Gentlewoman ſick there, and taking me with him; as we went neer the neat houſes, he made his ſervant fetch him a Muskmillion, which he had a more than ordinary deſire for, and the Meſſenger returning with one that was large, and not altogether ſo good as I have ſeen; I offer'd to diſſwade him from it, but not prevailing he eat very much of it, which I was diſ-ſatisfied to ſee, and he was himſelf afterwards ſatisfied, was the Original cauſe of his Mortal ſeizure; And I doubt not but thoſe *Chymical Phyſitians* that abided the *Peſt*, by their publique and free practice amongſt all Patients, eaſily ſaw that any light ſurfeit, was the in-let and reteiner, of that nimble devouring mortal Gueſt the Plague; and ſuch a Plague, that I think could not be fiercer or more deſtructive.

He was very well pleaſed after he had eaten largely of the Muskmillion, and in the Afternoon he returned home, and continued well that day, and moſt part

part of the night; but next morning he seem'd somwhat discomposed, with some little indisposition in his stomach; That morning he was engaged to attend a person, as I remember, neer *Charing-Cross*, (for I was not that day with him as I usually was) to whom some application (I imagine) was made about a Botch, or Carbuncle; the Poysonous matter thereof, so unexpectedly flew about the Room, the Patient being very Corpulent, that I heard say, occasion'd the most horrid stench he ever smelt; so that being fasting, as he came back to the house, he found it very much disturb his stomach, and add to his former disorder.

Yet for all this, although minded and desired to take Medicines, to rectify and prevent; his business, so prest him, that he was forc't to put off and defer the taking any thing several dayes, as I think from Wednesday to Munday; And delayes in those cases, and at that time, those that understand it, well know was not very safe: But indeed the great burden and care of the sick, that was then

then upon him, would not permit him any leisure, till at last, he was so far spent and seized, that he was intangled and taken captive, by the ill effects and misery, of that malignant and Monstrous disease; which were Morosity, frowardness, inaptitude to be perswaded, remissness, aversness to all kind of remedies; so that he could not be ever prevail'd with, to take one Medicine of his own, or any bodies else, only the Munday before his death (he dying the Wednesday following in that notable week the Plague arose to the highest, and was innumerably Fatal) by the greatest intreaties possible, he yielded to have Dr. *Bolnest* sent for, who when he came admiring to see him so negligently, and wilfully resolved, urg'd his advise and Medicines; but no perswasions taking place, although I must confess, then, I believe he was past the help of all Medicines whatsoever; he continued till Tuesday night, but stirring about his Chamber: and that night wee forc't him to take a sweating medicine, left by that Dr. which course he patiently endured; next morning being Wednesday, he had an extraordinary appetite, and was very hungry, so that those things being given he desired; he eat and drank largely, and afterwards lookt cheerfully; but in a few hours, he saw his infallible Messengers, and in two hours more, he pleasantly, sensibly, and most willingly resigned himself into the hands of him who can best judge of his Merit, and is most able and Just to reward him.

This terrible sickness now prevailing to the Amazement of all, and so outragious, that woful and lamentable were the shreeks, the cryes, and groans of poor creatures, and some of their needs so great, that our house being shut up, we had much adoe to prevent the doors and windows from being broken open; (and indeed the Concourse of people at that time, our Family being sick likewise, was very offensive, and noxious to the Neighbourhood) so that a person of Honour then in Town, was by the importunity of several considerable

siderable Persons, petition'd for the opening of the house again, though some of us still sick therein, that the urgent necessities of the sick might have that relief they so much wanted; whose answer, as I have heard from some of those that waited on him was, that although he was willing enough, and would have given a Thousand pounds to have saved my Fathers life, yet the house being sick, the disobligation and danger would be so great to the adjacent streets and places, that he desired they would be contented till the Family were recovered; yet with what conveniencies I could, I convey'd Medicines to many of those that wanted.

The next Friday after the death of my Father, I fell ill my self of this Raging disease, and by the goodness of *God*, and the Medicines of my Father, directed by my own order and instruction, I recovered; Three of our Family more, were likewise presently smitten with the same stroke, but all of them I preserved with my Fathers Medicines.

My Mother after continuing very sorrowful, and dejected for her late loss; Her grief and fears, at last subjected her to such irregularities, and occasions of diseases, that she fell ill; but in all the time of her sickness, nor after, by what I could perceive, she had no sign, Symptome, or distinction of the Pest; neither could D. *Needham*, her then Physitian, discern it to be that disease: And there is no more doubt with me about it, but that she died at such a time That all diseases were then included in one; that being the most Malignant, contagious, and Mortal.

This trouble I have given the Reader and my self, in some degree to satisfie Mr. *Stubbe* that I am alive, and that we did not all *dye thereof*; and to rectifie the delusion and Imposture he puts on the World; and since he will give no better account, and make no true Representation of one single person, and his Medicines, within a few miles of him so clearly to be discern'd; what Judgement is to be made of his History, of the body of his inspiration, and positive

tive damnation of those *Famous Univerſal Authors*, generally Honoured, and followed through all parts of Chriſtendome, that were before his time, and ſo remote and very far diſtant from him.

Yet did he —— dye thereof, ſaith the great Oracle Mr. *Stubbe*; and 'tis well for his Cauſe he did ſo; for if he had lived, Mr. *Medicus*, I muſt ſay your friend Dr. *Thompſon* in that particular, when he tells you he believed he would have been a thorn in the ſides of your Aſſociates; I have reaſon to know it was rationally aim'd, and ſo he would certainly have ſtuck more faſt to your ſides, than ever Mr. *Stubbe* did to his Maſter *V.* and prov'd ſuch a thorn, that all the *generous Medicaments* of our lowd *Campanell*, No nor the brighteſt Lancet he was ever maſter of, No, nor yet his Glorious *Viper Wine* it ſelf, ſhould never have been able to have eradicated: And were it my mind, I could likewiſe tell this great *talker of Phyſick,* what preparation he had made for that purpoſe, but I do not know that I owe him ſo much ſervice, neither do I ſee

that

Medicatrix, or the *Woman Physician*. 63

that I am oblig'd to gratifie him with that Rarity.

And now by the expreſs I have given of this *Chymicall Phyſitian*, in anſwer to the Lofty charge, but implicite nothing M. *Stubbe* ſo plauſibly inſinuates, and victoriouſly flatters himſelf, as if he had exceeding cauſe to clap his wings, and Crow, or cock his Hatt and take the Chair; it may by every common capacity be judg'd, wherein he was ſo very criminal in his words, Medicines and promiſe in the Peſt; and what an unpardonable act of offence he committed againſt Mr. *Stubbe*, in mentioning his thoughts, and the aſſurance he had reaſon to believe of theſe Medicines, he had acquired for this fatal deſtroying diſeaſe; or rather Divine Judgment, and imediate hand of *God*, which I think is a better definition, than any Philoſopher will, it may be allow.

And what would the *Phyſician at Warwick* have ſaid leſs, if he had been ſure of ſuch Medicines, and in probability of ſuch an occaſion for Experiment; And what would he have done

more

more, if he and his *Generous Medicaments* had not fled; and left the poor City to shift, and then come after like a boasting Coward, and cry, if I had been there, or rather durst have been there —— 'tis like you had been dead too.

He would have done strange wonders no doubt, thinking it easie with the *Frenchman* it may be, *Faire escran contre le vent sur les Alpes.* For he tells us, as I remember in one of his Books, discoursing of the *Plague*, which I verily believe is a Disease he knows nothing of, That he made a Trial of some of his Medicines at *Fullam*, in the beginning of this *Plague*, and he found pretty good effect thereby. Yes so good, as generously to run away, and leave his Patients when the Disease came to a true *Pest*; for I doubt not but this famous trial, and great adventure he made at that time, he calls the beginning of the *Plague* was long enough before it, when perhaps 'twas little more then the *Scurvy*, and scarce amounted to the degree of an ordinary *Feaver*.

But

But the Tinkling *Campanell* may now see, this Gentleman was as good as his promise, he did stick to the Afflicted City, and did administer publickly and freely, where the Doctors of the Common Road durst not venture themselves; as for example, Mr. *Stubbe* for one; And he may likewise see, he was not deceived in the Confidence and Soveraignty of those Medicines; and what Assistance, Service and Preservation they afforded; although not Thousands, yet it seems many Hundreds; and what an earnest that was for Thousands, if he had liv'd out the Calamity, any moderate and impartial Reader will presume; but if this severe Critick will be more nice as to the word, which none but a perfect Caviller will bluster withall; he thereby only exprest, that he doubted not but to preserve very many Lives thereby, which he did to Admiration; and would have made up even the very particular number and word he catches at, if he had been spared himself.

F   And

And further, to juſtifie thoſe very Medicines for that cruel Sickneſs, that Mr. *Stubbe* may have no true diſ-ſatisfaction for not anſwering his masked Objection, *Yet did he —— dye thereof*; I doubt he forgets, *It is appointed for all Men once to dye*; and it may be never read the *Duke* of *Gniſes* Motto, *Chacun a ſon tour*, if he will blame him for dying, I know not who 'tis he muſt diſpute withall; he muſt either accuſe his Charity, for his neglecting and looſing his own Life for the preſervation of his Neighbours, or he muſt fight with Providence, and contend the Almighty; for the beſt Vizard Mr. *Stubbe* is maſter of, cannot obſcure thoſe Medicines he then uſed, they are not at all leſſen'd, nor the Authors Confidence in them impeached, becauſe he never took them; if he would or could, in any reaſonable time have taken them, he had been as eaſily ſaved as I was my ſelf, and as eaſily as he was three times himſelf before; and as eaſily as he preſerved Hundreds of others. But if it were no more then this one inſtance, it were enough to extoll a Medicine,

Four

our in his Family, only had the Plague that took his Medicines, and they were all recovered, and I think yet alive; He himself, and if this Caviller will have it my Mother also, took them not, they died. But Mr. *Stubbe* had shew'd himself more Candid and Discreet, if he had considered, That in such great Cases, and in so mortal and sharp a Stroke, where so much need and necessity requires plenty of Physicians, there are then the fewest to be found; That the great burden then resting upon a few, if that paucity have any ability or charity, they must every moment extend it; by which extraordinary and perpetual care and diligence in managing the sick;

Those Men, though never so well stored with the most infallible perfection of Art, may at last, by a long and continued course of Administration, be wearied, spend their strength, and exhaust their Spirits; Nature in such case will fail, 'tis not immutable; and a Physician may thus have good Medicines, and save his Patients, but I think not consequently himself, whose business it is, publickly

lickly and conſtantly to expoſe himſelf to all kinds of buſineſs, as he did, without a Man will make it his only endeavour to keep himſelf alive, and help no Body elſe, (and then what makes ſuch a Phyſician in a place of danger, where he dare not do any good.) Theſe neceſſities being the prevailing neglect of his Life, and then total extinction, not deficiency or incapacity of the Medicines he commended therein.

So that 'tis impoſſible for any Man to enſure his own Life in ſuch particular Profeſſions, and in ſuch eminent Contagions, and fatal Diſeaſes, though he may his Patients very often. So many are the Arrows to be avoided, ſo many the Accidents to be prevented: And if Mr. *Stubbe* will ſay he will abide in, and outlive a *Plague*, he muſt then be able to ſay, he is not ſubject to a *Plague*, or elſe I doubt, he is as liable to that unavoidable deſtruction as other Men. But the Miſt caſt by this malicious diſguiſer, is of courſe diſperſed, and I am ſatisfied. This therefore only remains, for a concluſion of this firſt part of my
Vin-

Vindication, which is, It is an experimental truth, and well known, that those that cannot do good themselves, hate that any body else should.

And therefore let me take liberty to tell Mr. *Henry Stubbe* a *Physician at Warwick*, that in spite of his Malice, This Gentleman, whose worth he so wilfully would bouse, ended his Life with that Honour, never by him to be purchas'd, and that is, He Lived and was a faithful Servant to his King, He was and dyed a faithful Servant to this Country.

The Second Part

SECT. I.

A Revival of Dr. O Dowdes Medicine. The Authors Opinion of Learning.

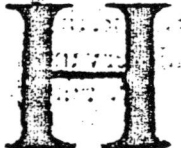Aving by the many urgent occasions, & importunate calls given me by Mr. *Stubbe*, (in all his Papers that I have seen yet) uncivilly reflecting on the Ashes of my Father, discharged some of my Resolves in answer to the truth of that particular History in the former discourse, I shall now in this, endeavour by a more general Survey, and positive Test to find out, whether Mr. *Stubbe* be so omniscient as he pretends; so able a Physician as he desires to be thought; and so fit to judge others, and regulate the whole World in matters of Physick as he says; which qualification in him I much question'd, And which by me, (since he hath forc'd me to it) shall now be determin'd: And further, I shall hereby satisfie Mr. *Stubbe*, That *although he did die thereof*, his Medicines did not *die thereof*, nor therein, which is no wellcom news to him, and such

his dis-ingenious and inhumane Brethren, that care not what becomes of Sick, or any thing else, so they can support their own Grandeur, Profit and Interest; They would have been glad his Medicines had *died thereof* too, I am sure; for good reasons I know, to the Honour, or rather, Shame of their Art be it spoken. But in few words, in being his Medicines are, improved too; and like to be much more so; and for satisfaction of which, Mr. *Stubbe* shall anon have the first refusal.

And rather then such effectual saving Medicines should not have been preserv'd; And had there been no probability of continuing and reviving them, I would have took some poor Schollar from an University, and furnisht him with that Knowledge, and those Medicinal Perfections (if there be no other then I fear Mr. *Stubbe* is accomplished withal) that place would never have endued him with, or otherwise. I would publickly, to the view of all Readers, (as my Father once design'd) have discover'd those Medicines, and the true Preparations and Management, together with the Method and Use thereof; that Mr. *Stubbe* his Cause might then have appeared unmask'd. And that the whole World might have seen the Ignorance and miserable Condition some Physicians keep them in; and what advantage and benefit they are generally destitute of; And the glory and difference between the great Se-

cretr,

crets, and sublime acquirements of a *Chymical Physician*, which I shall presently call a *Medicinalist*, and his Adaptation to attend and Cure the Sick, and their Diseases: And that *Physician* that can brag barely of Reading an Author, but knows not how to procure a Medicine, or recover a Disease; and such a one I shall presently call a *Verbalist*.

But least I go too far before I am fully understood, (having a *Vulpone* to deal withall) I must undeceive him, and prevent his doubling in what I perceive he makes it his business to perswade; and that is, That Learning is damnified and villified by his Adversaries; but this is a meer Juggle and fictitious design, only to oppose Ingenuity: such another Wheedle, as the only Argument he brings, and hopes will back him with some pretence against the *Royal Society*, and all ingenious and absolute necessary improvements, (without which, this Lame, Decrepid, halting Age, will not be reliev'd) That ingenious Scrutinies, and the conversation of such *Societies*, is the way to introduce *Popery*, which in another place I will again Note.

But Mr. *Stubbe* must take this notice, once for all to save trouble; That I have no reason, nor shall have any occasion, to reflect upon, or dis-praise the true design of Learning, and its requisite Method, and such Education in my following intrudements: And therefore in that

that expectance he will not be gratified, but as much the contrary, as his own *Generous Medicaments* are to Diseases: Neither do I think there is any person, though never so illiterate and rude, that can bear a hatred too, or despise so desireable and fit a qualification, as the proper intent, and just ends of Litterature.

And this will be no quarrel between the *Medicus* and me, we shall not differ herein; nor I believe he need not contest with any body else so much about it as he seems to do, were it not a subtlety, and so specious to oblige his Readers opinion of his undertakings.

For as to my own concern, and my particular Judgment of it, I freely declare I admire it; and that it is an Education very conducible, and proper for every person that can with any conveniency attain to it: It is an excellent Ornament and Accomplishment, and a Capacity suitable to prepare a Man, with the more ease, for any Profession; as also the enquiries and obtainments any Art dictates, and the true end thereof proposes: And if I my self had never so many Children, if I could possibly do it, I would breed them Schollars; so that I shall sufficiently take off the prejudice of Mr. *Stubbe*, and forewarn him hereby, when I do say, That I esteem real Learning, and the Foundation, Promoters, and Doctors thereof: And if there be any difference between us about it, it must be, That although I highly Honour,

and

and commend this kind of Education and Ornament; Yet I do say, Learning in it self, is only preparatory, not perfect, a proper progress and tendency, in order to the *Art of Physick*, not the Perfection and Consummation of that Art: A Man may read an Author, and yet not understand a Medicine; and I am confident an Able, knowing Author, never yet publisht a good effectual Medicine, as daily experience will best decide: No, this were to make a Divine Art cheap and contemptible; and to create and nourish more Sloth and Laziness then there is already: *Authors* I conceive direct and instruct their Students, only by pointing out the Way; not by walking to the Journeys end.

And as I am not satisfied, That every Author that writes of *Medicines* understands them; so I am as well assured, That a Man may sleep many years at the Fountain of Learning, and yet awake no *Physician*: *Medicines* are the Marrow and full Perfection of a *Physician*, and those are hard to be attain'd: They are many of them (that are excellent and worth a value) of some years preparation, and I doubt not but must be of many more for Invention: Learning will fit a Man for that Profession, but a diligent and indefatigable Elaboration must perfect it. *Medicines* when obtained, one may in a reasonable time learn to apply; but how to obtain those Medicines, I verily think is a question beyond Dr. *Stubbes's* Study. Sect.

SECT. II.

Since the Fall, the Body is subject to Diseases.
The Explanation of, and difference between, a Verbalist *and a* Medicinalist.
The Subject and End of Physick.
The subtlety of Mr. Stubbes's *Argument against the* Royal Society, *pretending Popery the Consequence.*
Plutarch's *Opinion of the decay of Virtue.*

WE are very sensible, That although Man was Created little lower then the Angels, and in a happy Station during his Innocency; yet no sooner was the Divine Commands prevaricated, and Disobedience appear'd; But the Almighty Curse fell upon him and his Posterity; and so subjected both Soul & Body to miseries Spiritual and Temporal: And although the rigour and severity of the first Covenant is Qualified and Redeemed by the infinite Grace and Mercy of the Second; and so the future happiness of Mankind is again thereby secured, and both Soul and Body made capable likewise of Eternal Glory hereafter.

Yet by this Fall, as the Body became subject to decay, so it continues liable to the Effects of Sin, the many Infirmities, Calamities, and Diseases that we see daily attend it.

Notwithstanding which, such is the Goodness and Mercy of our compassionate Creator, that even in this, we are not left Remediless, but he hath allowed us means for Comfort; *For of the most High cometh Healing: And the Lord hath Created Medicines out of the Earth:* And he that is wise may find them, but not without experiment. How precious a thing Life is, the Devil describes; (who 'tis like knows the value of one) when he says, *Skin for Skin and all that a Man hath will be give for his Life:* How sweet and pleasant a thing it is for the Body to be kept free from Sickness in this Life; any one that hath had a *Quartan Ague,* the Circuit of a year, a Fit of the *Gout,* the Age of a Moon, or a Fit of the *Stone,* the space of a Week, can competently judge.

The Body being thus obnoxious to Diseases, Health so great a Jewel, Life inestimable, and Medicines possible to be attained, that may answer the Necessities of Nature: What greater inducement can there be then this, for Physicians to employ themselves in the commendable Scrutinies of those proper qualifications, that may suit with the only design of Mans preservation? Yet pride and interest prevails amongst Men so much, that they will not let Truth appear; They rather spend their whole time in disputing and talking of a Disease, then looking after a Remedy to Cure it: Rather invent Names for one another, then

Me-

Medicines. By the Catalogue of Titles, one would think there were no Medicine wanting; as to read of an *Aristotelian*, a *Mountebank*, a *Quack-Salver*, a *Galenist*, a *Methodist*, a *Pseudo-Chymist*, a *Semi-Chymist*, a *Galeno-Chymist*, a *Pythagorean*, a *Sceptick*, a *Paracelsian*, a *Cartesian*, an *Alchymist*, a *Chymist*, an *Helmontian*, a *Baconical Disciple*, &c. who would not think, but that all Diseases are Curable? who would think there were a Disease in a Kingdom? and who will not say, but that here are Names promise more then some of their *generous Medicaments*? But I see Diseases are never the more recovered by variety of Names, and therefore to avoid Confusion, since this Age will not be confin'd, but are full of Verbal Inventions; I shall adventure to use two words only to serve my purpose; and to that distinction, I assign all degrees of Physical Practicers, viz. a *Verbalist*; by which I mean a wording Conjectural *Physician*, or rather one that pretends to be All-knowing in *Physick*, and yet is ignorant in the Cure of a Disease: The other is, a *Medicinalist*; and by that, I mean such a *Chymical Physician* that hath attained the highest degree of Medicines, and can Cure any Disease as far as the power of Art comprehends: for since Miracles are ceas'd, words cure no Diseases; Therefore good Noble saving Medicines, must be the Complement of Study and Operation; and none can properly judge of this, but those that enjoy them. The

The Body of Man (being liable to Diseases) is the *Subject* of Physick. To preserve the health thereof when it is in present enjoyment, and to restore and heal it, when it is Sick, is the chief and great *End* of Physick. In these few words is the Body of Physick contained; This is the sum of the *Art of Physick*, which so many Authors, in so many Volumes, and Books innumerable, whereby the whole World is fill'd, have made so much noise about, and not yet attain'd.

But now, Mr. *Stubbe* in this happy Age appears, and bids the Universe be of good Comfort; For he will regulate all Errors, supply all defects in Physick, and plant the World in knowledge for the future, and so set the Sick and Diseased free by his *Generous Medicaments*; the chief of which, I perceive, is his Lancett, and that he doth not a little brandish, and thereby seems to compleat himself with the Garland of *Victoria*.

In order to this, he Condemns and Crucifies all other Societies, Methods and Courses of Ingenuity, Persons and Promoters of necessary Acquirements, but what he is pleas'd to adore and worship himself: In fine, he refuses *Chymistry*, Operation, the true knowledge and preparation of a *Medicine*, demonstration, and *Experiment*; without which, the Sick will continue still as miserable and indigent,

gent, as this kind of Physician is ignorant.

This is a Project I take to be an absolute self Interest, although he is more subtile than (if possible) to own the least thought, or letter that may argue this; No, he abominates such an Act, as much as he doth the *Royal Society*, as much as he doth the tender of a *Medicinall Challenge*, or Touchstone of his Abilities: Therefore he takes another course, and renders himself very plausible, and his cause very indisputable; and this he doth, by Ringing his *little Bell* for the common people, and laying the old bait for the more Learned.

The *Medicus* at *Warwick*, whom I look upon to be a sole *Verbalist*; well knowing the Constitution of this Kingdome, by the experience he hath had under his Master Sir *H. V.* in the late times of Murder, and Rebellion; as well as by other satisfaction, and what a Bug-bear the name of *Popery* is to the Generality of the common people; and how ready, unanimously they will be to catch at a thing that sounds of that, and to oppose any thing that hath but the least colour of the Religion, or letter of the Name; although they know not why nor wherefore, (though they may have reason) but follow *Tradition* like their Tutor the *Verbalist*.

The *Medicus* being well assured of this; as well knows, he shall be sure to procure at least this advantage to his disguised design; that
the

the common people will quickly hearken to his Bell, and applaud his goodness ; let it be what it will, though to their own destruction, so long as it bears the gloss of a *papall* prevention : He thus begins to Tinckle, the consequence of the *Royal Society*, Experiment, Ingenuity, the most laudable and commendable, Nay, absolute necessary improvement of Knowledge is dangerous, and the Fore-runner of Popery; For, *never was there any sort of people that by so many Artifices, endeavour'd to insinuate themselves, and their Religion, into all places and Countries, as that of the Papists : There is not shape or disguise which they will not assume, no humour which they will not comply with ; not an action of theirs but ought to be suspected*; but he *speaks not this to reflect upon the Royal Society, who have found so great encouragement from that Party, by the concurrence of their Persons and purses ; and so freely keep correspondence with them from beyond Seas*: No Good-man; I believe he knows not what he speaks, for this is no Reflection.———*to see how friendly the Protestants and Papists converse together in this Assembly* :——*it must needs raise their hopes of bringing things to a closer Union, when they perceive the strangeness that ought to be, and hath been betwixt them taken off, and to read adresses*———*How much an Oratour gains upon his Auditors when he hath made them attentive, and what a step that is to gaining upon their Esteem, and*

and how conducing that is towards the perswading them to what he intends, I well understand: I do believe you do, otherwise you would never have ventur'd on those Plots you have laid to attain your desires; and you have made the best use of it you are able; but I cannot say you have met with your expectation: You depended much on your Oratory, else Mr. *Stubbe* had never been in Print; But you dare not appear to justifie the truth of your Doctrines, and I may say of you, as *Cicero* said of *Crassus*, you knew well enough the people would be glad to hear it, and therefore you spake it.

But what benefit and advantage Popery may derive from this, that our Nobility and Gentry, our Divines and Layety, laying aside all memory of the French and Irish Massacre, and Marian Persecutions, the Gun-powder Treason, the Firing of London, and forgetting all animosities and apprehensions of future dangers, (well rung Campanel, ring again.) Converse freely with, and write obligeingly to them, Testifie a great esteem of them. I deny that Consequence in Point of Religion, that because a Society takes the benefit of any Mans parts towards the improving an Art, or promoting any curious Invention, they must presently be Converts to their Religion, and esteem that. No, no Mr. *Stubbe*, the Political preservation of the Protestant Religion, is not your great and true design.

sign; but 'tis the opposition and destruction of all other Ingenuity, Knowledge, and promotion but what your own secular interest, and the private interest of your party obliges you too. *And from the dis-use of all harsh but too true Censures, come at length to lay aside all rancour and bitterness of thoughts*: What kind of Christian is our *Campanell*? would he have the Protestants turn Papists in earnest, and assure it by a bloody retaliation! *I say how great benefit Popery may draw hence, I cannot well comprehend*: Nor I neither. *Yet I guess in part from what the Historian sets down*, out of which his Collection is to this purpose, that a communication, and conversation with a Papist, is the way to be infected and to espouse not an Art, but the Religion of the Artist: But at this time our *Medicus*, I presume, desires to be thought a Polititian, and not a Phisitian; And if the case be so dangerous that the fight of a Papist, or any of a contrary Religion will infect a Man, and hazard his Faith by being in his company, without it may be knowing whether he be a Turk or a Jew, a Rebel or a Royalist, a Protestant or a Papist, which is not impossible; for Mr. *Stubbe* may imagine, that Religion is not the only Enquiry of every Artist in this age: How secure are Mr. *Stubbs* his Societies, whose *Protector* he would ambitiously be thought; what would quickly become of the Kingdome? Merchants would

would soone grow poor, Sea-Men beg, and the Nation starve, no Ship must go to *France*, *Spain*, to the *Indies*, or any Forreign parts; But the whole Trade of the Kingdom must be prohibited, all Commerce whatsoever overthrown and destroyed; or else we must be all Mahometans, Turks, Infidels, Jews, Papists, and Rebells, or what not.

But it is like Mr. *Stubbs* his Royal adversaries, are able to defend themselves without my help, and no doubt have (although I have not yet had time to see any of their writings) or easily may, soon take off these Political objections: So that I only mention this, to shew what Introduction this Politician hath contrived; what method he useth, and what sound his *Bell* makes to Alarum his vulgars, and call them to his Aid in carrying on his true design, for the preservation of himself, and his adherents, though the conclusion be to the prejudice and destruction of his common congregation. This is one of his wiles to get footing, and some colour for the defence and preservation of his interessed Project, beginning with those that are most likely to be ensnar'd, and so proceeds: I recommend this observation to the intelligible, and end this Plot with the opinion of *Plutarch*, a better States-man than Mr. *Stubbe*. *That Vertue it self, which is the greatest and sweetest Riches a*

Man can hvve, decayeth oftentimes through sickness, or else through Physick, and Potions. Let this be considered, and then our Polititian may be answered, that *there are more wayes to the Wood than one*; For a Kingdome may as well suffer by the Potion of a *Verbalist*, as the Sermon of a *Jesuit*.

<small>Plut. *in the Life of* Solon Fol. 89.</small>

SECT. III.

The Argument M. Stubbe *brings against the* Royal Society, *and the Ingenuity of this Age, that Learning is besieged; Answered. His Political design discovered to be his Interest.*

THe *Campanell* baits his next hook with the suggestion that Learning is besieged, and that the Foundation thereof will be injured; The Pillars of Divinity debilitated in their Education & Discipline; Physicians not so litterally quallifi'd, and the Booksellers Trade consequently not so good; and by this Train, he seems to be Cock-sure of blowing up all Men that oppose his Interest, and will not let him say and do what he pleaseth, and so endeavours hereby to oblige the rest of the Kingdome to his assistance, and begs their encouragement for his cause, and calls to them to behold what a discovery he hath made, and which

sometime

Medicatrix, or the *Woman Physician*.

sometime or never would have come to pass, if he had not found it out; and so Proclaims he can make no other Estimate of England, but that even the poor remains of Religion and Learning amongst us were so eminently endangered, that he could not expect their long continuance, nor with patience think how to survive them. Alas good Gentlemen! what a perplexity he is fallen into.

Therefore if this be the Case, what Man of Learning, and one that values it at so great a Rate as he pretends, would not make a good use of it, when it is in its splendour, and so preserve its future Glory, by manifesting its true Excellency, and necessary use; by the Fruits and Products thereof.

This great care of Learning in General, so much assured by our *Campanell*, to be the great and ultimate aim of his publick Quarrels; Wants no inducement in it self, to invite a general concurrence of Opinion, that some advantage and benefit is thereby intended: But for my part I am not yet convinc't, that our *Medicus*, notwithstanding all these shews, is any other than another *Demetrius*, and although his cry may seem to be otherwise, yet in reality the true cause is the same.

The name of Learning in all Ages, hath contracted a venerable Esteem; and therefore the continuance, Preservation, and Promotion thereof, still retains a commendation, and encou-

encouragement, in such a Patron as is found adequate, to that necessary end, and unbyas'd prosecution.

And so this subtle, and plausible pretence of Mr. *Stubbe*, he well hop'd was a most taking Method to engage a considerable Approbation; but I think if a due consideration be made, this will appear but a delusion, and that his *tinkling* is not to be nourisht, but rather his deceptive vail to be drawn off, and his mask'd cunning discovered; which I believe, notwithstanding all his Glorious perswasions will appear, to be little less than to support sloth, and idleness, and still keep the World in ignorance; and I question whether in conclusion he will not rather by his stirring and scribling, bring an accusation against Learning and the interest of his Party, than by his defence give a preservation to it.

As to the Noble and Honourable foundation, Ornament, and design of Learning it self, I know no man bears it any prejudice, but Mr. *Stubbs* himself; all admire, and desire really, and in earnest to cherish, and substantially to improve it; and that is more ingenuity and candour than its own *Champion* and *Protector* thereof bears: So that in this truth he that kindled the fire must put it out; and if he will contend (notwithstanding his prevallent Oratory) it must be with the Air; for I believe in this he hath hitherto met with no adversary. But

But the Learning of a *Physitian*, being that he so zealously renders himself concern'd for, I shall address my self to that particular which serves my purpose, as well as his Fallacy; And therefore I must take liberty to charge him with *Two things* I am dissatisyed in; and those are the motives of my stedfast perswasion, that Mr. *Stubbe* is not so justly bent in his writings to secure the necessity of Learning, as he fancies the world believes of him.

Because first, if Learning were that he chiefly aims at to Promote; why doth he then put such slanders and contempt on those *Learned Physicians*, that have been eminently adorned, with that qualification he so much commends?

Next, if he be so great a lover of Literature, and it be so absolutely requisite, what is the reason his very own *Authors* in *Physick*, he is so much devoted too, have not answered that end to this day? And why doth not he that owns himself the only Protector of Learning, and sole Dictator in Physick, make out, and plainly demonstrate unto the World, that Learning is of that use in Physick he avows? especially when it is a matter of that weight, and fatal consequence, that his Cause solely depends upon it, and is the period thereof, if not thereby determin'd.

Paracelsus, I believe, bears as great a Name, and is as Famous all over the World, as Mr. *Stubbe*, and I have heard reputed as good a Schollar

Scollar; yet in our *Campanels* esteem, he is more Ruftical than any Plow-boy, more contemptible than ever *Jack Adams* was; in fine, his beft Title is but a *Rhodomontader*.

Helmont, who by all Men that ever I heard difcourfe of him, reported him to be as great a Philofopher, as able a Phyfitian, and as profound a Shollar, as any in Print; receives no other Epitaph from Mr. *Stubbe*, then that he was *the moft infolent, but worft of Phyficians*. But for all that, it feems this defpifed ignorant *Phyfician* hath made fhift to convert the World; fo that at laft, all are like to come under his Difcipline.

More famous Men of Learning I could mention, under the contempt of Mr. *Stubbe*, but thefe (for brevities fake) are obvious and enough.

But it may be Mr. *Stubbe* will be ingenious, and confefs what made him accufe thefe Men; that it was his malice, and not their defect of Learning: Well, if that were the reafon, we will proceed to his own Fathers, and thofe he extolls for this neceffary accomplifhment.

Ga en, under whofe Banner this *Campanell* fights, hath been accounted a Prince of Learning; yet 'tis faid, by fome Men that write of him, he underftood not fo much as *Rofe-water*, he could not Cure the *Gout*, the *Stone*, the beft *Medicine* he had for an *Ague, Small-Pox*, a *Feaver*, was but his *Lancett*; many Petty Difeafes *seases* he call'd *incurable*. His Disciples ever since, and most of them that call themselves Schollars, such as our *Verbalist*, can talk well and Learnedly of any Disease; and if words would heal, they were really the only Physicians in the World; but when the performance is demanded, and their real abilities tryed, I need not say how many considerable Diseases are Cured, and languishing Sick restored.

So that the advantage and benefit of Learning by this means remains still questionable, and the true purpose and faith of Mr. *Stubbe* disputable. By this means Learning appears to the World to be but a preparatory way and method in order to the finding out the *Art of Physick*, not the Consummation and Complement of the knowledge of *Medicine*: So that Litterature in its self is declared deficient in Medicine, and not able to answer the necessity of the Sick, or the final perfection of the *Physical Scholar*: And therefore I conceive this Age doth not endeavour to derogate from it; but to add to it; and to furnish and compleat it with what undeniable conveniencies and full knowledge it now wants.

And hitherto Mr. *Stubbes*'s enterprise favours more of interest and policy then otherwise; neither is he so good as his promise, in defending his Societies as perfect in Physick; and all others ignorant and incapable of taking care of the Sick, or curing a Disease, because

cause he hath not yet given this proof to the World which is expected; so that for the present he hath rather brought an accusation against Litterature, then maintain'd a vindication of it. But perhaps this he will do hereafter, or else farewell *Champion at Warwick*; for he hath conjur'd up such a Ghost that will not easily disappear.

SECT. IV.

The Author allows what Honour is due to Mr. Stubbe.
A Coward not fit to wear a Garland.
Learning abused.
Two Miracles appear in Physick.
The History and Mystery of Van Helmonts not being known in the Street where he liv'd, contriv'd by the Plot of Dr. Kraft, and drawn in Colours by Stubbe.
Chymical Medicines *ont of Mr. Stubbes's reach.*
Who is quallified to Cure a Disease.
A Medicinal *Challenge to the* Champion at Warwick. *with a Discourse of several Diseases,* &c.
His former Evasion.
His bold questioning the Royal *promotion of this Age.*

I have no desire nor intention to detract from, or degrade Mr. *Stubbe* in any thing that is properly due to him; nor shall I deny him any
acknow-

acknowledgement he can juftly claim, Therefore I believe he may be enough of that name which is called a Schollar ; but that will not ferve his turn in thofe publick attempts he hath made in Phyfick, without he can juftifie his proceedings by demonftrative Actions, as well as words. He that will appear a *Champion* in any caufe, muft be generally Arm'd, and provided fo, that he may be able to defend any ftroke, and avoid any wound his Enemy can give him ; and in a Battle the inequality of Swords, the goodnefs of Guns, or how a Soldier comes to be well mounted, is not then to be difputed ; But their caufe to be maintain'd, their Adverfaries oppos'd, their valour evidenc'd, and and themfelves defended : otherwife that fide that proves victorious, will have fome reafon to be gratified with the thoughts, at leaft, of being the beft Soldiers.

That *General* that will bid defiance to his Enemy, challenge him to the Field, encourage and imbolden his Army, direct what courfe they fhall take to overcome their *Combatants*, tell them how eafily 'tis to be done, what exploits he will do, and lead them on in perfon himfelf, nay, dye with them if occafion require ; And when the Enemy approaches, and the Trumpet Sounds before the Fight begins ; This brave *Commander* turns his Back, leaves his Men, and rides quite away ; fhall this piece of Valour be called a Conqueror, or is he fit to wear a *Garland* ?

I have often enough said, that Learning is an useful Ornament, but not the perfection of knowledge in Physick; and therefore that necessary Introduction is more abused then used by the *Physician*, as I fear too sensibly appears in these times.

For a Man to come and talk of Physick, to call himself a *Teacher* of it, and stand up to guide the whole World therein, in such an ingenious, knowing and intelligible Age as this is, without any other abilities to back him, then words, seems to me not only a Riddle, but almost a Miracle; and I thought if there had been any wonders with us at this day, they had been only these two, That in so many hundred years the Art of *Learned Physick* is no more improved; *Physicians* that desire to be *Honoured* with the name of *Learning*, are no more able in their *Science*, then their Masters of Old were near Two Thousand years before them.

And that *Chymistry* so much Clouded and Murdered, in so few years should flourish, grow so famous, and so universally prevail, generally esteem'd, and produce so much benefit.

Learning is abused, or else, I am sure it is of little or no value in *Medicine*, or to be sought after by the *Physical Student*; and by this means the Proverb will be truly verified, *Il vaut mieux tomber entre les mains d'un Medecin heureux, que d'un Medecin Scavant.*

And if this be all the benefit that Mr. *Stubbe* can brag of in reading an Author, notwithstanding his reaping the profit, that of a Thousand years skill, and in viewing and learning as many Authors of Medicine, he cannot yet cure a considerable Disease; I see no reason he hath to plume himself with the Glory of his *Teachers*; or to magnifie himself with the assurance, that 'tis best to continue in the Footsteps, and walk in the Path of these Ancients; because the Travellers are many, and so the Path consequently well trodden; for it seems they never came to their Journeys end. But 'tis no matter for that, Mr. *Stubbe* is sure, and in the right, he cannot erre, because he follows what the *Italian* Proverb commends, and loves *to go that way which the Men go*; and what way is that? even the same that our *English* Proverb discommends, and that is, *That way which Asses go*. Mr. *Medicus*, if this be your excellent way, I will promise you, if I can avoid it. *Jen' iray pas Jur vos brisees*.

And if words be the only attainment of our *Campanells* Studies, I cannot apprehend him to be capable of being a *Medicinal Judge*, or so omniscient as to condemn *Helmont*, and all *Chymical Physicians*, Fools; though *Verbalists* I know are suitable enough furnisht to invent abuses of what ingenuity and abilities other Men have; as it particularly is reported by Travellers, it happened in the Story of *Helmont*,

mont, That Mr. *Stubbe* rejoyces in reciting the account, Dr. *Kraft* his Brother in folly contriv'd, to oblige his *Tribe* withall: *Kraft* vainly plotting to suppress the fame and thundring noise of *Helmont*, makes this report to his Fraternity, *That he was in* Brussells, *and enquired after* Van Helmont, *and demanding of some persons which had liv'd long in the same Street that he did, where his House was? they could not tell him; and protested, they had never heard of his name: whereat he was surpriz'd;* and so am I, to think that Dr. *Kraft* should be so Idle, as to believe, he should be believed; and that this trick would take, for the destruction of *Helmont*; which as I have heard the truth of, from some Travellers that have made it their business, to enquire after this malicious representment; and that have been as far as *Jamaica* or *Barbados*, which are the utmost Travels I perceive Mr. *Stubbe* can boast of; And in few words, they found this Trincket of *Kraft*, to be only an enquiry made by him in a Family of Forreigners, newly come out of *France*, of mean people, and not settled many days in the house, they took; nor its possible had never heard, nor had occasion to enquire, after the name of *Helmont*, before they knew they were certainly in *Brussells*: And the answer of these was, its affirmed, a sufficient satisfaction for Dr. *Kraft* to gratifie his design, and record the notorious History to all Ages. And

And this is enough to compleat Mr. *Stubbe*, and make him vapour, that by this one Blow *Van Helmont* hath lost his Head; and his Authority aud Credit is hereby taken off, and that *he was no intelligent person; and that it is plain, he was a Man of no Practice*, and consequently no fitting Judge of a Medicine; for he says, *nothing is firm in Physick, but what is confirm'd by a happy experience: and 'tis an Imbecillity of Judgment (saith the great Stagirite) to desert experience, and adhere to reason.* How! is it possible that our *Medicus* writes these words, and as his own Opinion too? I am then in better hopes of making good my design then I thought; and have a little reason to fancy, the *Campanell* and I shall end the dispute by Experiment.

So it seems, Dr. *Kraft* by this one Cratchet, hath been the Bane of poor *Helmont*; and blown him quite up, for ever more being so much as nam'd.

But if you desire to know the reason why the great *Helmont* is now known all over the World; That he is now the only admir'd Man, by as great Schollars as Mr. *Stubbe*, That so many Men follow his *Doctrine*, and grow eminent and able *Physicians* thereby. And if you desire to know the reason why *Helmont* in his Life, challeng'd all the *Physicians of Europe*, that oppos'd *Chymistry*, to Cure any Disease with them, and they would not engage him;

him; And if yon desire to know how many Troops of Sick People repair'd to him in one year: And if you will know what made Mr. *Stubbes*'s Brethren use all the Art they could to prevent *V. Helmonts* Writings from being publick: If you would lastly know, whether our *Campanell* be able to make good by Experiment, that this great and excellent Physician *Van Helmont*, which he so much scorneth, had no Medicine, who must inform you? not Mr. *Stubbe* I dare warrant you; no, here Mr. *Stubbe* begs your pardon, and takes leave, Truth and Ingenuity must not appear; that were the way to destroy all his Interest, and render him a greater Friend to the Kingdom then he intends to be.

Thus it may easily be discerned, with what virtues a *Verbalist* is endowed; what is the great gerfection of their boastings; And that Mr. *Stubbe* doth not lessen *Chymical Medicines*, because they are advantagious, and most beneficial to the Sick, and as they are *proper Remedies* truly to recover Diseases; but because Mr. *Stubbe* is exactly in the Case of *Esops* Fox, *the Grapes were Sower* because they were out of his reach, so that if he *had them he would not eat them*: So these rare Medicines that are in the hands but of a few Men, are too high for Mr. *Stubbes*'s procurement, (although he brags *he hath experienc'd as Generous Medicaments as any of the Chymists can boast of*:)

Medicatrix, or the *Woman Physician.* 97

of:) but with what confidence this Man of words, can utter such an affirmation, let the *Virtuosi* and Dr. *Thompson* declare.) And therefore Pish, throw those Medicines away, they are to be despised, of no value; and if I had them, I would not use them: or like the tir'd Huntsman upon a Cold scent, and after a lost Hare; cries out, *Hang her, let it go, 'tis but dry Meat.*

Nor do I conceive he abominates *Paracelsus*, *Helmont*, or any of the *Alchymists*, so much for disability of Parts, want of Learning, great Knowledge, &c. but because they directed the World, and taught them that there was a better, a speedier, and more effectual way to Cure Diseases; then the *Monopoly* of *interessed Physicians* practic'd, and it may be understood: *their Medicines* heal'd Diseases; and so *Galen* and his followers were like to be forsaken, the easie pratling accomplishment, and the profit of a few Professors like to be prejudic'd: O *Demetrius, Demetrius*, Great is thy Goddess *Diana*! 'Tis no matter for Millions of poor Afflicted and Diseased Creatures; so a handful of Men, and their Profession be maintain'd and continu'd; their inability and pride who dares question?

But Mr. *Stubbe*, to capacitate himself, that he may be thought proper to sit at the Stern, and Steer the whole Helme of Physick, gives his Opinion thus, *He is most accomplish'd that*

H *under*

understands Humane Nature best, and the operation——of some hard words, *is the person to be employed in* Physick: *not one that can produce a Catalogue of Diseases*, though he Cured them all; *not one that can boast of effectual, pleasant, and universal Medicaments, is to be regarded, 'tis not the most acute experimental Philosopher,* (no, I thought you had commended Experience just now) *that is the best Practitioner: Many Theorems are plausible, which Practice refutes:* (Yea, why therefore I thought Experiment had been the only sure way to Evince; but it may be I understand not the word *Theorem* aright.) *This was the death of Van Helmont,* at Threescore or Fourscore years old, if it were so; *Thus* Des Cartes *dyed of a Pleurisie, because he refused to be let Blood*; I know not whether he did or no, nor you neither; But if he did, I presume, he thought that Remedy as bad as his Disease; and if he had no other Medicine to save him, I doubt not but he foresaw his End; and that 'twas as good dye by a Disease as a Lancett: And I am of that Opinion my self, if I can procure no Medicine to relieve me, the *Lancett* never will. And Phlebotomy in a *Pleurisie* is as deservedly under my Pish, as *Chymical Medicines* are yours.

'*Tis not great Ingenuity of parts, employed in Florid or different Studies, that makes any Man a competent Judge of a Disease, or the operation of a Medicament:* 'Tis not this, nor 'tis not that, what it is, I think he cannot tell, and he himself is neither Fish nor Flesh. *Il n'est ni figue ni raisin.*

Therefore since you make it so hard a matter to distinguish, who are proper to cure a Disease, and to carry the name of *Medicinalists*, I will tell you, 'Tis those that can get good Medicines, and when they have so done, know how effectually to use them; This in few words, and plain English, is the Sum Total of a *Physician*; and I think as much to the purpose, as all Mr. *Stubbes's* Volumes contain; And with this, Mr. *Medicus* and I will end the Quarrel.

And in pursuit thereof, I do say, That a *Verbalist*, a bare *Physician*, stuft with words, without good Medicines, is no more to be regarded, then one of the Patients in *Bedlam*; one that will boldly challenge the whole World, and resolves to be their Judge and Tutor too, and yet refuse to be tryed for a satisfaction of his Abilities, to manage such Imployments, is not fit for such a Seat.

Therefore I say, a *Verbalist* is not fit to be decreed a *Physician* to the *Universe*: And how we shall be assured Mr. *Stubbe* is the only Man fit for this Lofty purpose, since Words only will not do, for I see no Actions, without which, I am not oblig'd to believe what account *Stubbe*, and such give on their own behalf.

Therefore that I may come to the true [worth]
of Mr. *Stubbes*'s worth; and that I may give
him an opportunity to juſtifie his words by
convincing Actions; and divulge himſelf [to]
the Kingdom, That he is that able Phyſician
and true Friend to ſick Mortals as he pre-
tendeth; and all others he abuſeth, to be rejected and contemned, as he hath propoſed:
I thus challenge him by a Medicinal Experiment, in all thoſe great Diſeaſes fit for a Phyſicians true notice and buſineſs to conteſt[.]
And it is not to be done any other way then
this, *Galen*, *Kraſt* & *Stubbe* ſay Aye; *Helmont*
and the *Virtuoſi*, and *O Dowde* too, ſay no[:]
and where doth the truth appear all this
while? *la verité ſe perd.*

Mr. *Stubbe* was of one Opinion in the beginning of this Kings Reign, he is now of
another; and how ſhall I be ſatisfied he will
not change his mind again if he lives till the
next; Fancies, Opinions, and Whimſies, are
not to be nouriſht in *Medicine*, The excellency of that *Art* muſt be made good by Fact,
and proved by Experience; and this Mr.
Stubbe now and then allows highly of: This
is an Age that believes no Authors, nor any
Medicines, but what are ſeen and known to
be true, and juſtified by Fact. Therefore,
Firſt of all, I ſhall oppoſe him in thoſe particular Diſeaſes he commends Phlebotomy in;
and ſince the *Verbaliſts* and *Medicinaliſts* cannot

not agree themselves yet of a Diseases, nor its Cure; All that Ratling the *Gunpowder* makes in his Books, with the Authors he summons up, signifie nothing, so those flourishes are still in dispute.

He begins first with the Plague, and says, *If Presumption and Arrogance could have entombed the Pest, the most insolent, but worst of Physicians, that is,* Van Helmont *had secured Mankind against its ill effects.* But this charge I imagine arises to so inconsiderable a matter, that it argues more malice then sense; for since *Van Helmont* never told Mr. *Stubbe* his Medicines, he can blame him for no other cause; And the *Medicinalists* are too cunning for that, I presume, which makes Mr. *Medicus* the more angry against them.

As to what else Mr. *Stubbe* recites of his Authors, what they did in *Plagues,* what they say the Disease is, and that Phlebotomy is many times used in that Sickness, &c. It matters not; for he only writes by report, he confesses he never saw that Disease, nor never will, I believe, if he can help it; and therefore to what end doth he summon up his Authors, and their Writings? For first, if they had good Medicines, they run away, and will not stay in such Calamitous times to administer them, but leave Prescriptions and Directions with Nurses, and petty Agents, to take care of the Sick in those great Exigents; when

there

there is more need of all the affistance and perfonable attendance of a Phyfician himfelf: So that in fuch Cafes the Patients are likely to be bravely preferved. He may vapour of curing his *Viper-Catcher*, but not of curing the *Plague*.

And then to what end fhould Mr. *Stubbs* difcourfe of this Difeafe, and its Cure, that never faw it; doth he think Men will believe he underftands it, and will truft to his words or his Authors, or their Medicines, when they dare not truft themfelves? This falls of courfe and is not of confideration in this defign.

And I have fufficiently difcours'd of th laft great *Peft* before; and that I was in it and then I faw Phlebotomy of no ufe, I vifite and cured Patients of it my felf, and hav much reafon by good Experience to know th Method and Medicines for the *Plague*; An fince Mr. *Stubbe* knows nothing of it, but what he hath read or heard, and run away from it; He can be no *Champion* in that Divine Battle.

But having gone beyond the bounds of this Tract I firft intended, I fhall briefly take notice of thofe particular Difeafes, in which he commends and juftifies Phlebotomy as abfolutely neceffary; and without which thofe Difeafes cannot be Cured, which are the *Small Pox*, *Scurvey*, *Pleurifies*, and *Feavers*, &c and then come to the Effential decifion of th controverfie.

Th

The *Small Pox* is a Disease Mr. *Stubbe* applauds Phlebotomy in, *and avows it commonly prudent, and many times positively necessary to be used, as in the begining of that Disease, and after their Eruption:* This averment I confess heretofore might have been of some colour, when Physicians, and the World were in ignorance; but now it will by no means be allowed to pass Oraculous; nay, though *he hath said it*; for not only Nurses, but the very Common People, the Patients by woful experience, condemn and reject it. But Mr. *Stubbe* goes on to declare himself largely in it, to be a proper Remedy, and to be confidently administred in several degrees and times of that Disease; and recites many Authors to help him out, that they were in the days of Old of that Practice and Opinion, and so still to be followed; And by way of a miraculous addition to his knowledge, he cries out, that he is able now to inform the World what he knew not before; And that is, *That Phlebotomy in the Small Pox, even after they are come out, is the Old English Practice,* witness, *Johannes Anglicus,* and *Gilbertus Anglicus,* almost three hundred years ago: What Fashion was three hundred years ago, matters not now; The *English* have more Wit now; They might loose their Lives then, because their *Physicians* knew not how to Cure them; But this Age knows better things; we can save our Lives, and Cure a Disease, and that without *Phlebotomy*; so we are like to leave that desperate fashion; for we have better in vogue; what English *John* and *Gilbert* did Hundreds of years ago, or any other Authors in those cases, was because they knew no better; And what *Henry* did at *Jamaica*, or doth now at *Warwick*, is no matter, since I perceive he understands no more, then they did; what excellent use and benefit the Lancett is of in the *Small Pox*, we have had sufficient testimonies thereof in this Age, and that by lamentable consequences; being an Observation common to all sorts of People.

And Mr. *Stubbe* had best enquire, what effect Phlebotomy had on a Person of Great Fortune and Quality that fell sick of the *Small Pox* this last Summer in the *Pell Mell*, not many days before his intended Nuptials; for although 'tis reported he was blooded in his Sickness, *Yet did he dye thereof.*

If the Lancett be so effectual to the preservation of the Sick in this common and frequent Disease, as he would have it, how comes the Bills to be so full of Dead Children, &c. as sometimes a hundred or more in a week.

So that 'tis not what Mr. *Stubbes* or his Authors have said or done, but what they ought to have said or done; and we are oblig'd by the necessities of the Sick to do.

But to avoid Mr. *Stubbes*'s multiplicity and showers of words, which are to no purpose, because Phlebotomy is by the best *Chymical Physicians* denied in this Disease, And therefore it still remains a question to this day; and what hath Mr. *Stubbe* done towards a confutation? nothing at all but by words: And so we shall never have any Judgement of the truth, nor any end of the Contest.

But to prosecute my *Verbalist*, I do totally deny and reject Phlebotomy in the *Small Pox*, and that it is of no use or value with the *Medicinalist*, And I will tell Mr. *Medicus* stranger wonders yet; Those that have Skill, and good Medicines, will not only secure, and with Gods Blessing as far as possible for Art, preserve the Life of the Patient in the *Small Pox*, without taking away one drop of Blood, but prevent all the many dangerous accidents, the Patient undergoes for want of Assistance; when the Physician many times Gapes, and looks on to see what nature will do it self, and cannot, or will not, give that help Nature demands, and the pressing occasions require; and more, Skill and Good Medicines will manage the Patient in this Sickness so, that he may avoid most commonly ever being confin'd to his Bed, and those tedious decumbitures, they are of course otherwise obnoxious too; as likewise the nice danger of taking Cold these Sick are subject too, and so proves often a mortal prejudice, will by this means be prevented; And what is more rare

yet,

yet, Skill and good Medicines will preserve and free the greatest Beauty, the finest Face, and most curious Skin from any mark, disfigure, or pit of this *Beauty destroying Disease*.

But methinks I hear critical Mr. *Stubbe* say, why then, sure you will have all the Ladies in Town your Patients: I doubt not, but I shall have some in these Cases, and many others, since Mr. *Medicus* hath forc'd me to tell the World, in answer to him, what Remedies I can afford them, and what good I can do them, not by him to be pretended too, much less perform'd, notwithstanding all his Oratory and Trincketts: And all this great business is done by a few poor Chymical Medicines, such as he calls Purgatives, Diaphoreticks and Cordials, though of greater virtue.

These things I have said now for the good of the Sick, and against Mr. *Medicus* and Phlebotomy; and how will Mr. *Stubbe* disprove me, and why am not I to be believ'd as well as Mr. *Stubbe*, since I do not know that I am guilty of Falshood; I have had Twelve years Experience, and in that time, (I must desire Mr. *Medicus* not to be offended) I have met with those Cases the *Physician at Warwick*, I am confident in all his Practice never saw; And for *Medicines*, I am sure I have Ten times better, and more *Generous* then ever he had, hath, or ever will have.

But

But the *Campanell* and I hitherto speak only good words, therefore that we may proceed to more satisfaction, I do say, what I have said I can do, and am ready to do, and will justifie and maintain by experimental Actions, which Mr. *Stubbe* hath only yet avowed; and only says, *He hath wrote nothing in reference to the Plague, Small Pox,* &c. *but what he is perswaded to be true*: But what assurance will this give to the Learned *Chymists*, or dying Patients; I am perswaded *Henry Stubbe* is no Physician, but I dare not say it, because it may be I am not sure of it; but I will now have more reason to be assured of it.

For I do hereby take liberty to tell Mr. *Henry Stubbe a Physician at Warwick*, That I will Cure the Disease of the *Small Pox* with him without Phlebotomy, or taking one drop of Blood from the Patient: And I will Cure the Patient with that safety and advantage, I have before set down; and more, that my Antagonist may have no objection, I will not say Ten; but I will Cure two for one with him in this Disease; that is, I will Cure two Patients of the *Small Pox* by my Method and Medicines, without Phlebotomy, for his one that he shall Cure by Phlebotomy and his Method; and if he desires it, I will give him greater odds yet, rather then decline the Trial.

In the mean time I will give him one eminent example amongst many, and that is,
That

That not long since, in one Gentlemans Family, eight persons fell ill of the *Small Pox*; and by Medicines only I recovered them all, and freed them likewise every one from Marks and Disfigures.

I have the longer insisted on this Disease, because it is of great concern; The Lives of the Kingdom and Posterity is in question thereby; for most at some time or other have it, and there are very few that escape it: and 'tis a Disease Mr. *Stubbe* glorifies his Lancett in, and brings all his strength to support and maintain, if words will prevail; besides, since it is a Disease on which the truth and efficacy of his Asseverations rests; The proof on which his Phlebotomical Medicament, and the Justice of his Cause depends; if he pleaseth, by this proffer I have made, we will decide the matter.

But the rest he names being of less Consequence, and standing on the same Narrative and avow, I shall but mention, and give him the same offer.

The *Pleurisie* is a Disease he extolls Phlebotomy in; but there he shuffles so pittifully, and is so engag'd, being hunted by his adversary, that he knows not how to get out; and then runs away to his Authors, to tell what they did a Thousand years ago; but dares not come to make out what he avers by Fact; and I perceive hath learnt no more of this Disease,

nor

nor made a further progress therein, then to know *which Arm to Bleed*. Lastly, he will neither believe his Adversaries affirmations, nor come to the proof of the contrary; and seems to reflect on my Father, by telling his Enemy, he should have Printed an account of Cures, as he did, although they had been fictitious: But once for all, let me tell this *Quacking* Parrot, and *Chego* Doctor, That the Ingenuity and Medicines of *O Dowde*, were and are beyond the Pride, the ridiculous Malice, and poor ignorant knowledge of *Stubbe*; And more, as to the Disease of a *Pleurisie*, if Mr. *Stubbe* is Master of no other Medicine then Phlebotomy, and cannot Cure it without a Lancett, I must say he is ———— not a Physician; more fit to direct Farriers then Physical Students; I laugh to think such a Man should have the Confidence to proffer Judgement and Regulation to *Chymical Physicians* and the Sick *Universe*. And in full answer to him, as to this Disease, I do hereby proffer him to Cure the *Pleurisie*, and give *Five* Patients in *Ten* odds, without any use of the Lancett; and he shall have liberty to manage his *Phlebotomical Art*.

The *Scurvey* he mentions in the number of the rest, as if Blood-letting were its proper remedy too; but I am not certain he understands what that Disease is; For he says, *he is weary with Writing, and the Sicknesses of that season*

season would not permit his leisure (which I wonder at) *to debate the Scurvey*; But 'tis no matter for that, I deny his Assertion, that Phlebotomy is a proper Remedy for the *Scurvey*; and more, I say it is not to be used in that Case, where the Patient is afflicted with that real and true Disease, and the Physician stored with good *Medicines*; And in this Disease I challenge him as in the *Small Pox*, to give him odds, and will Cure two Patients without the Lancett, for one of his with.

These are the principal Diseases he avows Blood-letting in, but hitherto hath not proved it true; He approves of it also in most Diseases: But in *Feavers* and acute Diseases, I must not omit to startle him a little more, He in one place of his Books (for 'twere a tedious work to mark all that I comprehend) is very witty, and fancies he over-runs the *Royal Society*, by quibling on their *Commanding Medicaments,* (*which over-rule Nature*) *and the followers of* V. Helmont, *who teach, that 'tis an imbecillity of a Physician to attend or permit any — or a concoction of a Disease, we are willing to be tryed by that Rule*; Done; I deny that any *Medicinalist* will wait for the Concoction of a Disease, by natures own attempt and ability, but prevent that hazard by Art.

Therefore I deny Phlebotomy herein likewise, or that there is any such thing to be attended for by a good *Physician*, he calls by the hard name of a *Crisis*, or *Concoction of the Sickness* and Diseased matter: And thereto I call him to Experiment.

The inflamed troubled motions, and disturbed Circulation of the Blood, in acute or sharp Diseases, as in a violent Feaver, is to be abated and allayed without the Lancett, in less then the space of Four and Twenty hours, and then the Patient need not fear a Flame of danger, though Mr. *Medicus* nor his Lancett be not at hand.

He saith *Phlebotomy is not a direct Method in all Diseases*, no, I believe not, but an indirect; and the effect thereby produced accidental, and at best but in part, and what then, since there is no need at all of it, and good Medicines will do it without any hazard, danger, or so much trouble, long Torments and Charge, as his Phlebotomical course administers

But in *Apoplexies*, *Squinancies*, and sometimes in *Feavers*, he is used solely or principally to relye upon Phlebotomy. If he be so, I doubt his Patients have no great reason to adore him: but even in these Diseases, I deny his direct and principal Method, And I affirm there is no such thing as Phlebotomy, without some extraordinary accident intervene, which rarely or never happens.

Therefore I see no reason why the *Medicus* should Glory so much in the Art of Phlebotomy, since I have read a *Sea-Horse* was his first
Master;

Master; and it is of so little use: And since I must tell him by the way, That (in this Age) if the greatest Physical Schollar now in *Europe* were to get him a name of esteem by being stil'd a *Phlebotomist*, he would be much frustrated. Nay, if an Angel should appear with that Doctrine at this day, he would not be received; for the Eyes of the World are now open, the Sun Shines, and *Experientia docet*.

But because he speaks so very passionately, and as positively, though not so discreetly of an Apoplexy, I must mention a passage of his in one of his Books, concerning the Cure thereof; and give him one eminent Instance to the contrary, amongst many I could name: His words are to this purpose; *for any Man to think that such a Distemper as an Apoplexy can be Cured without Phlebotomy is direct Madness.* I see, this Man and I shall differ as long as we Live; for its a most certain truth, That it is a direct Madness not to think the contrary: *For all other Evacuations* (———— nor is the *Apoplectick in a condition to swallow*) *or Stool, Urine, or Sweat and Expectoration, are either useless, or too tedious to depend upon in such indispositions.* How? For shame Mr. *Stubbe* leave Writing of Physick at least: And to let you see you are mistaken in your Judgement, I do not only say, this dangerous Disease is to be Cured, and always Cured with Good Medicines without Phlebotomy; and that the

Patient

Patient in this Case is both able to receive an interiour Medicine, and Nature likewise able at the same time, to evacuate and discharge the Stomack and Midriff, as the Brain, of her Enemy. But that Good Medicines are not so useless, nor half so tedious and hazardous as his Method with Phlebotomy, I will give him one Example in full answer to him, and all his *Assertions*, which was a Cure performed on an *Apopletick* person, to the view and notice of all the Country round him; The Patient was one *Major Abrell*, a Gentleman of Good Fortune, and well known in the County where he lives, who fell ill one Night of an *Apoplexy*, I being then in the Country within two or three Miles of him, his Lady sent earnestly to press my coming to him; but because I was at that time indisposed, and not willing to take the trouble of the Country in such affairs, I desired to be excused, and advised their sending for some other: Yet I was presently after importun'd by several Messengers one after another from her, with earnest intreaties, and the promise of any Reward (if I would accept it) because his Case seem'd so dangerous, and having many Children, his Estate unsetled: But I denied and refused as before, till at last by their undeniable importunity, and the perswasions of some of my own Relations in the the Family with me, I went, and found him in his

I Bed,

Bed, in a desperate and sad Condition, having lain so for several hours, Speechless and Insensible, his Mouth displac'd by a strong Convulse and Foming thereat, with difficulty of Breathing, and a Ratling in his Throat, as if ready to be choaked: This grievous Spectacle was beheld and attended by his own weeping Family, and many sorrowful Friends: His Chamber and House being well furnisht with Neighbours and Visitants. So soon as I had told them what was to be done, I ordered the Patient to be placed in that posture as I thought fit, for the reception of that Medicine I had carefully and particularly prepared for him; and his Mouth being with some trouble opened, I gave him a small quantity of this Liquid Medicine, some of which took place, and immediately, in as little time as I could walk the Room too and fro, the Convulse ceased: And in less then a Quarter of an hour, Nature began to be enliven'd, assisted, and rouzed up. And the Patient moved, discharging half a Pint or more, (in a short space) of the offensive and Apoplectick matter; and in an hour, he began to look about, and came to utter many words, and in half an hour more spoke sensibly: Now having secured his Life from any fear of danger, I left him, leaving my directions.

In the Afternoon (this being about Nine of the Clock in the Forenoon) he sent me word,

word, he was pretty well, and before Night (I was inform'd after) he rose out of his Bed, and sate up: And with 3 or 4 Medicines more which I sent him, he was recovered perfect well; and his Head and Body, not only cleansed and disburthened of this ill Guest, but of some other troublesome indispositions he had for some years been oppressed with.

And now Mr. *Stubbe* may see what *a direct Madness it is to think, that an Apoplexy can be Cured without Phlebotomy:* And whether this course where there are such Noble, Amicable, Safe, effectual Remedies to be had, is not better, less tedious, more certain and quick to prevent the great hazard and danger of delay in this Sickness, then his impertinent Lancett, Shavings, burnt Feathers, Snuffe, Tickling the Nose, Pinching the Fingers and Toes, Hooping in the Ears, Touching the Lute, Frictions, Ligatures, and a long List more.

And as I have by this example contradicted the bold erronious Doctrine of the *Physician at Warwick*; so I think, I have likewise impeached an infallibility of one of his own great Authors too; And that is *Wirtzung*, who in his *General Practice of Physick,* treating of an *Apoplexy,* and the Patient saith, *It is to be taken for a most sure and infallible sign thereof, if the Fome at the Mouth, be it by no means possible to be Cured*; so that all Physicians herein agree, That nothing can be done, but only to satisfie his

Friends,

Friends, yet without all hope of Recovery. My Patient was thus afflicted, yet he did not *dye thereof.*

But I must try our *Champion* further in some other Diseases. The *Gout* is a Disease the *Medicus* seems to be altogether as much to seek in, as the *Apoplexy*; And therefore like a Learned *Omniscient in Physick*, he inveighs against *Paracelsus* and others, and says, *What Man could have dyed or languished under the Gout —— if the Rhodomontades of* Paracelsus, *and —— had contained any Solidity?* Why is there any body that doth dye or languish of the Gout? If there be, I will instruct Mr. *Stubbe* a little better in the reason of it, for I see I must be his *Tutor*, as well as his *Opposer*; and I am sorry to see any Man abuse that he so highly Commends, and lays so much Claim too.

Those Men that dye and languish of this Disease, do not dye nor languish, because there is no Remedy for it; but because Remedies are scarce, and few Physicians Master of them: 'Tis not because there are no Medicines to Cure it, for there are Medicines that will certainly relieve the Patient; but because 'tis the ill fortune of those Men, not to meet with, or imploy such *Medicinalists* that have these efficacious Medicines. Therefore 'tis no argument of value to say, many Men are not, or cannot be relieved of the *Gout*. Nor, if the *Gout* could be helped, such a Great Man, This, or That

That Rich Man, would surely have help, that have used so many Receipts, and tryed so many Receipts, and tryed so many Physicians and Great Schollars too, and refuse no Charge to procure Relief.

If Mr. *Stubbe* cannot Cure this Disease, it doth not follow, that nobody else can; and if many Men of Fame and Learning do not know all Medicines, yet doth not follow that there are no Medicines; for we see Learning, though so useful, yet it may be mis-imploy'd; and a Man may be a Schollar, and yet not Cure the Gout, nor many other great Diseases: And we know how oftentimes, many Men have great Learning, and come to be famous in Repute, and yet not be able to Cure Diseases so well as Physicians of less esteem.

And many times the Patient is quite tir'd out with the Drenches and Fruitless Application of such helpless Physicians as *Stubbe*, insomuch, that they will not admit of those Medicines and Method that would succour them: so that the loss of their Faith, is often the loss of their Lives.

These things avail not, since there are such Medicines invented, and in use, though not in all, but a few hands; and Great and Rich Patients, as others, are not always happy in their Choice of Physicians, or Lot of Medicines; so that it only argues the excellency and rarity of a Medicine, not the impossibility.

In few words, such Medicines I have, and I offer him in this Disease, as in others, the experiment for Conviction: And in the mean time I must tell him, what it seems he understands not; That any severe fit of the Gout may be taken off, and the Patient relieved in 3 or 4 days of Medicine, and less if necessity urgeth: This I can do, and then what will be expected from the Oracle of Physick, famous Mr. *Stubbe*.

But what do I mention these things to the Physician of *Warwick*, *Paracelsus*, *Helmont*, the *Virtuosi*, and all such, are but Fools to him; for he can talk bravely, write and say any thing: And alas! They can but only write and say, and do what they write and say.

And amongst all the Accusations of *Paracelsus*, I wonder Authentick Mr. *Stubbe* hath not summon'd in the too severe History of Dr. *Fuller*, which I expected; but it may be that Book was burnt in the Fire with the rest of his Library: And so I end this Disease, as I desire to be understood, That I intend to justifie Good Medicines, and the truth, but need not humane infirmities, since they are as natural to Mr. *Stubbe* as they were to *Paracelsus*: And since amongst all my Conversation with the Learned, the greatest maxim of verity I have observed is, *humanum est errare*.

But if notwithstanding Mr. *Stubbe's* loud ringing, Diseases are never the more Cured, what

what shall we do with the over-spreading Disease, now so Raging, called the *Venereal Lues*, or *French Evil*, which sweeps away so many, and is like to be very destructive to Posterity: This is a *Plague*, which without an extraordinary prevention, will certainly be more mortal then that of 1665: of this Disease The Patient is said to be Cured; his Relapse is the Scurvey, his Death the Consumption: But of this Disease the Patient is not Cured; His Relapse is the first Disease, and his Death the same: Of this Disease the Father is Sick, the Son dyes, the Grand-child is infected; and where is the *Physician at Warwick*? If he would consult the Kingdoms Interest, so far, as to search out true effectual Remedies for this destroying Calamity; It would be a greater Service then ever he hath either attempted, or done it yet: His *Universal Medicament* the *Lancett* will not do this, but it may be he is of the mind of some others of his Profession, who think its enough, to wrap themselves with the Cloak of Learning, and that is a protection sufficient; and in this Disease will not undertake the Cure, pretending, its an *ill Sickness*, and the Patients deserve not to be Cured, because they know not how to do it: so the Sick must perish. This indeed shews rare Charity, and notable Ability, But these Men (I perceive) are such, as in few years more, must either learn to catch this vouring Malady, or leave off practising Physick.

Great are the Tortures poor Patients are forc'd to undergo, in the common course of this Cure, as well as tedious, troublesome, and loathsome Administrations; And when all this is past, the benefit generally received thereby, is little more then a Palliation and Stop to the virulent fruits of it, not a total and clear eradication of the Cause: And when few months or years after, the Disease returns, and the Patient is new afflicted, he is then soothed up 'tis the *Scurvey*, the *Kings-Evil*, the *Gout*, &c. or what Mr. *Stubbes* pleaseth; and so the Patient must be contented with a Physical Life, but a Languishing Body, without he happens to meet with better assistance.

Yet this is not the greatest mischief neither, for by this means, not only the Patient, but Families and Posterity are in danger of Ruine: to ascertain which truth, there wants not evident examples.

It is very much to be admired, that amongst so much Learning, there are so few Good Medicines used in this Disease, and so weak and mean a course generally taken for the recovery of this filthy Evil, since it is a Sickness both very easily and pleasantly, and as truly healed; and the Body made free from the impurities and dangerous consequences thereof, with as little

little trouble, and less prejudice, then many ordinary Diseases; and without the horrid Drenches, Fluxing, Salivation or Nodding as they call it, Tubbing and Bathing, Mercurial Unctions, Lotions, Cerecloths, Emplaisters, &c. And any endless, frivolous, impertinent Dietary observation.

I could in this Disease, as in many others, quote eminent Cases, and bring in question the skill and great Knowledge of as Learned and famous Physicians as he at *Warwick*; but I omit, being *ambitious* at this time only to oppose Mr. *Stubbe*, and to inform him, That when these *Frenchified Patients* are beyond his Art, they are then in the power and deliverance of Good Medicines; and of this he may be more assured by *Experiment*.

I am told the *Medicus* cannot Cure a poor *Quartan Ague*, under the Revolution and Course of a years *Medicaments*, and sometimes not that neither; but forc'd to let both the Patient and his quivering Disease take their fortune; I know it is a truth, that General Practicers of Physick cannot Cure an *Ague*; But for Learned Mr. *Stubbe*, the great Physician at *Warwick*, the Mouth and Oracle of Physick, not to have such *Generous Medicaments* as will reach a *Quartan Ague*, the most contemptible Disease that happens to a Physicians care, I cannot believe: 'Tis enough for the Men of Old to be ignorant in the Cure of

this

this petty creeping Disease, I hope litteral Mr. Stubbe scorns to be so Idle, and to have spent his time, and employ'd his Learning to so little purpose, as not to be able dexterously to Cure an *Ague.* If this should happen to be his misfortune, if he pleases to come to me, I will instruct him how he shall be able to do all this in 4 or 5 days.

I deny *Phlebotomy* to be of any use in this Disease likewise, where the Physicians is furnisht with Good Medicines and Skill to apply them: And let Mr. *Stubbe* produce me as many Ague-sick people, *Quartan's,* or else, if they are not quite spent and decayed by this Disease, as he pleaseth; let the continuance of that Disease be of what time it will, I will not exceed six days of Medicine, and recover them by removing the true Cause of the sickness, and what is more, without the foolish *Jesuits Powder* too, though as much in Fashion as the *Physician at Warwick* : And to an *Experiment* of this, I likewise Challenge Mr. *Stubbe* ; and so I end these kind of Diseases our *Medicus* commands and avows the necessity of Blood-letting in, with this conclusion, That whosoever is Lavish in Blood-letting, and depends upon that for the Cure of a Disease, let his Schollarship or Fame be what it will, it is a most certain sign, that man is in want of Good *Medicines*: Those that understand the Glory of a Good *Medicine,* know I guess aright; those that do not 'tis no matter: The Patient will sometime or other have reason to believe and remember, That purifying and preserving the blood and vital Spirits in the body, and vainly taking them out of the body, are distinct things.

But if the *Ague* be so hard to Cure, what will our *Champion* do to clear himself of the great Diseases of the *Apoplexy,* the *Gout,* the *Venereal Lues,* or *Il mal Francese,* that destroying Disease of this Age; as also the *Stone,* the *Falling-sickness, Dropsies, Consumptions,* and such like, which for brevities sake I must omit more distinctly naming now: And to sum up my Challenge to M. *Stubbe,* thus I say, That I will Cure any of these Diseases before-named; and more, those that he cannot, if it be in the power of natural means to relieve them, (for I hope he will not tender me impossibilities.) And that all things may be certainly proposed in few words, to ascertain the method and course of this Challenge, *Mr. Stubbe* shall have the first refusal and *experiment* of such of these Diseases, and so many Patients as he shall choose to himself; and those that he cannot recover in such a reasonable time as shall be by judicious and proper Physicians thought fit, I will: To this purpose the Battel may be set in order; And to this offer I challenge *Mr. Henry Stubbe a Physician at Warwick.*

But I must here observe, That when my *Verbalist* comes to be proved, that the truth of his bold and impudent Assertions may appear, he leaves his Enemy Conqueror, and thinks it enough to say, as he doth to one of his Adversaries that follows him home to the test of his worth: *he valued not his proffer'd Essay, because he was so inconsiderable:* I presume, meaning he was but a single person.

Yet when he comes to bring Arguments to beg others to oppose his Adversary, and having slipt his own Neck out of the Collar, He says, *Though the man be despicable, the president is not.* If this be not as subtle a *Mountebank* as ever stag'd *Moor-fields,* I am content to forfeit my Judgement; Therefore it may easily be satisfied what force his own Objection bears, when he is truly searcht into; 'tis very true what *Mr. Stubbe* saith, the matter is not inconsiderable, and he will do well to defend and protect it, for he hath left it at present very disputable. And if he had ever thought this pretence of consideration, why did not he accept his Friend *O Dowdes* proffer in his Life, when he offer'd to Cure any Disease, with the best Professors of his Gang, for Five Hundred pounds, then *Mr. Stubbe* was no Champion, though now he is a most excellent Sir *John Falstaffe*. But I confess, I admire this *Medicus* as *Cicero* is said to be admired,

more

more for his tongue then his heart; for I see his words and actions are as different, as *a Frenchmans words and his writings: Platonick Lover* like, who is described by our *English saying, to be one that is still saying Grace, and never falls to his Meat*: He says well, if all that he says were true, And although he thinks he hath said enough, in saying, *his Patients depose for their Cures*; yet I am never the more convinced by that, unless he will tell me, when he will raise them up again; and that is a Prophetick inspiration, I fear this divine Physician is not yet Glorified with.

Now I return to my *Chymical Vindication*, and to tell *Mr. Stubbe*, that it rests much upon him to come to an experimental Essay: And that I may aggravate him the more, I will acquaint him with what he would willingly (no doubt) be ignorant of; and that is, the sick Patients are dissatisfied, because he will not justifie what he dares invent and publish: He brags he is a great Schollar, and hath arriv'd to the period of Learning, if so, let him evince that excellency, since its denied: and if those Persons and Medicines he decries as contemptible, excell and surpass all his knowledge, where doth the *odium* fall? He accuseth the ingenuity and *Royal promotion* of this Age, as that which infringeth and bears upon his interested Physical Profession; and such attempts, though never so necessary and profitable to the Universe, ought to be consulted by opposition and diminution of its growth and fertility; Yet if the *Innovation*, as he terms it, of this Royally ingenious Age, be found more serviceable and available, more real and beneficial to King and People, then other more private interests, though more ancient pretences: what would this *Incendiary* drive at?

But now I think on't, the passage I have hinted, is of some consequence, and not to be omitted, least he adventure upon the like confidence for the future; and therefore I shall mention it: In his *Preface* to the *Colledge of Physicians*, fawning and dissembling with them; He writes, *But the Innovations of late years have*

have taken off much from your *Renown* and *Authority*, and both *extenuated* and *impaired your Credit*: Well! what then; *which is so much the more to be resented, in that it arose not from any evil effect of our late Civil Wars, but the Insolence and Extravagance of more modern attempts: Giving encouragement* to more able Practicers then himself: Have a care; but let me ask *Mr. Stubbe* one question, is he a Prince or a Subject? And let me ask the Reader two, did ever the Sun shine? was ever the *Physician at Warwick* Servant to *Sir H.V.* if the Reader saith yes, I say, this is as plain as either: I confess, I have much ado to forbear our *English Campanell*, but at present I will not be severe, only remember him, That he owns himself, he once deserv'd to loose his Head; Let me now tell him, such another Scribble will make him forfeit his Hand; Certainly this man fancies the People of this Kingdom have lost their Eyes, and their Understanding: I acknowledge, the late *Civil Wars*, as he calls them, might do much towards both; but however, I think there is enough left to discern him to be———. *En la terre des aveugles, le borgne est Roy*; and in such a Countrey *Stubbe* would fitly make a *President*.

But I have given *Mr. Stubbe* my medicinal Tender, which if he refuses, I see not what he hath done more in justification of his design, then what one in a *Bib* and *Long Coat* might have performed.

If he refuses this, I hope he will be contented to loose the name, not only of the *Judge of Physick*, but of a *Physician* too; and that his Profession may be any thing but a *Real Medicinalist*, and a *Friend to the Kingdom*.

Then I hope the World will have some reason to see, whether he be a *Medicus* or a *Politicus*, and whose interest is to be consulted.

Then he must own, the medicines of *S. Helmont*, *O Dowde*, and such ——— are able to make better Physicians then *Galen, Kraft, M.* or *Stubbe* and such ———
Then it must appear, what great reason Mr. *Stubbe* hath

hath to Fetter contrary Practicers, more knowing and assistant then he. If this be not done, our *Champion* may Talke and Write till his Lungs are lacerated, and his Pen proves a veficatory to his Fingers, and he will never be believed in *Medicinal affairs*; For what honour can he expect, That will write, say and avow those things he cannot, or will not make out and justifie: since what Physicians speak and write signifie little, if it cannot be attested by fact, in case their affirmations are denyed.

In fine, if Mr. *Stubbe* refuses this fair end of our *Phlebotomical* and *Chymical* dispute, which is not to be denyed by one that protests so much Love to the sick: I must then make bold to tell him, That he will do prudently hereafter, to let the Dead sleep quietly in their Graves; For notwithstanding his Bravado, the Successors of *O Dowde* do gainsay and object against the ignorant *Mal*-practice of *Stubbe*, and such ——— And I shall believe *Van Helmonts* recital out of another Author, is true, and in some degree verified in this *Verbalist*; many have not attained unto wisdom, because they thought that they had attained unto it: And I shall likewise then conclude, *Mr. Stubbes's Generous Medicaments*, are of no greater extent then the Pills of *Poge's* Servant; And that he is some *Ignes fatuus*, or *Will of the Wispe*, and till such misleading Meteors are more in request, I acquiesce my Pen.

POST-

POSTSCRIPT.

I Have thought it reasonable to say, That by the Vindication and Offer I have made in the foregoing Tract, I hold my self discharged of the Duty of a Child, in that behalf before incumbent on me: And in the next place, unless Mr. Stubbe will accept my offer, I conceive Alchymical Medicines, and the Medicinalist, are thereby unfetter'd, and free'd from his desir'd Bondage.

If the Physician at Warwick thinks it not above him, but will come to an experimental Tryal, let a judicious way and method be propos'd for it, (if not that I have mention'd) in order to what I have said, and I am and shall be ready to maintain what I have denyed, and to confirm what I have affirmed, by the greatest assurance of truth, and that is Experiment. And I will also, before our Engagement in every Disease, discourse him therein, and give a rational and proper account of the same, and when I have so done, I will Cure the Disease, and allow him odds, &c. (if desired) as I have before expressed: For he shall find me principl'd with Queen Elizabeths Motto, semper eadem.

And whether this be not a fair and civil proposal, I demand the Judgement of every ingenious Reader.

But if he thinks to avoid this just Charge, and the true merit of his Doctrine, by Scurrility, Railings and Abuses (because I see he is so apt, right or wrong, to abuse living or dead) and so

think

POSTSCRIPT

think to hide his Errors, and cloud the truth by such degenerate mean shifts.

I shall then conclude that course to be not like a Schollar, a Physician, a Gentleman, or any thing that can be called ingenious; but rather some kind of Politicus, and so beneath my notice: And I doubt not, but all Men will count him Ridiculous, and void of any true honour, no way fit to regulate the Kingdom.

Yet if this should prove the Case, I will not forsake him; But am resolv'd to beg that leave, which I believe I shall not be denyed; And he shall be sure then to receive that Return and Reply I have reserved for him: And more then that, I will with the Astrologer, once a year imploy my Printer.

Last of all, if he looks upon it to be more Prudent and Physical to remain scornfully Silent, I cannot say further.

I forgot to give Mr. Stubbe my Opinion of his famous Cure on the Viper-Catcher; but because he is so great an Opiniator, as to think, whatever he doth himself is above all others, and that in this Act, he hath been so miraculously successful, that by much intreaty, he hath condescended to give the World a Relation of his Method, as a great kindness, and unutterable instruction; I shall in short, inform the ingenious Reader my Judgement therein, And that is, That I find nothing of Rarity in his Physical prescription for a Viper-bite; but what (I must believe) every Perite and modern Mole-catcher in the Country comprehends.

That the Sick may have some more advantage by this then Letters and Words, let them read my following Advertisement.

AN

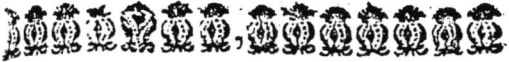

An Advertisement of Dr. O. Dowdes Medicines, and the Authors.

Since Letters and Words Cure no Diseases, no not the Ague by spell, And that the Sick may have some other benefit then Talk and Scribble, I will advertise: That as the great and only end of *Physick*, is to preserve the Body in Health, and to restore it to Health when lost: And being Mistress of that Knowledge and Medicines as hath inabled me to perform all this as far as the best of Medicines will reach. I thought my self oblig'd to give this notice to Poor as well as Rich, and for publick good in general: That all the several Medicines of my Father, together with many others now in my Custody, may at any time be had from me, by those, whose occasions require them.

I shall here name some of my Medicines, and only mention some of the most considerable Diseases, and leave the Reader to believe those of the lesser Ranck and meaner Degree, are more easily Remedied, and may likewise have Medicines accordingly.

In the Small Pox my Purging Essence, a Febrile Antidote, a Vital Tincture, my Dyaphoretick

An Advertisement.

phoretick Elixir, *an* Aural Cordial, *and with other* Medicines *are proper as the Age of the Patient,* Nature, Time, *and Degree of the Disease (when consider'd) require :* Whereby the Stomack, Bowels, *and* Internal Parts *may be* cleansed, scoured, *and discharged of the* Malignant, Turbulent Matter : Nature *assisted in its* Motion, Eruption *and* Maturation. *The* Pores of the Body *opened; the Center, principal parts, and* Vitals *preserved and fortified;* Expulsion *of the remaining* Humours *gently promoted; the* Malignity *mortified, driven forth and forc'd (without any return) to the Skin,* Habit *and Circumference of the Body, the* Fever *moderated, and the* Acrimony *and* Virulency *of the* Peccant Matter *Corrected,* Mitigated, *and Allayed, and so taken off, that no Pit or Disfigure of Face or Skin, shall ever happen; especially if the Patient in any reasonable time have this Assistance; besides the Sick will very rarely have occasion to keep the Bed, above a day or Two, sometimes not at all.*

And these Medicines, *and my Method in this Disease, are so easie, safe, and effectual, and the Patient put to so little trouble or hazard, that I never yet to this day knew any Person that either my* Father *or self, gave Medicine too, that dyed of this Disease:* Many Patients *and many eminent Accidents I could mention; but that this place is too narrow for that purpose :. But because this is an universal Disease, and so many lives daily*

An Advertisement.

daily indanger'd thereby; I will so far discharge my Charity to the Sick, and urge my Knowledge herein, as to advise all those that shall at any time be concerned in this Sickness, That as they tender, the Lives and Welfare of themselves, their Children and Friends; they shun and avoid Blooding, as they would their most mortal Enemy; and for assurance I write no more then what I know, I am and will be ready to justifie the Truth hereof, by just Tryals against the best Phlebotomist this Nation affords.

In the Gout (severally nam'd as the place is affected, as the Hand-Gout, the Hip-Gout, the Knee-Gout, the Gout in the Feet, &c.) A Medicinal Milk, an Aural Tincture, Two sorts of Radiant Pills, A Purging Potion, an Extract against the Gout, A Cordial Potion, and for outward application, Two Unguents, the one White, the other Green, and my Golden Balsamick Spirits: By which Medicines the sharp acrid Humours, congealing between the Joynts, coagulating and alienating the Juices thereof, perverting their natural use and design, and thereby causing so much Anguish, Torment, and Pain to the Patient, are carryed away and removed; all the most remote parts of the Body cleansed, and Nature disburthened of this vexatious Malady, and restored; and any of these Fits taken quite off in Three or Four days, though never so severe; and although all other Aplications have failed, and the Patient lain

many

An Advertisement.

many Weeks or Months under this tedious Dolour.

In the Consumption (which is a Disease many Physicians go the wrong way to Cure, just as a Chirurgion that endeavours to heal up, or close an old Wound or Sore, before the bottom thereof be firm and sound; so in the Consumption, they endeavour to Cure it by administring Nutriment and Restoratives before the Flux of Humours be prevented, and the fixed matter removed) A Pulmonick Essence, a Pectoral Electuary, a Cleansing & Coroborating Extract, Balsamick Drops: By which Medicines the cause of those salt, sharp, fretting Humours will be attempered and dislodged; the Phlegmatick, and Corosive Matter digested and removed: The Lungs, Vitals, wasting and decaying parts strengthned, fortified, and healed; and Radical Moisture restored.

In the Stone, An Anodine Potion, Purging Pills, an Elixir of Gold, a Red Tincture, The Diuretick Water of Alchymists: By these Medicines which are very precious, and never fail in this Disease; the Reins, Urinary Passages, and Bladder, are cleansed from all slimy, glutenous, muceus, stony matter, and all Obstructions; as also, from any Sand, Gravel or Stones, that are bred and lodge in the Kidneys, and Bladder, and all such Gravel and Stones, are thereby dissolved, broken, expel'd, and cast out, and the Patient set free from these Infirmities

An Advertisement.

ties and Torture, when left remediless by others.

In the Scurvy, *A* Stomack Extract; *A* Scorbutick Medicine, *A* Cleansing Potion, *A* Volatile Cordial Elixir : By these Medicines the whole Body will be throughly cleansed, and the Scorbutick Corruption carryed away, the Blood purefied, and its Circulation rightly procured, the several digestions rectified, Nature assisted, enlivened and strengthned; and the Patient healed.

In Agues, *as* Quotidian, Tertian, Quartan, &c. *A* Splenetick Essence, my Purgative Pills, *A* Diaphoretick Elixir, and sometimes a Sudorifick Medicine, *A* Vital Potion : By these Medicines the Stomack, Spleen and adjacent parts are purged, and cleared of all tough, indigested Matter, all Obstructions opened, the Aguish Matter evacuated, and evaporated; the gross fixed Humours in the Blood gently cleansed away, the Circulation rectified, and Blood spiritualiz'd; the Fits cease and are taken quite away, the Stomack, Spleen, digestive Offices, and weakned parts restored, strengthned and confirmed, and the Body easily and safely made whole, and all this by 3 or 4 or half a Dozen Medicines; and with as much certainty as any thing a woman can promise, although the Disease be of long Continuance, and never so deeply rooted.

In Dropsies (called the Water Dropsie, the Timpany or Windy Dropsie, the Third sort, when moist bad Humours are said to be dispersed throughout all parts of the Body) *An* Hydropick Medicine,

An Advertisement.

Medicine, *A* Stomack Extract, *A* Sudorifick Elixir, Purging Pills, *A* Diuretick Elixir, *A* Cordial Drink : *By these Medicines the Pores, Vents of the Body, and Urinary Passages will be opened and cleansed, and all Obstructions removed, the Watry and ill Humours dryed up and evaporated, carryed off and purged out by Urine and Seige ; the Blood restituted by a lively fermentation, and the several debilitated and oppressed parts supported and comforted with vigour and strength, for its present and future preservation: I have commonly Cured these Diseases, when the Patients have been left for a Death-bed preparation by others, and shall at any time undertake and secure the same, if the principal parts and strength are not absolutely decayed and exhausted.*

In the Venereal Disease *called the* French-evil *or* Pox *(which is not proper here to be discours'd more of then what follows) An* Aperitive Medicine, *the* Elixir of Life, *my* Solary Pills, *An* Imperial Pill, *A* Diaphoretick Elixir, *A* Cordial Potion : *By which Medicines the Patient will be pleasantly, safely and easily Cured ; this foul Disease throughly eradicated, without any Reliques, dangerous future accidents and returns, all the impurities carryed away and ejected, and the Body made as pure, healthy and sound, as if it had never been prison'd with it. In few words, for the good of languishing miserable Patients under this horrid venomous and raging Disease, which is seldom truly Cured (though not for*

their

An Advertisement.

their presumption or incouragement in filthy evil actions) I can (as I have done) recover this Sickness, when the Patient is given over by other Physicians, and any Hospital in or about this City, provided what any Reader will allow, that the Vital and Principal Parts are not rotted and consumed &c. by the delay and course of a Seven years prescription or otherwise, and this without the abominable tormenting Method of Fluxing, Nodding or Salivation, Tubbing, Racking, unprepared Mercury Drenches and Pills, Mercurial Unguents, and Lotions, and the dangerous preposterous administrations, the common Practisers, and Pretenders to Physick use.

In the Falling-Sickness, The Essence of Exalted Gold, A Capital Elixir, an Epileptick Extract, A Central Electuary, A Powder, Pectoral Pills, an Epileptick Antidote, A Vital Elixir: By these Medicines the Stomack, Midriffe, and Center of the Body where this Disease is first and chiefly seated, and by after causes the Brain dejected, Spirits, Sense, and Passages of the Head obstructed, oppressed and impeded, will be cleared of the stupefactive poisonous Matter, and this unsensitive dangerous Disease taken quite away, without any return: And the Stomack, &c. set right, Head & Spirits Quickned, assisted, rais'd up, and comforted, Sense and Motion made more active, vigorous, and fitly restored: This Incurable Disease lookt upon so by most, although of many years standing, if the Patient will be at the charge may be perfectly recovered in few Weeks.

In

An Advertisement.

In the Griping of the Guts, A vomiting and purging Medicine, Purging Pills, A Digestive Electuary, A Vegetable Tincture, A Stomack Extract, Spirits of Sulphur Spiritualiz'd, A Diaphoretick Cordial : *By these Medicines the Stomack and Digestions will be cleansed, and set in order, and the Cause removed, the Blood, Bowels, and other parts of the Body rectified and freed, and the sharp, slimy, tormenting, scorbutick, vexatious pain, and Humours carryed away, transpired, and sweated out, and the alienation, impurities and errours of the Nutrimental Juices amended and corrected, and the Patient in few days well and throughly healed.*

The rest I must omit, as Pleurisies *and* Apoplexies *before named, and other Diseases being too many here to discourse, as* Fevers, Pallies, Convulsions, Jaundise, Rickets, Worms, Lethargies, Vertigo's, Phrensies, Bloody-Flux, Impostumations, Ulcers *in* Kidneys *and* Bladder, Collicks, Ptisicks, Leprosies *before too far gone*, &c. *in every one of which the Patient may have suitable Medicines.*

Diseases attending Women.

AS Histerical Fits, *or Fits of the Mother*, Green-sickness, Wastings, Barrenness, Obstructions, Fluxes *of several Kinds*, &c. *The Distases incident to this Sex are many, and not proper here largely to be discoursed on; therefore I purposely omit them, and shall only say, they may have effectual Remedies from me in their respective Infirmities, likewise, as well as in the rest that I have before mentioned*

From the Feathers in the *Old Pell-mell*
near St. *James's* 1. *Decem.* 1674.   F I N I S.

The Mid-wives just Petition (*Wing* M2005) is reproduced by permission of the Clark Library. The text block of the original measures 111 × 160 mm.

The Mid-wives just
PETITION:
OR,
A complaint of divers good Gentlewomen of that faculty.

Shewing to the whole Christian world their just cause of their sufferings in these distracted Times, for their want of TRADING.

VVhich said complaint they tendered to the House on Monday last, being the 23. of *Ian.* 1643.

With some other notes worthy of observation.

Printed at London, 1643.

The Midwives just Petition, or a complaint of divers Gentlewomen of that faculty, &c.

Humbly Shewing,

THat whereas many miseries do attend upon a Civill War, there is none greater than the breaking of that conjunction which matrimony hath once confirmed, So that womens husbands being absent at the Wars, they cannot enjoy that necessary comfort and benevolence which they expect from them, this, if well considered, is a shrewd matter and doth give beginning to a naturall depopulation of towns and Cities, when the causes of populous fertillity are any wayes hindered, whereby all places, especially this famous City, must needes become very thin of people, and great want of men fit for employment both for Church and State, and all corporations must necessarily from thence ensue, for men grow not up on a suddain, there must be a seed time before harvest, bearing of children before their birth, as we very well know, who in that kind have been great assistants unto women, and constant deliverers of much good to the Common-wealth.

And whereas we are called Mid-wives by our profession, wee knowing the cases of women better than any other, as being more experienced in what they sensibly suffer since the wars began, living the religious lives of some cloysterd Nuns contrary to their own naturall affections, if they could by any means help it without wronging their husbands: Our Petition shall therfore consist of many branches, whereby the injuries of women in this present age may be clearely discerned, for it is a great wrong that women should want their husbands and live without comfort, whereby we Midwives are also undone, for as women are helpers unto men, so are we unto women in all their extreamities, for which we were formerly well paid, and highly respected in our parishes for our great skill and mid-night industry, but now our Art doth fail us, and little gettings have we in this age barren of all naturall joyes, and onely fruitfull in bloudy calamities, we desire therefore that for the better propagating of our owne benefit, and the generall good of all women, wives may no longer spare their husbands to be devoured by the sword, but may keep them fast locked within their own loving armes day and night, perfecting their embraces in such a manner as is not to be expressed freely, but may be easily conceived by the strong fancy of any understanding women; We Mid-wives must be as secret as night and close in all conceits, but wee know assuredly that this would bring about much content, while our selves should feast high at Christnings, and nurses also should more frequently be paid for their monthly keeping of women, we have with much horror and astonishment heard of Kenton Battayle, wherein many worthy members and men of great ability were lost to the number of 7563. who were buried thereabouts by the Church-wardens, Clerkes, and Sextons of the adjacent Parishes, as they have lately delivered upon their severall oaths, which doth make us humble Petitioners, that blood may not hereafter be shed in such a manner; for many men, hopefull to have begot a race of souldiers, were there killed on a sudden before they had performed any thing to the benefit of Midwives, which was a great losse and hinderance to the Commonwealth; whereby some maydes were deprived of promised marriage, and wives by the hand of death were quickly Widdowed, and with them the hope of posterity was also extinguished, it is therefore hereafter to be desired that Warre may not eate up and devoure the youth of this Kingdome, but that men may performe the blessing given to *Adam* by encreasing and multiplying,

thereby

thereby to repayre the great havock and losse which this unnaturall War doth make in England. Heretofore the happinesse of the English women was compared unto heaven, but now they have just cause to tremble at the report of every gunne, which can send a speedy death to their instruments of conjunction and delight, without whom they are but halfe themselves, and being indeed nothing in themselves, from them they receive perfection, weight, and number, and grow as rich in children as they are in beauty, while wee Mid-wives shall fare and feede the better for their frequent christnings and gossipings.

We take notice what divellish new Engines for Warre are daily invented by the Cyclops and such like Artists, to destroy one another; namely the Poleax, Petronels, Carbines, Firelocks, Snap-hances, Pistols, nay cases of Pistols, Granadoes, and their hand Granadoes, and the Morter peices, and your terrible two-edged swords, able to affright poor women to see such naked weapons; then the Cavalliers, and your Dragoneers, and your Ingineers, which are those persons which exercised those weapons: such instruments were never used, or scarce seene in England, and all out of jealousies, doubts and feares; because you men will not confide in one another: All these weapons are but to destroy brave man which should be preserved and kept for better uses and purposes: It were farre better for those men that they followed their owne trade, and the old game of England at home with their wives; then for them to runne abroad to be a common souldier, and stand Sentinel two or three hours in the cold for a little Suffolk cheese and a peice of browne bread, and at length kill one another for eight pence a day, with the night to boot too: and it may be lose a limbe or some other good joynt: when indeed and in very good sooth they

they need not stand at home so long by nineteene parts, and have more thanks (if not a reward) for their paines.

It were nothing so irkesome to us poor Midwives that our trade is now decayed, if the sword in the scabbard were used and employed against a Forreigne Enemy; it would not then be halfe so grievous, for the old proverbe saith, what the eye sees not, the heart greives not at. But we poor Midwives both see, and our hearts know it and now our tongues confesse it; that it is a lamentable case when the sonne shall goe out against the father; father against the sonne; brother against brother, and kinsman against kinsman, this wee speake is grievous to bee thought on; and we condole even to the lower-most angle of our triangular hearts.

Wee desire therefore that a period may be set to these unhappy differences, and that the generall and naturall Standard may no longer lye couchant; but that women may be fruitfull vines, that there may be no armes, but such as will lovingly embrace women, and because wee know that some upon different occasions desire to absent themselves from their best beloved, having first plundred their chests and took away that they have, we desire that such men may be compelled forthwith to returne to their wives, or beare on their heads the fortune which they have most worthily deserved, being guilty of that punishment by their long absence.

And whereas all are not Penelopes that can withstand the siege of a strong temptation, but must yeeld up the Fort to the flattering enemie of their long preserved chastity, it is better to keepe then to make that fraile sex honest: let not therefore the drumme wound the ayre no more with false stroakes, nor the pike bee bathed in the bloud of guiltlesse men, let not the sword ravish from our
bosomes

bosomes the delight of our lives: this word husband speaking benefit and comfort both to Wives and Mid-wives, since our felicity cannot subsist without the others fertility and trusefullnesse, and therefore let us Mid-wives whom it most nearely concernes, desire that some order may be taken, that the old song of England may not be againe revived, *few men of London*; And that the delicate sex of women may not lye in their beddes like cold marble images cut out by some Artificers hand, but being full of warme spirit, and life, they may obliege the world to them by repairing the losses of this War, and have husbands as formerly at their command to maintaine them bravely, and bring them yearely under the delivering power of the Mid-wife, which cannot be done unlesse the Wars cease, and men returne againe unto their wives.

Moreover we have just cause to feare those dreadfull prophesies which point so directly at this age, foretelling that there should be a great scarcity of men, and such abundance of women farre exceeding the other, both in strength and number, so that a hundred should run after one, being a fearefull prodigy in nature, and a dearth to be more feared, then that of Corne or any other commodity: Coals are not so necessary as husbands warme in bed, and comfortable at board, and therefore in this sad age it is fit to take a view of the calamities of women in other nations, for if men be scarce, all other plenty is nothing to women, they consumate our happinesse, and make us richer then all the precious stones of the Indyes, therefore most deplorable will the continuall losse of more Souldiers be, since they might live to comfort us, and declare their undainted valour in the soft and delightfull field of love: And whereas most certaine intelligence brought unto us, that many notorious Papists, doe resort to the Queenes Standard, lately by her erected at

Mother Shiptons Prophesie.

New-

New-castle: we desire likewise that our Standard may once again be set up in our City and Suburbs; for we mid-wives know that women are not so cold or out of soule, but that they can endure a fight bravely under a Standard, and can use a weapon as well as men if they get it in their handling, let their courage therefore teach them to fight for their owne priviledges, and if they prove the weaker vessels, yet wee Mid-wives desire that the distresses of widowed women bee looked upon with a charitable construction, not doubting but by all good willers to their sex, their Petition shall be regarded as the publique voyce of their long conceal'd affections, shewing also how greatly necessitated they have bin in their husbands absence, whose happy returne shall satisfie their longing, and gives us the Midwives of London great cause to rejoyce. And we shall humbly pray, &c.

FINIS.

DATE DUE